T0227222

Acute Respiratory Distress Syndrome

Editors

MICHAEL A. MATTHAY
KATHLEEN D. LIU

CRITICAL CARE CLINICS

www.criticalcare.theclinics.com

Consulting Editor
GREGORY S. MARTIN

October 2021 • Volume 37 • Number 4

ELSEVIER

1600 John F. Kennedy Boulevard • Suite 1800 • Philadelphia, Pennsylvania, 19103-2899

http://www.theclinics.com

CRITICAL CARE CLINICS Volume 37, Number 4
October 2021 ISSN 0749-0704, ISBN-13: 978-0-323-79464-0

Editor: Joanna Collett
Developmental Editor: Hannah Almira Lopez

Critical Care Clinics (ISSN: 0749-0704) is published quarterly by Elsevier Inc., 360 Park Avenue South, New York, NY 10010-1710. Months of issue are January, April, July, and October. Business and Editorial Offices: 1600 John F. Kennedy Blvd., Suite 1800, Philadelphia, PA 19103-2899. Customer Service Office: 6277 Sea Harbor Drive, Orlando, FL 32887-4800. Periodicals postage paid at New York, NY and additional mailing offices. Subscription prices are $258.00 per year for US individuals, $890.00 per year for US institutions, $100.00 per year for US students and residents, $287.00 per year for Canadian individuals, $952.00 per year for Canadian institutions, $328.00 per year for international individuals, $952.00 per year for international institutions, $100.00 per year for Canadian students/residents, and $150.00 per year for foreign students/residents. To receive student/resident rate, orders must be accompanied by name of affiliated institution, date of term, and the signature of program/residency coordinator on institution letterhead. Orders will be billed at individual rate until proof of status is received. Foreign air speed delivery is included in all *Clinics* subscription prices. All prices are subject to change without notice. POSTMASTER: Send address changes to *Critical Care Clinics*, Elsevier Periodicals Customer Service, 11830 Westline Industrial Drive, St. Louis, MO 63146. **Customer Service: 1-800-654-2452 (US). From outside of the US, call 1-314-447-8871. Fax: 1-314-447-8029. E-mail: journalscustomerservice-usa@elsevier.com (for print support) or journalsonlinesupport-usa@elsevier.com (for online support).**

Reprints. For copies of 100 or more of articles in this publication, please contact the Commercial Reprints Department, Elsevier Inc., 360 Park Avenue South, New York, NY 10010-1710. Tel.: 212-633-3874; Fax: 212-633-3820; E-mail: reprints@elsevier.com.

Critical Care Clinics is also published in Spanish by Editorial Inter-Medica, Junin 917, 1er A, 1113, Buenos Aires, Argentina.

Critical Care Clinics is covered in *MEDLINE/PubMed (Index Medicus), EMBASE/Excerpta Medica, Current Concepts/Clinical Medicine, ISI/BIOMED,* and *Chemical Abstracts.*

Contributors

CONSULTING EDITOR

GREGORY S. MARTIN, MD, MSC
Professor, Division of Pulmonary, Allergy, Critical Care and Sleep Medicine, Research Director, Emory Critical Care Center, Director, Emory/Georgia Tech Predictive Health Institute, Co-Director, Atlanta Center for Microsystems Engineered Point-of-Care Technologies (ACME POCT), President, Society of Critical Care Medicine, Atlanta, Georgia, USA

EDITORS

MICHAEL A. MATTHAY, MD
Professor of Medicine and Anesthesia, Senior Associate, Cardiovascular Research Institute, Associate Director Critical Care Medicine, Departments of Medicine and Anesthesia, Cardiovascular Research Institute, University of California, San Francisco, San Francisco, California, USA

KATHLEEN D. LIU, MD, PhD, MAS
Professor of Medicine and Anesthesia, Director, Medical Intensive Care Unit, Departments of Medicine and Anesthesia, University of California, San Francisco, San Francisco, California, USA

AUTHORS

J. MATTHEW ALDRICH, MD
Department of Anesthesia and Perioperative Care, Critical Care Medicine, University of California, San Francisco, San Francisco, California, USA

LANAZHA T. BELFIELD, PhD
Section of Pulmonary, Critical Care, Allergy and Critical Care, Wake Forest University School of Medicine, Winston-Salem, North Carolina, USA

LIEUWE D. BOS, MD, PhD
Department of Respiratory Medicine, Infection and Immunity, Amsterdam University Medical Center, AMC, Amsterdam, the Netherlands

SAMUEL M. BROWN, MD, MS
Division of Pulmonary and Critical Care Medicine, Department of Medicine, University of Utah School of Medicine, Salt Lake City, Utah, USA; Division of Pulmonary and Critical Care Medicine, Department of Medicine, Intermountain Medical Center, Murray, Utah, USA

STEVEN Y. CHANG, MD, PhD
David Geffen School of Medicine at UCLA, Los Angeles, California, USA

MELISSA H. COLEMAN, MD
Division of Cardiothoracic Surgery, Department of Surgery, Critical Care Medicine, University of California, San Francisco, San Francisco, California, USA

KEITH CORL, MD, ScM
Division of Pulmonary, Critical Care and Sleep Medicine, Rhode Island Hospital,
Providence, Rhode Island, USA

SARAH FAUBEL, MD
Professor of Medicine, Division of Renal Diseases and Hypertension, Department of
Internal Medicine, University of Colorado, Anschutz Medical Campus, Aurora, Colorado,
USA

D. CLARK FILES, MD
Section of Pulmonary, Critical Care, Allergy and Critical Care, Wake Forest University
School of Medicine, Winston-Salem, North Carolina, USA

HEATHER M. GIANNINI, MD, MS
University of Pennsylvania, Perelman School of Medicine, Philadelphia, Pennsylvania,
USA

KATHRYN W. HENDRICKSON, MD
Division of Pulmonary and Critical Care Medicine, Department of Medicine, University of
Utah School of Medicine, Salt Lake City, Utah, USA; Division of Pulmonary and Critical
Care Medicine, Department of Medicine, Intermountain Medical Center, Murray, Utah,
USA

MAYA E. KOTAS, MD, PhD
Division of Pulmonary, Critical Care, Allergy and Sleep Medicine, Department of Medicine,
University of California, San Francisco, San Francisco, California, USA

JENNIFER T.W. KRALL, MD
Section of Pulmonary, Critical Care, Allergy and Critical Care, Wake Forest University
School of Medicine, Winston-Salem, North Carolina, USA

JISOO LEE, MD
Division of Pulmonary, Critical Care and Sleep Medicine, Rhode Island Hospital,
Providence, Rhode Island, USA

MITCHELL M. LEVY, MD, MCCM, FCCP
Division of Pulmonary, Critical Care and Sleep Medicine, Rhode Island Hospital,
Providence, Rhode Island, USA

MICHAEL A. MATTHAY, MD
Professor of Medicine and Anesthesia, Senior Associate, Cardiovascular Research
Institute, Associate Director Critical Care Medicine, Departments of Medicine and
Anesthesia, Cardiovascular Research Institute, University of California, San Francisco,
San Francisco, California, USA

NUALA J. MEYER, MD, MS
Associate Professor, University of Pennsylvania, Perelman School of Medicine,
Philadelphia, Pennsylvania, USA

ELIZABETH A. MIDDLETON, MD
Assistant Professor of Medicine, Division of Pulmonary and Critical Care Medicine,
Department of Internal Medicine, Program in Molecular Medicine, University of Utah
School of Medicine, Eccles Institute of Human Genetics, Salt Lake City, Utah, USA

JESSICA A. PALAKSHAPPA, MD, MS
Section of Pulmonary, Critical Care, Allergy and Critical Care, Wake Forest University
School of Medicine, Winston-Salem, North Carolina, USA

BRYAN D. PARK, MD
Division of Pulmonary Sciences and Critical Care Medicine, Department of Internal Medicine, University of Colorado, Anschutz Medical Campus, Aurora, Colorado, USA

ITHAN D. PELTAN, MD, MSc
Division of Pulmonary and Critical Care Medicine, Department of Medicine, University of Utah School of Medicine, Salt Lake City, Utah, USA; Pulmonary Division, Department of Medicine, Intermountain Medical Center, Murray, Utah, USA

NIDA QADIR, MD
David Geffen School of Medicine at UCLA, Los Angeles, California, USA

PRATIK SINHA, MB ChB, PhD
Division of Clinical and Translational Research, Department of Anesthesia, Washington University School of Medicine, St Louis, Missouri, USA

ERIK RICHARD SWENSON, MD
Professor of Medicine, Physiology and Biophysics, Department of Medicine, Division of Pulmonary and Critical Care Medicine, University of Washington, Medical Service, Veterans Affairs Puget Sound Health Care System, Seattle, Washington, USA

KAI ERIK SWENSON, MD
Division of Pulmonary and Critical Care Medicine, Massachusetts General Hospital, Division of Pulmonary, Critical Care, and Sleep Medicine, Beth Israel Deaconess Medical Center, Boston, Massachusetts, USA

B. TAYLOR THOMPSON, MD
Division of Pulmonary and Critical Care Medicine, Department of Medicine, Massachusetts General Hospital, Harvard Medical School, Boston, Massachusetts, USA

KATHERINE D. WICK, MD
Department of Anesthesia, Cardiovascular Research Institute, University of California, San Francisco, San Francisco, California, USA

GUY A. ZIMMERMAN, MD
Professor of Medicine, Division of Pulmonary and Critical Care Medicine, Department of Internal Medicine, Program in Molecular Medicine, University of Utah School of Medicine, Eccles Institute of Human Genetics, Salt Lake City, Utah, USA

Contents

> Acute respiratory distress syndrome (ARDS) is a heterogeneous syndrome
> of high morbidity and mortality with global impact. Current epidemiologic
> estimates are imprecise given differences in patient populations, risk fac-
> tors, resources, and practice styles around the world. Despite improve-
> ment in supportive care which has improved mortality, effective targeted
> therapies remain elusive. The Coronavirus Disease 2019 pandemic has re-
> sulted in a large number of ARDS cases that, despite less heterogeneity
> than multietiologic ARDS populations, still exhibit wide variation in physi-
> ology and outcomes. Intensive care unit rates of death have varied widely
> in studies to date because of a variety of patient and hospital-level factors.
> Despite some controversy, the best management of these patients is likely
> the same supportive measures shown to be effective in classical ARDS.
> Further epidemiologic studies are needed to help characterize the epide-
> miology of ARDS subphenotypes to facilitate identification of targeted
> therapies.

> The acute respiratory distress syndrome (ARDS) remains a major cause of
> morbidity and mortality in the intensive care unit. Improving outcomes de-
> pends on not only evidence-based care once ARDS has already devel-
> oped but also preventing ARDS incidence. Several environmental
> exposures have now been shown to increase the risk of ARDS and related
> adverse outcomes. How environmental factors impact the risk of devel-
> oping ARDS is a growing and important field of research that should inform
> the care of individual patients as well as public health policy.

> Acute respiratory distress syndrome is a common condition among criti-
> cally ill patients, but remains under-recognized and undertreated. Under-
> recognition may result from confusion over the clinical inclusion criteria,
> as well as a misunderstanding of the complex relationship between the
> clinical syndrome, the variable histopathologic patterns, and the myriad
> clinical disorders that cause acute respiratory distress syndrome. The
> identification of the clinical syndrome and determination of the causal
> diagnosis are both required to optimize patient outcomes. Here we review

Clinical risk factors alone fail to fully explain acute respiratory distress syndrome (ARDS) risk or ARDS death, suggesting that individual risk factors contribute. The goals of genomic ARDS studies include better mechanistic understanding, identifying dysregulated pathways that may be amenable to pharmacologic targeting, using genomic causal inference techniques to find measurable traits with meaning, and deconvoluting ARDS heterogeneity by proving reproducible subpopulations that may share a unique biology. This article discusses the latest advances in ARDS genomics, provides historical perspective, and highlights some of the ways that the coronavirus disease 2019 (COVID-19) pandemic is accelerating genomic ARDS research.

Acute kidney injury (AKI) complicates approximately a third of all acute respiratory distress syndrome (ARDS) cases, and the combination of the two drastically worsens prognosis. Recent advances in ARDS supportive care have led to improved outcomes; however, much less is known on how to prevent and support patients with AKI and ARDS together. Understanding the dynamic relationship between the kidneys and lungs is crucial for the practicing intensivist to prevent injury. This article summarizes key concepts for the critical care physician managing a patient with ARDS complicated by AKI. Also provided is a discussion of AKI in the COVID-19 era.

This review describes the management of mechanical ventilation in patients with acute respiratory distress syndrome, including in those with coronavirus disease 2019. Low tidal volume ventilation with a moderate to high positive end-expiratory pressure remains the foundation of an evidence-based approach. We consider strategies for setting positive end-expiratory pressure levels, the use of recruitment maneuvers, and the potential role of driving pressure. Rescue therapies including prone positioning and extracorporeal membrane oxygenation are also discussed.

The optimal fluid management for acute respiratory distress syndrome (ARDS) remains unknown. Liberal fluid management may improve cardiac function and end-organ perfusion, but may lead to increased pulmonary edema and inhibit gas exchange. Trials suggest that conservative fluid management leads to better clinical outcomes, although prospective randomized, controlled trials have not demonstrated mortality benefit. Recent discoveries suggest there is large heterogeneity in ARDS, and varying phenotypes of ARDS respond differently to fluid treatments. Future advances

CRITICAL CARE CLINICS

SERIES OF RELATED INTEREST

Hematology/Oncology Clinics
https://www.hemonc.theclinics.com/

THE CLINICS ARE AVAILABLE ONLINE!
Access your subscription at:
www.theclinics.com

Preface

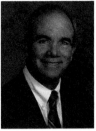

Michael A. Matthay, MD   Kathleen D. Liu, MD, PhD, MAS
Editors

We are pleased to introduce this issue of *Critical Care Clinics*, focused on acute respiratory distress syndrome (ARDS). Although planned before the COVID-19 pandemic, this issue is particularly timely given the world events of the past 18 months. The articles in this issue address several key topics in the field of ARDS with both a clinical and a research focus, as well as define some of the important questions that need to be answered for our understanding of the pathogenesis and treatment of ARDS to advance. Some of the articles include studies on COVID-19 ARDS, noting that this field is changing rapidly. This preface provides a brief overview of each of the articles and then our brief perspective on some of the opportunities for progress in ARDS.

The articles cover much that we have learned in the last few years. The issue starts with an article on epidemiology that identifies patients who are at higher risk and discusses the recent COVID-19 pandemic. This is followed by an article on environmental factors that emphasizes the impact of inhaled factors, including cigarette smoke, air pollution, and vaping, and an article that reviews the clinical diagnosis, including how to exclude mimics such as heart failure and volume overload. Next, there is a detailed article on the physiology of ARDS, including up-to-date information (at the time of publication) on how COVID-19 is similar to and different from classical ARDS. This is followed by two complementary articles on pathogenesis, one focused on clinically relevant experimental studies and one focused on recent advances in our understanding of the biologic and clinical heterogeneity of ARDS in critically ill patients, including those with COVID-19. The field of genetics and ARDS is just beginning to provide important insights into disease risk and pathogenesis, which is covered in the next article. Nonpulmonary organ failure is an important risk factor for adverse outcomes in ARDS, and there has been significant interest in organ cross-talk in the pathogenesis of ARDS and multiorgan failure. One of the organs of particular interest in clinical and experimental studies is the kidney, and our current understanding is well covered in an article on acute kidney injury and ARDS. The next three articles cover important aspects of the treatment of ARDS. At present, our most important management strategies for ARDS are supportive care therapies, including lung protective ventilation and a fluid conservative management strategy. Beyond

https://doi.org/10.1016/j.ccc.2021.06.001
0749-0704/21/© 2021 Published by Elsevier Inc.
criticalcare.theclinics.com

lung protective ventilation, a number of ventilator strategies have been tested in randomized clinical trials, and these are reviewed, along with potential indications for extracorporeal membrane oxygenation. Fluid therapy, including fluid selection, is a critical part of ARDS management, and current management based on clinical trials is discussed in detail. With regards to pharmacologic therapies for ARDS, numerous agents have been tested yet been unsuccessful. However, some of these agents might be reconsidered for testing with the use of both predictive and prognostic enrichment strategies. Last, but not least, studying the long-term outcomes of ARDS is a rapidly growing field; this is an area that was recognized as important and now in the COVID-19 era is even more appreciated for its importance clinically and for future research studies.

In addition to all these topics, we would like to emphasize how ARDS has clearly become even more recognized since COVID-19 as a major cause of morbidity and mortality that needs new strategies for testing novel therapeutics. The importance of novel approaches has been emphasized in several recent articles.[1,2] A number of platform trials have rapidly tested therapies in the setting of COVID-19. Specifically, I-SPY COVID has tested a number of novel and repurposed agents that could rapidly be manufactured/supplied at large scale using a phase 2 design to rapidly identify candidate agents with the potential for large therapeutic benefit in the setting of severe COVID-19. The open-label RECOVERY and REMAP-CAP platform trials have identified pharmacologic therapies with significant benefit in subpopulations of COVID-19, including dexamethasone and tocilizumab.[3,4] In addition, there is a good rationale for expanding the current Berlin definition of ARDS to include high-flow nasal cannula oxygen,[5] as well as developing additional criteria that would allow the definition to be adapted to resource-limited areas so the recognition of ARDS can be global, facilitating early recognition and early treatments for both classical ARDS and COVID-19–related ARDS.

Michael A. Matthay, MD
Department of Medicine
Department of Anesthesia
Cardiovascular Research Institute
University of California, San Francisco
505 Parnassus Avenue, M-917
San Francisco, CA 94143, USA

Kathleen D. Liu, MD, PhD, MAS
Departments of Medicine and Anesthesia
University of California, San Francisco
505 Parnassus Avenue, M-917
San Francisco, CA 94143, USA

E-mail addresses:
Michael.matthay@ucsf.edu (M.A. Matthay)
kathleen.liu@ucsf.edu (K.D. Liu)

REFERENCES

1. Matthay MA, Arabi YM, Siegel ER, et al. Phenotypes and personalized medicine in the acute respiratory distress syndrome. Intensive Care Med 2020;46:2136–52.

2. Ware LB, Matthay MA, Mebazaa A. Designing an ARDS trial for 2020 and beyond: focus on enrichment strategies. Intensive Care Med 2020;46:2153–6.

3. Group RC, Horby P, Lim WS, et al. Dexamethasone in hospitalized patients with Covid-19. N Engl J Med 2021;384:693–704.
4. Investigators R-C, Gordon AC, Mouncey PR, et al. Interleukin-6 receptor antagonists in critically ill patients with Covid-19. N Engl J Med 2012;384: 1491–502.
5. Matthay MA, Thompson BT, Ware LB. The Berlin definition of acute respiratory distress syndrome: should patients receiving high-flow nasal oxygen be included? Lancet Respir Med 2021. https://doi.org/10.1016/S2213-2600(21)00105-3.

The Epidemiology of Acute Respiratory Distress Syndrome Before and After Coronavirus Disease 2019

Kathryn W. Hendrickson, MD[a,b], Ithan D. Peltan, MD, MSc[a,c], Samuel M. Brown, MD, MS[a,b,*]

KEYWORDS

- ARDS • Epidemiology • Incidence • Subtypes • Mortality • COVID-19

KEY POINTS

- Acute respiratory distress syndrome (ARDS) is heterogeneous.
- ARDS has high incidence among intensive care unit patients.
- ARDS has high morbidity and mortality.
- Improved supportive care has decreased ARDS incidence and mortality.
- Coronavirus Disease 2019–associated ARDS is a syndrome within the known ARDS spectrum.

INTRODUCTION

Acute respiratory distress syndrome (ARDS) occurs when a diverse array of triggers cause acute, bilateral pulmonary inflammation and increased pulmonary capillary permeability leading to acute hypoxemic respiratory failure. Pulmonary biopsy (or autopsy) classically demonstrates diffuse alveolar damage (DAD).[1] Recognizing that ARDS is a syndrome and that research and benchmarking require reproducible definitions, a 2011 consensus conference in Berlin proposed a practical, updated definition (the "Berlin Definition"),[2] In summary, this requires,

[a] Division of Pulmonary and Critical Care Medicine, Department of Medicine, University of Utah School of Medicine, 26 North 1900 East, Salt Lake City, UT 84112, USA; [b] Division of Pulmonary and Critical Care Medicine, Department of Medicine, Intermountain Medical Center; [c] Pulmonary Division, Department of Medicine, Intermountain Medical Center, 5121 South Cottonwood Street, Murray, UT 84107, USA
* Corresponding author. Pulmonary Division, Department of Medicine, Intermountain Medical Center, 5121 South Cottonwood Street, Murray, UT 84107.
E-mail address: Samuel.Brown@imail.org

Crit Care Clin 37 (2021) 703–716
https://doi.org/10.1016/j.ccc.2021.05.001
0749-0704/21/© 2021 Elsevier Inc. All rights reserved.

1. An acute process developing within 1 week of a known clinical insult or new or worsening respiratory symptoms;
2. Radiographic images showing bilateral opacities not fully explained by effusions, lobar or lung collapse, or nodules; and
3. Impairment in oxygenation as measured by a Pao_2/Fio_2 $\leq$300 mm Hg in the presence of a positive end-expiratory pressure (PEEP) of at least 5 cm H2O.

Despite many advances in the understanding of ARDS, morbidity and mortality remain high with few targeted therapies. In this epidemiologic review, we consider the etiology, subtypes and phenotypes, incidence, mortality, long-term outcomes, and the relationship(s) between Coronavirus Disease 2019 (COVID-19) and prepandemic ARDS.

ETIOLOGY

Admitting that patients would not have survived long enough to be diagnosed with ARDS before the widespread use of intensive care unit (ICU) ventilators for hypoxemic respiratory failure, Ashbaugh and colleagues first reported on ARDS as a distinct syndrome in a 1967 series of 12 patients.[3] Despite suffering from heterogeneous primary insults, the patients all developed similar patterns of acute-onset respiratory failure with bilateral infiltrates and decreased pulmonary compliance accompanied by autopsy findings of acute inflammation and hyaline membranes.[3]

This initial report captured the heterogeneity of ARDS that continues to present challenges in diagnosis and treatment. Pneumonia is the most common trigger for ARDS, although nonpulmonary sepsis, aspiration pneumonitis, and trauma are also common. An assortment of less common triggers have been identified including pancreatitis and blood transfusion. Clinical syndromes compatible with ARDS but with no identifiable trigger are referred to as acute interstitial pneumonia (AIP) or sometimes Hamman-Rich syndrome rather than ARDS and may represent a response to an array of sometimes overlapping pulmonary insults.[1,4–15] In both ARDS and, presumptively, AIP, an insult elicits an inflammatory response which leads to increased-permeability pulmonary edema creating the hypoxemia and bilateral opacities on imaging required for diagnosis.[16,17] In its most severe forms, DAD results pathologically.

ARDS resulting from direct pulmonary insult such as pneumonia manifests pathologically as alveolar collapse, fibrinous exudate, and edema of the alveolar walls to a greater degree than ARDS resulting from nonpulmonary causes such as pancreatitis.[18] This may represent a spectrum of severity or alternative pathophysiological processes. What is less clear is why some patients with inciting conditions develop ARDS while others do not, and whether differences in genotype, phenotype, or therapeutic context play a role remains unclear.

Chronic conditions including obesity and diabetes have been associated with a decreased incidence of ARDS. In diabetes, some hypothesize that this observed association reflects a decreased inflammatory response among diabetics.[19,20] A potential association with obesity is less clear.[21–23] Importantly, collider bias may in fact account for the observed associations.[24]

On the contrary, chronic alcohol use has been associated with higher risk of ARDS. Kaphalia and Calhoun[25] found that chronic alcohol use leads to pulmonary immune dysfunction, epithelial dysfunction, and the inability to handle reactive oxygen species leading to the high permeability pulmonary edema and hyaline membrane formation seen in ARDS. Smoking is also associated with higher risks of ARDS. Not only are patients who smoke more likely to get pneumonia they also have higher rates of ARDS triggered by nonpulmonary causes.[26,27] Cigarette smoking may thus increase the risk of the inflammatory cascade that results in ARDS. Interestingly, ozone exposure (but no other known pollutants) is also associated with increased risk of ARDS.[28] Consistently, older age,[8] non-white race (likely a surrogate for "social determinants of disease"),[29] and some genetic variants[30] have been described as host factors associated with risk of developing ARDS.

Although age is a risk factor for developing ARDS, it has not consistently been found to be associated with increased mortality. The multinational LUNG-SAFE (The Large Observational Study to Understand the Global Impact of Severe Acute Respiratory Failure) study showed older age to be a risk factor for mortality[31]; however, when controlling for risk, severity, and comorbidity, the independent relationship between age and mortality in ARDS is not consistent.[8] The association of race and ethnicity with ARDS mortality was studied in a retrospective cohort study in 2009 using patient data from three ARDS network randomized control trials. Black race and Hispanic ethnicity were found to have not only higher rates of ARDS than white individuals but higher mortality as well. The causes of race- and ethnicity-related differences are not well understood and likely vary between groups but, in all cases, likely derive substantially from "social determinants of disease" rather than genetic factors. For instance, the fact that higher mortality in Black patients resolves with adjustment for illness severity suggests barriers that hinder Black individuals from seeking early care, physician delay in diagnosis, and other factors worsen the severity mix in these groups.[29]

SUBTYPES

A defining characteristic of ARDS is its heterogeneity, from Ashbaugh's initial publication to the present day.[32,33] Traditional categorizations (as, eg, in the Berlin definition) are based on severity of hypoxemia, which correlates with mortality and the extent of DAD on pathologic examination.[34,35] The effects of some potential ARDS therapies may also vary with hypoxemia severity. For example, in 2018, Guo and colleagues[36] published a systemic review and meta-analysis showing a likely trend toward improved outcomes in patients receiving a high-PEEP protocol. For patients with a Pao_2/Fio_2 (P/F) ratio ≤ 200, there was a slightly lower risk of death; however, in patients with a P/F ratio 201 to 300, there was a possible higher risk of death. Of note this mortality benefit has not been seen in any individual randomized control trials[37–39] and remains a controversial topic. Another example is the 2019 study of therapeutic neuromuscular blockade to improve outcomes in ARDS. Although a previous trial hinted at decreased mortality in patients with P/F ratio less than 130,[40] this larger trial concluded no mortality benefit.[41]

ARDS can also be subdivided based on the initial insult, whether pulmonary (pneumonia, pulmonary contusion, and aspiration) or extrapulmonary (nonthoracic trauma, nonpulmonary sepsis, and transfusion).[7,42,43] Several pathologic, biologic, and physiologic differences have been identified on this basis.[18,44–47] However, in practice, it is difficult to differentiate between the two groups based on substantial overlap.[13] These pathologic, biologic, and physiologic differences are heavily influenced by underlying lung function and architecture, smoking status, chronic diseases, and other conditions, which inflate the heterogeneity of ARDS. No mortality difference has been found between the two groups, likely related to the complexities of the overlap between the two groups.[48]

More recently, "machine learning"-style techniques have been used to identify distinct subtypes. Post-hoc analysis (using latent class analysis) of the ARMA (ARDSnet: Ventilation with Lower Tidal Volumes as Compared with Traditional Tidal Volumes for Acute Lung Injury and the Acute Respiratory Distress Syndrome) and ALVEOLI (Assessment of Low Tidal Volume and Elevated End-Expiratory Pressure to Obviate Lung Injury) trials revealed two phenotypes of ARDS.[37,49] Relative to phenotype 1, phenotype 2 was hyperinflammatory, with higher plasma levels of inflammatory biomarkers, a higher prevalence of vasopressor use, lower serum bicarbonate, and a higher prevalence of sepsis found in phenotype 2 than in phenotype 1.[50] Critically, in terms of its clinical utility, this hyperinflammatory phenotype was also associated with higher mortality. Phenotype may also predict response to therapies: A post-hoc analysis of a randomized controlled trial of statin therapy for ARDS suggested benefit for hyperinflammatory patients.[51] It will be important with the expanding use of novel statistical techniques for subtyping to ground them in reality and validate them in both prospective cohorts and within prespecified subgroups in prospective trials.

INCIDENCE

The incidence of ARDS varies globally by over 400%.[52] It is important to acknowledge in this context that ARDS as a syndrome reflects both patient physiology and clinical context. For example, where patients with hypoxemic respiratory failure are not routinely intubated (as may occur in certain institutional settings in USA/Europe or in low- and middle-income country settings with limited supplies of ventilators and/or resources and personnel for ICU-level care), ARDS incidence may appear lower than it actually is. Similarly, routine use of high-tidal-volume ventilation among patients at risk may increase the incidence of ARDS in a given setting. With those caveats in mind, incidence ranges from 10.1/100,000/y in Brazil in 2014 to 82/100,000/y in the United States in 2005 (**Table 1**).[5,7,8,10] Between-study differences in case ascertainment and local context may drive these observed differences.[53,54] Some studies, for instance, relied on clinician diagnosis while others used billing codes, both of which may be inaccurate. Both methods are likely to undercount ARDS cases, as only 60% of ARDS cases were appropriately identified by clinicians in one large study.[1] Differences in the prevalence of ARDS risk factors may account for some of the variation as well.

Likely the highest quality evidence on ARDS incidence and management patterns originates from LUNG-SAFE, a prevalence study conducted during a 4-week period in 459 ICUs in 50 countries. Overall, 10% of all ICU patients and 23% of mechanically ventilated patients met ARDS criteria, yielding an ICU incidence of 5.5 cases per ICU bed per year.

In 2011, the Prevention and Early Treatment of Acute Lung Injury (PETAL) Network developed the Lung Injury Prediction Score (LIPS) to help identify patients in the emergency department with high risk of developing ARDS. ARDS predictors included in the final score both triggers (ie, shock, aspiration, lung contusion) and risk modifiers (ie, smoking, diabetes mellitus, acidosis). This tool also works in hospitalized patients as a quick and effective way of identifying high-risk patients.[55–57] Hopes that this score would help enrich enrollment in trials of therapeutics to decrease incidence and death from ARDS, however, have so far not borne fruit. For instance, the LIPS-A trial, in which aspirin was tested as a possible intervention in this subgroup of patients, showed no difference in rates of ARDS and rates of death after receiving aspirin versus placebo.[58]

Between 2001 and 2008, rates of ARDS fell by half in two ICUs in Rochester, Minnesota, in a population-based, retrospective cohort study of the epidemiology of ARDS patients admitted during that time period. Severity of acute illness, greater number of comorbidities, and major predisposing conditions in patients with ARDS increased while mortality stayed the same during this time. Interestingly, the reduction in incidence occurred exclusively in patients with hospital-acquired ARDS. As noted by the authors, during this time, a separate hospital-wide program to limit risk factors for ARDS was undertaken which can explain this reduction in hospital-acquired ARDS. This indicates that ARDS may, in part, be a preventable hospital-acquired

Table 1
Main epidemiologic studies on ARDS incidence after AECC definition

Authors, Year of Publication [Reference]	Study Period	Country or Countries	Incidence of All ARDS Categories (per 100,000 Person-Years-Population-Based Studies) or Percentage (%, Hospitalization-Based Studies)	Incidence of Moderate and Severe ARDS Categories (per 100,000 Person-Years-Population-Based Studies) or Percentage (%, Hospitalization-Based Studies)
Sigurdsson et al,[15] 2013	1988–2010	Iceland		3.65–9.63
Nolan et al,[4] 1997	1990–1994	Australia		7.3–9.3
Luhr et al,[5] 1999	1997	Scandinavia (Sweden, Denmark, Iceland, Norway)	17.9	13.5
Bersten et al,[6] 2002	1999	Australia (South, Western, and Tasmania)	34	28
Brun-Buisson et al,[13] 2004	1999	Europe	7.1% (of all ICU admissions)	6.1% (of all ICU admissions)
Rubenfeld et al,[7] 2005	1999–2000	King County, WA, USA	78.9	58.7
Manzano et al,[8] 2005	2001	Granada, Spain	25.5	23
Sakr et al,[92] 2005	2002	Europe	12.5% (of all ICU admissions), 19.1% (of all mechanically ventilated patients)	10.6% (of all ICU admissions), 16.5% (of all mechanically ventilated patients)
Li et al,[9] 2011	2001–2008	Olmsted County, MN		81 (in 2001), 38.3 (in 2008)
The Irish Critical Care Trials Group,[14] 2008	2006	Ireland	19%	
Caser et al,[10] 2014	2006–2007	Vitoria Region, Brazil	10.1	6.3
Linko et al,[11] 2009	2007	Finland	10.6	5
Villar et al,[12] 2011	2008–2009	Spain		7.2
Bellani et al,[1] 2016	2014	50 Countries	10.4% of all ICU admissions, 5.5 cases per ICU bed per year	

ARDS was defined using the Berlin definition nomenclature: All ARDS categories include mild, moderate, and severe ARDS.

complication.[9] Multiple additional studies have shown that using LTVV in all visitors to the hospital and ICU have decreased incidence of ARDS arguing for the use of LTVV in all patients and not only on those with respiratory failure.[59,60]

ACUTE RESPIRATORY DISTRESS SYNDROME-ASSOCIATED MORTALITY

Despite improved mortality rates, ARDS continues to be a syndrome of high mortality. As noted previously, P/F ratio correlates with ARDS outcome, prompting the authors of the Berlin Criteria to maintain the traditional severity categories in their updated consensus definition. Mortality in cohorts analyzed by the Berlin Criteria authors was 34.9% (95% confidence interval [CI]: 24%-30%) in mild ARDS, 40.3% (95% CI: 29%-34%) in moderate ARDS, and 46.1% (95% CI: 29%-34%) in severe ARDS, as defined by P/F thresholds of 300, 200, and 100.[2] The LUNG-SAFE study reported similar findings, with 28-day mortality of 29.6% (95% CI: 26.2%-33.0%) in mild ARDS, 35.2% (95% CI: 32.4%-38.1%) in moderate ARDS, and 40.9% (95% CI: 36.8%-45.1%) in severe ARDS using the same P/F thresholds used in the Berlin definition.[1]

Reported ARDS mortality has decreased over recent decades. Compared to the late 1990s, when independent studies reported ARDS mortality of 58% to 59%,[4,13] mortality in contemporary studies is much lower (**Figs. 1** and **2**). ARDS mortality in 2014 in LUNG-SAFE was 10.4%,[1] and 28% in the LOTUS-FRUIT U.S. multicenter study conducted by the PETAL Network in 2019.[61] While imperfect,[62] death certificate data also suggest decreasing risk of death for ARDS patients, with annual attributable mortality in one U.S. death certificate analysis decreasing from 5.01 per 100,000 people in 1999 to 2.82 per 100,000 population in 2013.[63] While changes in ascertainment (diagnosing more patients with less-severe ARDS) and decreasing use of mechanical ventilation for patients near the end of life may contribute to this trend, it appears likely that increasing the use of LTVV since the publication of the seminal ARMA trial in 2000 is a key factor driving improved outcomes in ARDS.[49] In fact, among patients who do

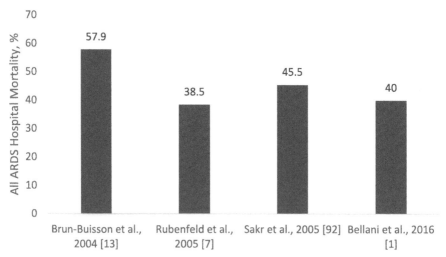

Fig. 1. Estimated overall hospital mortality rates for patients with ARDS of any severity. Hospital mortality reported in the main epidemiologic studies in all ARDS categories (mild, moderate, and severe). On the X-axis, the studies are chronologically ordered based on the study period.

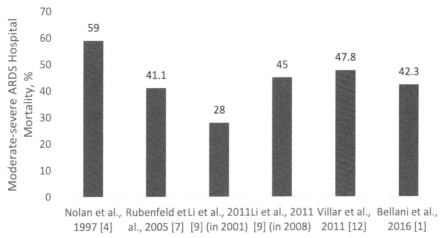

Fig. 2. Estimated mortality rates for patients with moderate-severe ARDS. Hospital mortality reported in the subgroups of moderate-severe ARDS. Moderate-severe ARDS hospital mortality in the study by Li *and colleagues* [2011] is reported in two different years of study, 2001 and 2008. On the X-axis, the studies are chronologically ordered based on the study period.

receive low tidal volume ventilation, there has been no change in mortality.[64] It is also important to note that, in some settings, apparent stability of crude ARDS mortality may mask changes in case mix (increasing illness severity and comorbidities) and therefore improving risk-adjusted mortality.[9]

LONG-TERM OUTCOMES

Despite the significant lung injury experienced during the course of a patient's illness with ARDS, postillness pulmonary function tests showed normalization at 5 years after ICU.[65] Despite this normalization in lung function, reported quality-of-life scores and exercise tolerance, measured by 6-minute walk test, remain lower than average at 5 years. Multiple factors likely contribute to this including persistent weakness and neuropsychologic impairments. These neuropsychologic issues are heterogeneous and affect both the patient and their caregivers.[65] These patients also accrue larger health care costs after hospitalization because of increased utilization of the health care system. ARDS is one of the most common reasons for admission to a long-term ventilator rehabilitation unit.[66]

COVID-19

The severe acute respiratory distress syndrome-associated coronavirus-2 was first identified in December 2019 in Wuhan, Hubei, China, as the agent causing what is now called COVID-19.[67] COVID-19 was officially declared a pandemic by the World Health Organization on March 11, 2020. As of November 21, 2020, 57,274,018 confirmed cases have been reported with 1,368,000 deaths worldwide.[68] While it is increasingly clear that COVID-19 is a multisystem disease, the primary manifestation is a viral pneumonia that, in some patients, progresses to ARDS, often complicated by protracted illness or death.

Mortality estimates for COVID-19-associated ARDS vary widely, ranging from 3.4% to 88.3% (**Table 2**).[69–74] These estimates are affected by the studied population,

Table 2
Twenty-eight-day mortality rate data of patients with ARDS from COVID-19

Authors, Year of Publication [Reference]	Study Period	City, Country	Mortality
Yang et al,[69] 2020	12/24/2019–01/26/2020	Wuhan, China	61.5%
Wang et al,[70] 2020	01/25/2020–02/25/2020	Shanghai, China	88.3%
Grasselli et al,[71] 2020	02/20/2020–03/18/2020	Milan, Italy	26%
Ferrando et al,[72] 2020	03/12/2020–06/01/2020	Spain and Andora	36%
Bhatraju et al,[74] 2020	02/24/2020–03/09/2020	Seattle, USA	50%*
Gupta et al,[73] 2020	03/04/2020–04/04/2020	Various cities, USA	6.6%-80.8% (35.4%)

All patients were admitted to the ICU with ARDS due to COVID-19. All mortalities are 28-d mortality except the study by *Batraju et al which includes a 14-d mortality.

health system factors (thresholds for hospitalization varied across cohorts substantially), therapeutic context (Early in the pandemic, large numbers of potentially toxic therapies were administered in cocktails.), institutional context (the degree to which the studied health care systems were strained by the pandemic surge), and patient-level risk factors (some sites predominantly cared for patients in nursing homes). For example, patients admitted to hospitals with fewer ICU beds had higher risk of death likely because of less training and comfort of caregivers in treating ARDS as well as limited resources in these settings, particularly in the pandemic context. Critically, some early mortality studies had insufficient follow-up to provide accurate estimates of morality, excluding patients without a final outcome (discharge or death) and thereby inflating mortality estimates by excluding patients alive and still in the hospital.

The question of whether and how COVID-19-associated ARDS differs from prior forms of ARDS has been surprisingly contentious.[75] Early anxiety about abrupt decompensation specific to this condition, the risk of aerosolization and consequent transmission to caregivers with high-flow nasal cannula oxygen, and lack of effective therapeutics all played a role, as did clinician perceptions that some patients with COVID-19 exhibit "happy hypoxemia" and/or higher-than-expected lung compliance for their degree of hypoxemia.[76] The opinion that ARDS resulting from COVID-19 might be exceptional and clinicians' frustration over the lack of proven treatments were sometimes associated with calls for application of therapies previously shown ineffective in general ARDS and even for the use of high-tidal-volume ventilation. Spring and summer 2020 witnessed a vigorous debate on the issues, with some thought leaders arguing for novel supportive care, and others arguing that standard supportive care for ARDS represented the best approach.[77,78]

While some prognostic factors differ and time from COVID-19 symptom onset to full ARDS is sometimes slightly longer than with some classic ARDS etiologies,[79] most evidence to date suggests that ARDS in COVID-19 lacks important differences from the syndrome generally. Contradicting the postulated "L-type" (high compliance) and "H-type" (low compliance) dichotomy advanced by some as unique to COVID-19 ARDS,[76,80] the spectrum of lung compliance in COVID-19 ARDS appears similar to that observed in prior studies of general ARDS.[81] Pathologic analysis also shows findings similar to ARDS generally, demonstrating hyaline membrane formation, edema, and DAD.[82] We therefore manage COVID-19 ARDS with the package of evidence-based care that we apply to ARDS generally, including strict adherence to low-tidal-volume ventilation,[49] consideration of prone positioning,[83] and high PEEP for more severe ARDS,[36] conservative fluid management,[84] protocolized spontaneous breathing and awakening trial,[85] and early mobilization.[86] It is nevertheless plausible that, given its homogeneous trigger and potentially more homogeneous inflammatory phenotype, ARDS resulting from COVID-19 could respond to therapies that failed trials enrolling patients with a heterogeneous array of triggers and endotypes. The apparent efficacy of steroid therapy in several (imperfect) trials,[87,88] a treatment for which trials in general ARDS population had repeatedly yielded conflicting evidence,[89–91] may be one early example of this phenomenon.

SUMMARY

ARDS remains a common, deadly problem among critically ill patients around the world. It is a syndrome of significant heterogeneity, with sub-phenotypes requiring further characterization and tools for prompt clinical identification. COVID-19 has brought new challenges including a large, and relatively homogeneous, population of ARDS patients but does not seem to cause a truly unique respiratory failure syndrome distinct from ARDS generally nor even engender a truly homogenous subtype of ARDS. Further advances in ARDS care will likely require improved understanding of the epidemiology of this syndrome and its subtypes as well as innovative trials of focused therapeutics. Given the high mortality of the syndrome and its long-term morbidity, ongoing study into treatment and care of patients with ARDS is paramount.

CLINICS CARE POINTS

- Although acute respiratory distress syndrome (ARDS) has a high incidence among intensive care unit patients, with high morbidity and mortality, it remains underdiagnosed.
- The Berlin criteria were created to help clearly identify patients with ARDS.
- Supportive measures with low-tidal-volume ventilation, prone positioning, conservative fluid management strategies, high PEEP for severe disease, protocolized spontaneous breathing and awakening trials, and early mobilization have lowered the morbidity and mortality of ARDS and are the cornerstone of therapy.
- COVID-19-associated ARDS is a syndrome on the ARDS spectrum and should therefore be treated with the same strategies as classic ARDS while we await results of ongoing trials.

DISCLOSURE

K.W. Hendrickson declares no disclosures. I.D. Peltan reports receiving research support from the National Institutes of Health, Centers for Disease Control, Janssen Pharmaceuticals, and Immunexpress, Inc. and support to institution from Regeneron and Asahi Kasei Pharma. S.M. Brown-please see pdf in Other Content tab.

REFERENCES

1. Bellani G, et al. Epidemiology, patterns of care, and mortality for patients with acute respiratory distress syndrome in intensive care units in 50 countries. JAMA 2016;315(8):788–800.
2. Force ADT, et al. Acute respiratory distress syndrome: the Berlin definition. JAMA 2012;307(23):2526–33.
3. Ashbaugh DG, et al. Acute respiratory distress in adults. Lancet 1967;2(7511): 319–23.

4. Nolan S, et al. Acute respiratory distress syndrome in a community hospital ICU. Intensive Care Med 1997;23(5):530–8.
5. Luhr OR, et al. Incidence and mortality after acute respiratory failure and acute respiratory distress syndrome in Sweden, Denmark, and Iceland. The ARF Study Group. Am J Respir Crit Care Med 1999;159(6):1849–61.
6. Bersten AD, et al. Incidence and mortality of acute lung injury and the acute respiratory distress syndrome in three Australian States. Am J Respir Crit Care Med 2002;165(4):443–8.
7. Rubenfeld GD, et al. Incidence and outcomes of acute lung injury. N Engl J Med 2005;353(16):1685–93.
8. Manzano F, et al. Incidence of acute respiratory distress syndrome and its relation to age. J Crit Care 2005;20(3):274–80.
9. Li G, et al. Eight-year trend of acute respiratory distress syndrome: a population-based study in Olmsted County, Minnesota. Am J Respir Crit Care Med 2011; 183(1):59–66.
10. Caser EB, et al. Impact of distinct definitions of acute lung injury on its incidence and outcomes in Brazilian ICUs: prospective evaluation of 7,133 patients*. Crit Care Med 2014;42(3):574–82.
11. Linko R, et al. Acute respiratory failure in intensive care units. FINNALI: a prospective cohort study. Intensive Care Med 2009;35(8):1352–61.
12. Villar J, et al. The ALIEN study: incidence and outcome of acute respiratory distress syndrome in the era of lung protective ventilation. Intensive Care Med 2011;37(12):1932–41.
13. Brun-Buisson C, et al. Epidemiology and outcome of acute lung injury in European intensive care units. Results from the ALIVE study. Intensive Care Med 2004;30(1):51–61.
14. Irish Critical Care Trials, G. Acute lung injury and the acute respiratory distress syndrome in Ireland: a prospective audit of epidemiology and management. Crit Care 2008;12(1):R30.
15. Sigurdsson MI, et al. Acute respiratory distress syndrome: nationwide changes in incidence, treatment and mortality over 23 years. Acta Anaesthesiol Scand 2013; 57(1):37–45.
16. Bachofen M, Weibel ER. Structural alterations of lung parenchyma in the adult respiratory distress syndrome. Clin Chest Med 1982;3(1):35–56.
17. Tomashefski JF Jr. Pulmonary pathology of the adult respiratory distress syndrome. Clin Chest Med 1990;11(4):593–619.
18. Hoelz C, et al. Morphometric differences in pulmonary lesions in primary and secondary ARDS. A preliminary study in autopsies. Pathol Res Pract 2001;197(8): 521–30.
19. Moss M, et al. Diabetic patients have a decreased incidence of acute respiratory distress syndrome. Crit Care Med 2000;28(7):2187–92.
20. Rubenfeld GD, Herridge MS. Epidemiology and outcomes of acute lung injury. Chest 2007;131(2):554–62.
21. Ni YN, et al. Can body mass index predict clinical outcomes for patients with acute lung injury/acute respiratory distress syndrome? A meta-analysis. Crit Care 2017;21(1):36.
22. Zhi G, et al. Obesity paradox" in acute respiratory distress syndrome: asystematic review and meta-analysis. PLoS One 2016;11(9):e0163677.
23. McCallister JW, Adkins EJ, O'Brien JM Jr. Obesity and acute lung injury. Clin Chest Med 2009;30(3):495–508, viii.

24. Stensrud MJ, Valberg M, Aalen OO. Can collider bias explain paradoxical associations? Epidemiology 2017;28(4):e39–40.
25. Kaphalia L, Calhoun WJ. Alcoholic lung injury: metabolic, biochemical and immunological aspects. Toxicol Lett 2013;222(2):171–9.
26. Calfee CS, et al. Cigarette smoke exposure and the acute respiratory distress syndrome. Crit Care Med 2015;43(9):1790–7.
27. Hsieh SJ, et al. Prevalence and impact of active and passive cigarette smoking in acute respiratory distress syndrome. Crit Care Med 2014;42(9):2058–68.
28. Ware LB, et al. Long-term ozone exposure increases the risk of developing the acute respiratory distress syndrome. Am J Respir Crit Care Med 2016;193(10): 1143–50.
29. Erickson SE, et al. Racial and ethnic disparities in mortality from acute lung injury. Crit Care Med 2009;37(1):1–6.
30. Meyer NJ, Christie JD. Genetic heterogeneity and risk of acute respiratory distress syndrome. Semin Respir Crit Care Med 2013;34(4):459–74.
31. Laffey JG, et al. Potentially modifiable factors contributing to outcome from acute respiratory distress syndrome: the LUNG SAFE study. Intensive Care Med 2016; 42(12):1865–76.
32. Calfee CS, et al. Trauma-associated lung injury differs clinically and biologically from acute lung injury due to other clinical disorders. Crit Care Med 2007; 35(10):2243–50.
33. Tejera P, et al. Distinct and replicable genetic risk factors for acute respiratory distress syndrome of pulmonary or extrapulmonary origin. J Med Genet 2012; 49(11):671–80.
34. Villar J, et al. A universal definition of ARDS: the PaO2/FiO2 ratio under a standard ventilatory setting–a prospective, multicenter validation study. Intensive Care Med 2013;39(4):583–92.
35. Thille AW, et al. Comparison of the Berlin definition for acute respiratory distress syndrome with autopsy. Am J Respir Crit Care Med 2013;187(7):761–7.
36. Guo L, et al. Higher PEEP improves outcomes in ARDS patients with clinically objective positive oxygenation response to PEEP: a systematic review and meta-analysis. BMC Anesthesiol 2018;18(1):172.
37. Brower RG, et al. Higher versus lower positive end-expiratory pressures in patients with the acute respiratory distress syndrome. N Engl J Med 2004;351(4): 327–36.
38. Meade MO, et al. Ventilation strategy using low tidal volumes, recruitment maneuvers, and high positive end-expiratory pressure for acute lung injury and acute respiratory distress syndrome: a randomized controlled trial. JAMA 2008; 299(6):637–45.
39. Mercat A, et al. Positive end-expiratory pressure setting in adults with acute lung injury and acute respiratory distress syndrome: a randomized controlled trial. JAMA 2008;299(6):646–55.
40. Papazian L, et al. Neuromuscular blockers in early acute respiratory distress syndrome. N Engl J Med 2010;363(12):1107–16.
41. National Heart L, et al. Early neuromuscular blockade in the acute respiratory distress syndrome. N Engl J Med 2019;380(21):1997–2008.
42. Shaver CM, Bastarache JA. Clinical and biological heterogeneity in acute respiratory distress syndrome: direct versus indirect lung injury. Clin Chest Med 2014; 35(4):639–53.

43. Bernard GR, et al. The American-European Consensus Conference on ARDS. Definitions, mechanisms, relevant outcomes, and clinical trial coordination. Am J Respir Crit Care Med 1994;149(3 Pt 1):818–24.

44. Pelosi P, et al. Pulmonary and extrapulmonary acute respiratory distress syndrome are different. Eur Respir J Suppl 2003;42:48s–56s.

45. Gattinoni L, et al. Acute respiratory distress syndrome caused by pulmonary and extrapulmonary disease. Different syndromes? Am J Respir Crit Care Med 1998;158(1):3–11.

46. Albaiceta GM, et al. Differences in the deflation limb of the pressure-volume curves in acute respiratory distress syndrome from pulmonary and extrapulmonary origin. Intensive Care Med 2003;29(11):1943–9.

47. Calfee CS, et al. Distinct molecular phenotypes of direct vs indirect ARDS in single-center and multicenter studies. Chest 2015;147(6):1539–48.

48. Agarwal R, et al. Is the mortality higher in the pulmonary vs the extrapulmonary ARDS? A meta analysis. Chest 2008;133(6):1463–73.

49. Acute Respiratory Distress Syndrome, N, et al. Ventilation with lower tidal volumes as compared with traditional tidal volumes for acute lung injury and the acute respiratory distress syndrome. N Engl J Med 2000;342(18):1301–8.

50. Calfee CS, et al. Subphenotypes in acute respiratory distress syndrome: latent class analysis of data from two randomised controlled trials. Lancet Respir Med 2014;2(8):611–20.

51. Calfee CS, et al. Acute respiratory distress syndrome subphenotypes and differential response to simvastatin: secondary analysis of a randomised controlled trial. Lancet Respir Med 2018;6(9):691–8.

52. Pham T, Rubenfeld GD. Fifty years of research in ARDS. The epidemiology of acute respiratory distress syndrome. A 50th birthday review. Am J Respir Crit Care Med 2017;195(7):860–70.

53. Ferguson ND, et al. Acute respiratory distress syndrome: underrecognition by clinicians and diagnostic accuracy of three clinical definitions. Crit Care Med 2005;33(10):2228–34.

54. Frohlich S, et al. Acute respiratory distress syndrome: underrecognition by clinicians. J Crit Care 2013;28(5):663–8.

55. Gajic O, et al. Early identification of patients at risk of acute lung injury: evaluation of lung injury prediction score in a multicenter cohort study. Am J Respir Crit Care Med 2011;183(4):462–70.

56. Trillo-Alvarez C, et al. Acute lung injury prediction score: derivation and validation in a population-based sample. Eur Respir J 2011;37(3):604–9.

57. Soto GJ, et al. Lung injury prediction score in hospitalized patients at risk of acute respiratory distress syndrome. Crit Care Med 2016;44(12):2182–91.

58. Kor DJ, et al. Effect of aspirin on development of ARDS in at-risk patients presenting to the emergency department: the LIPS-A randomized clinical trial. JAMA 2016;315(22):2406–14.

59. Serpa Neto A, et al. Association between use of lung-protective ventilation with lower tidal volumes and clinical outcomes among patients without acute respiratory distress syndrome: a meta-analysis. JAMA 2012;308(16):1651–9.

60. Writing Group for the, P.I, et al. Effect of a low vs intermediate tidal volume strategy on ventilator-free days in intensive care unit patients without ARDS: a randomized clinical trial. JAMA 2018;320(18):1872–80.

61. Lanspa MJ, et al. Prospective assessment of the feasibility of a trial of low-tidal volume ventilation for patients with acute respiratory failure. Ann Am Thorac Soc 2019;16(3):356–62.

62. Falci L, et al. Examination of cause-of-death data quality among New York city deaths due to cancer, pneumonia, or diabetes from 2010 to 2014. Am J Epidemiol 2018;187(1):144–52.
63. Cochi SE, et al. Mortality trends of acute respiratory distress syndrome in the United States from 1999 to 2013. Ann Am Thorac Soc 2016;13(10):1742–51.
64. Walkey AJ, et al. Acute respiratory distress syndrome: epidemiology and management approaches. Clin Epidemiol 2012;4:159–69.
65. Herridge MS, et al. Functional disability 5 years after acute respiratory distress syndrome. N Engl J Med 2011;364(14):1293–304.
66. Mamary AJ, et al. Survival in patients receiving prolonged ventilation: factors that influence outcome. Clin Med Insights Circ Respir Pulm Med 2011;5:17–26.
67. Zhu N, et al. A novel coronavirus from patients with pneumonia in China, 2019. N Engl J Med 2020;382(8):727–33.
68. Available at: https://www.who.int/emergencies/diseases/novel-coronavirus-2019? gclid=EAlaIQobChMIoNWJg6m86wIVjcDACh2RZAFnEAAYASAAEgI7APD_BwE. Accessed August 27, 2020.
69. Yang X, et al. Clinical course and outcomes of critically ill patients with SARS-CoV-2 pneumonia in Wuhan, China: a single-centered, retrospective, observational study. Lancet Respir Med 2020;8(5):475–81.
70. Wang Y, et al. Clinical course and outcomes of 344 intensive care patients with COVID-19. Am J Respir Crit Care Med 2020;201(11):1430–4.
71. Grasselli G, et al. Baseline characteristics and outcomes of 1591 patients infected with SARS-CoV-2 admitted to ICUs of the Lombardy region, Italy. JAMA 2020;323(16):1574–81.
72. Ferrando C, et al. Clinical features, ventilatory management, and outcome of ARDS caused by COVID-19 are similar to other causes of ARDS. Intensive Care Med 2020;46(12):2200–11.
73. Gupta S, et al. Factors associated with death in critically ill patients with coronavirus disease 2019 in the US. JAMA Intern Med 2020;180(11):1436–47.
74. Bhatraju PK, et al. Covid-19 in critically ill patients in the seattle region - case series. N Engl J Med 2020;382(21):2012–22.
75. Barbeta E, et al. SARS-CoV-2-induced acute respiratory distress syndrome: pulmonary mechanics and gas-exchange abnormalities. Ann Am Thorac Soc 2020; 17(9):1164–8.
76. Marini JJ, Gattinoni L. Management of COVID-19 respiratory distress. JAMA 2020;323(22):2329–30.
77. Matthay MA, Aldrich JM, Gotts JE. Treatment for severe acute respiratory distress syndrome from COVID-19. Lancet Respir Med 2020;8(5):433–4.
78. Wiersinga WJ, et al. Pathophysiology, transmission, diagnosis, and treatment of coronavirus disease 2019 (COVID-19): a review. JAMA 2020;324(8):782–93.
79. Li X, Ma X. Acute respiratory failure in COVID-19: is it "typical" ARDS? Crit Care 2020;24(1):198.
80. Gattinoni L, et al. COVID-19 pneumonia: different respiratory treatments for different phenotypes? Intensive Care Med 2020;46(6):1099–102.
81. Panwar R, et al. Compliance phenotypes in early acute respiratory distress syndrome before the COVID-19 pandemic. Am J Respir Crit Care Med 2020;202(9): 1244–52.
82. Calabrese F, et al. Pulmonary pathology and COVID-19: lessons from autopsy. The experience of European Pulmonary Pathologists. Virchows Arch 2020; 477(3):359–72.

83. Guerin C, Reignier J, Richard JC. Prone positioning in the acute respiratory distress syndrome. N Engl J Med 2013;369(10):980–1.
84. National Heart L, et al. Comparison of two fluid-management strategies in acute lung injury. N Engl J Med 2006;354(24):2564–75.
85. Girard TD, et al. Efficacy and safety of a paired sedation and ventilator weaning protocol for mechanically ventilated patients in intensive care (Awakening and Breathing Controlled trial): a randomised controlled trial. Lancet 2008; 371(9607):126–34.
86. Taito S, et al. Early mobilization of mechanically ventilated patients in the intensive care unit. J Intensive Care 2016;4:50.
87. RECOVERY Collaborative Group, Horby P, Lim WS, et al. Dexamethasone in hospitalized patients with Covid-19. N Engl J Med 2021;384(8):693–704. https://doi.org/10.1056/NEJMoa2021436.
88. Prescott HC, Rice TW. Corticosteroids in COVID-19 ARDS: evidence and Hope during the pandemic. JAMA 2020;324(13):1292–5.
89. Schein RM, et al. Complement activation and corticosteroid therapy in the development of the adult respiratory distress syndrome. Chest 1987;91(6):850–4.
90. Peter JV, et al. Corticosteroids in the prevention and treatment of acute respiratory distress syndrome (ARDS) in adults: meta-analysis. BMJ 2008;336(7651): 1006–9.
91. Villar J, et al. Dexamethasone treatment for the acute respiratory distress syndrome: a multicentre, randomised controlled trial. Lancet Respir Med 2020; 8(3):267–76.
92. Sakr Y, et al. High tidal volume and positive fluid balance are associated with worse outcome in acute lung injury. Chest 2005;128(5):3098–108.

Environmental Factors

Katherine D. Wick, MD[a,b], Michael A. Matthay, MD[b,c,d],*

KEYWORDS

- Acute respiratory distress syndrome (ARDS) • Acute lung injury (ALI)
- Environmental pollution • Wildfires • Tobacco smoke • e-cigarettes
- e-cigarette and vaping-associated lung injury (EVALI)

KEY POINTS

- Preventable environmental exposures are associated with an increased risk of developing the acute respiratory distress syndrome (ARDS).
- Environmental pollution and cigarette smoke likely predispose the lung to injury from other causes, whereas e-cigarettes are a direct cause of lung injury.
- Evidence-based strategies of lung protective ventilation, fluid conservative strategy, and early prone positioning for Pao_2/Fio_2 less than 150 mm Hg are the cornerstones of management regardless of environmental factors.
- Both patient- and policy-level interventions are needed to reduce harm from these exposures.

INTRODUCTION

The acute respiratory distress syndrome (ARDS) affects at least 10% of patients in the intensive care unit (ICU) and carries a high mortality rate of approximately 40%.[1] There have been effective advances in supportive care, but there are as yet no consistently proven effective pharmacologic treatments for ARDS.[2] One approach to addressing this problem is to target the heterogeneity of ARDS by understanding patient factors that impact response to treatment once ARDS has already developed. For example, secondary analyses of randomized clinical trials demonstrate that ARDS subphenotypes respond differentially to simvastatin therapy.[3] Another important facet is early intervention in hospitalized patients at risk of ARDS.[4] However, clinicians and researchers should also focus on identifying preventable patient exposures that increase the risk for ARDS, as demonstrated by a growing body of research. Understanding and

[a] Department of Anesthesia, University of California, San Francisco, 513 Parnassus Avenue, HSE 760, San Francisco, CA 94143, USA; [b] Cardiovascular Research Institute, University of California, San Francisco, San Francisco, CA, USA; [c] Department of Medicine, University of California, San Francisco, 505 Parnassus Avenue, M-917, San Francisco, CA 94143, USA; [d] Department of Anesthesia, University of California, San Francisco, 505 Parnassus Avenue, M-917, San Francisco, CA 94143, USA
* Corresponding author. Department of Medicine, University of California, San Francisco, 505 Parnassus Avenue, M-917, San Francisco, CA 94143.
E-mail address: Michael.matthay@ucsf.edu

Crit Care Clin 37 (2021) 717–732
https://doi.org/10.1016/j.ccc.2021.05.002
0749-0704/21/© 2021 Elsevier Inc. All rights reserved.

addressing these exposures offers an opportunity for primary prevention (**Fig. 1**). This review summarizes the current literature on environmental exposures and ARDS development and outcomes, discusses underlying mechanisms, and outlines the implications for patient management and policy-guided solutions.

AIR POLLUTION

According to the World Health Organization, the pollutants with the greatest effect on human health are ozone, sulfur dioxide (SO_2), nitrogen dioxide (NO_2), and particulate matter (PM).[5] In 2014, PM less than 10 μm in diameter (PM 10) and less than 2.5 μm in diameter (PM 2.5) accounted for at least 3 million deaths and 85 disability-adjusted life years, primarily because of impacts on chronic cardiovascular and pulmonary conditions.[6] Recently, air pollution in the United States has begun increasing for the first time since 2016 (**Fig. 2**).[7] Ambient pollution is a risk factor not only for the development or worsening of chronic illnesses[8–10] but also for acute illness. For example, a case-control study of older adults in Canada found that long-term exposure to PM 2.5 and NO_2 was independently associated with an increased risk of hospitalization for community-acquired pneumonia.[11] Short-term exposure to increasing levels of PM 2.5 was also shown to increase the risk of hospital admission for cardiac and respiratory disease in the United States.[12]

Several recent studies have demonstrated that exposure to even low to moderate levels of ambient pollutants increases the risk of developing ARDS. In a prospectively enrolled cohort of patients with ARDS in the Southeastern United States, long-term ozone exposure was associated with the development of ARDS in a dose-dependent manner.[13] This association was most pronounced among patients with trauma as their primary risk factor. Although the association between ozone exposure and the development of ARDS remained significant when controlling for potential confounders including smoking status, there was a statistically significant interaction between ozone exposure and smoking. When patients were stratified by smoking status, ozone exposure

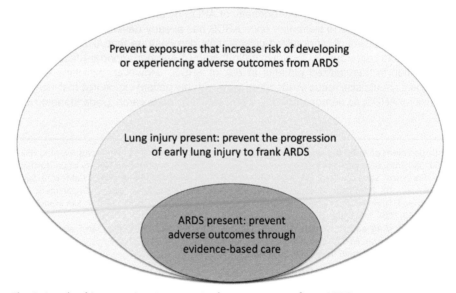

Fig. 1. Levels of intervention to prevent adverse outcomes from ARDS.

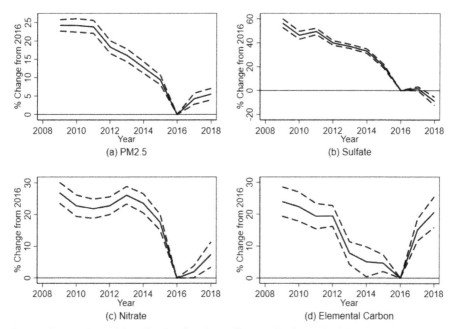

Fig. 2. Changes in ambient levels of major pollutants in the United States, 2008 to 2018. Dotted lines represent 95% confidence intervals. (*From* Clay K, Muller N. Recent increases in air pollution: Evidence and implications for mortality. 2019. https://doi.org/10.3386/w26381; with permission.)

remained significantly associated with ARDS only among smokers. The investigators concluded that cigarette smoking likely potentiates the risk from ozone exposure.[13]

A subsequent study of patients from a prospectively enrolled cohort in Philadelphia further investigated the relationship between exposure to pollutants and ARDS development among patients with trauma.[14] This study analyzed exposure to low to moderate levels of ozone, NO_2, SO_2, PM 2.5, and carbon monoxide (CO). Long-term exposure to each of the pollutants was independently associated with an increased odds of developing ARDS. Furthermore, even 6 weeks of exposure to NO_2, SO_2, and PM 2.5 increased the odds of developing ARDS.[14] Differences between the findings of the 2 studies might be accounted for by regional variation in levels of pollutants and air quality monitoring and by the shared risk factor of the population in the second study. Together these studies suggest that exposure to ambient pollution even at low to moderate levels for time periods as short as 6 weeks increases the risk of ARDS.

Large epidemiologic studies have also found associations between exposure to ambient pollution and an increased risk of developing ARDS. An observational study of more than 1 million hospitalizations between the years 2000 and 2012 among Medicare beneficiaries who developed ARDS used advanced modeling drawing on multiple data sources to predict average annual levels of ambient pollution across more than 30,000 zip codes.[15] The investigators found that the rate of ARDS hospitalizations increased with increasing levels of both PM 2.5 and ozone. These findings were consistent even in regions where pollutant levels were within national air quality standards. The effect of PM 2.5 was most pronounced among patients whose primary risk factor was sepsis. Ozone exposure had the greatest effect among patients with pneumonia or trauma as their primary risk factor. Although fully accounting for confounding factors in observational studies can be difficult, results were similar in a propensity-matched analysis that included variables such as demographic variations and percent of ever-smokers.[15] The results of this large study demonstrate that the association between ambient pollution and ARDS is present outside of the trauma population in patients who are older with comorbid conditions. Another retrospective cohort study of more than 90,000 patients found that increases in average annual PM 2.5 and ozone concentrations independently increased the odds of death from ARDS, suggesting that ambient pollution impacts not only ARDS incidence but also its outcomes.[16] High levels of ambient pollution have also been associated with incidence and adverse outcomes in the coronavirus disease 2019 (COVID-19) pandemic,[17,18] although further studies in this area are needed.

The preponderance of the literature examining the connection between ARDS and ambient pollution has revealed an association between long-term rather than short-term exposure to pollutants and ARDS incidence and outcomes. For example, the investigators who found a link between long-term ozone exposure and ARDS did not find the same association for 3-day exposure to environmental pollutants.[13] However, one study from Guangzhou, China, demonstrated an association between short-term PM exposure and incident ARDS.[19] This association may be related to the exceptionally poor air quality of the region[20] in contrast to the other studies, which focused on settings with low to moderate levels of pollutants. There is some evidence, however, that short-term exposure to low levels of ambient pollution is associated with adverse pulmonary outcomes in critically ill patients. A study from Antwerp, Belgium—an area with historically low levels of ambient pollution—found that short-term pollution exposure was associated with longer mechanical ventilation.[21] This study included a broad range of critically ill patients, some of whom did not have ARDS, but does suggest that a deleterious effect from short-term pollution exposure is not limited to areas with exceptionally poor air quality.

Various underlying biological mechanisms may explain the basis for the relationship between environmental pollution and ARDS. A meta-analysis of exposure studies in healthy volunteers found that ozone increases the number of bronchoalveolar lavage (BAL) neutrophils,[22] which are implicated in ARDS pathogenesis.[23] Ozone exposure also increased total protein levels in this analysis,[22] reflecting loss of alveolar epithelial/endothelial barrier integrity.[24] Many components of air pollution exert deleterious effects on pulmonary surfactant.[25] Urban air particles directly stimulate an inflammatory response by pulmonary macrophages in vitro.[26] PM has also been shown to increase markers of apoptosis, oxidative stress, and inflammation[27] and to directly cause lung injury in mouse models.[28] In humans, increased PM 2.5 levels are associated with circulating markers of endothelial injury,[29] which is one of the key pathophysiological mechanisms in the development of ARDS.[30] Although environmental pollutants alone may not be sufficient to induce severe pulmonary injury in humans, they likely increase susceptibility to other causes of ARDS such as respiratory infection[31] and prime the alveolus for damage in these settings.

WILDFIRES

Wildfire smoke is an increasingly prevalent source of environmental pollution. Climate change has led to more frequent wildfires over a longer season.[32] In the United States, PM air quality has improved over the past 3 decades except in areas that are prone to wildfires.[33] Wildfires are associated with acute increases in ozone and PM as well as other pollutants such as volatile organic compounds.[34] As noted earlier, previous studies of the relationship between ambient pollution and ARDS[13–16] have generally focused on the average exposure in various regions over time, rather than on events that might be expected to acutely increase ambient pollution. In addition, smoke from wildfires may have chemical properties that make its risk profile different from that of PM or smoke from other sources.[34,35] Although it is clear that wildfire-related pollution contributes to increased respiratory morbidity and health utilization overall,[36] the specific relationship between ARDS and exposure to pollutants generated by wildfire smoke has not been studied (in contrast to direct inhalational or thermal injury or burn-related ARDS in persons who are survivors of fire accidents,[37,38] which is outside of the scope of this review). In vitro evidence demonstrates that wood smoke exposure diminishes alveolar barrier function[39] and increases alveolar endothelial oxidative stress and apoptosis.[40] In mice, PM collected during wildfires induced a more proinflammatory response and greater oxidative stress than ambient PM collected in the absence of wildfires.[41] Woodfire smoke exposure has also been shown to induce a pulmonary and systemic inflammatory response in healthy volunteers.[42] It is mechanistically plausible that the increased inflammation, oxidative stress, and lung microvascular permeability in response to woodfire smoke demonstrated under experimental conditions would translate to an increased risk of ARDS. Future research should test whether ARDS incidence and outcomes change during or after wildfire events.

CIGARETTE SMOKE

The link between cigarette smoke and adverse health outcomes is well established, and reducing cigarette use has been a major focus of public health efforts over the past half century.[43] Although rates of tobacco smoking have generally declined globally, they remain unacceptably high, and cigarette smoking is a leading cause of avoidable death. For example, the 2015 Global Burden of Disease Study found that approximately 11% of women and 14% of men in the United States report daily smoking and that smoking accounted for 6.4 million deaths globally.[44] Alternative tobacco and nicotine delivery systems such as electronic cigarettes (e-cigarettes), or vapes, are increasingly popular, an especially concerning trend among children and adolescents.[45] Although their long-term health consequences are not well established, e-cigarettes cause a specific lung injury syndrome, e-cigarette- or vaping-associated lung injury (EVALI).[46] E-cigarettes will be discussed in detail in a separate section.

Although some retrospective studies have not found an association between cigarette smoking and ARDS,[47] many studies demonstrate that both active smoking and passive cigarette smoke exposure are associated with ARDS, especially among certain clinical populations. Importantly, this association is independent of alcohol use, which is frequently associated with smoking and is a known risk factor for ARDS.[48] A retrospective cohort study of patients in Northern California found that ARDS was more common among self-reported smokers in a dose-dependent manner. The investigators estimated that smoking carried an attributable risk in ARDS of 50%.[49] A 2014 study of 381 patients with ARDS previously enrolled in randomized clinical trials examined the relationship between tobacco exposure and ARDS.[50] Rather than relying on patient or surrogate reports, which lack sensitivity when compared with biomarkers for tobacco exposure,[51] urine levels of NNAL (4-(methylnitrosamino)-1-(3-pyridyl)-1-butanol) were used to determine smoking history. The rate of active smoking among patients with ARDS in this study was significantly higher than the population average (36% vs 20%, $P<.01$). Smokers were younger and had fewer comorbidities than nonsmokers despite similar ARDS severity. Although unadjusted mortality among smokers was significantly lower than in nonsmokers, there was no significant difference after adjusting for comorbidities and severity of illness,[50] suggesting that smokers develop ARDS when their illness is less severe than that of otherwise similar patients.

Prospective studies have also demonstrated an increased risk of ARDS among smokers. Current cigarette smoking (determined through medical chart review) conferred increased odds (odds ratio, 3.4; 95% confidence interval, 1.22–9.7; $P = .020$) for the development of transfusion-related acute lung injury (ALI) in a two-center prospective case-control study.[52] Donor smoking history increased the odds of grade 3 primary graft dysfunction in a multicenter prospectively enrolled cohort of lung transplant recipients.[53] A prospective study of the association between tobacco exposure and the development of ALI[54] after blunt trauma used plasma levels of cotinine to differentiate between active and passive smoke exposure and to quantify exposure levels.[55] Active smokers and passively exposed patients in this cohort from a single level 1 trauma center had similarly increased odds of developing ARDS independent of confounding factors, including alcohol use and trauma severity. Higher levels of plasma cotinine were associated with higher odds of developing ARDS.[55] Another prospective study of patients with trauma enrolled between 2005 and 2015 confirmed that cigarette smoke exposure remains an important risk factor for ARDS and highlighted a particularly elevated risk among passive smokers in later years.[56] In patients with trauma, impaired platelet aggregation likely mediates at least part of the effect of cigarette smoke exposure on ARDS risk.[57] In addition, cigarette smoke alters the microbiota in patients with trauma such that their pulmonary microbiome is enriched for specific pathologic bacteria that are associated with ARDS development.[58]

In a prospectively enrolled cohort with diverse predisposing risk factors for ARDS, active cigarette smoking both by self-report and urine NNAL was associated with an increased odds of ARDS among patients with nonpulmonary sepsis as their primary predisposing risk factor.[59] Patients with trauma and transfusion as their primary risk factor were not included in this study because of the previously established link between smoking and ARDS in these populations. Again, the mortality rate of active smokers was lower in an unadjusted analysis, but mortality was similar after adjusting for baseline severity of illness.[59] This finding is consistent with the previous one that smokers are at increased risk of developing ARDS when their underlying illness is comparatively less severe.

Similarly to ambient pollution, cigarette smoke exposure likely predisposes the lung to injury in the setting of a second insult such as trauma, multiple transfusions, or sepsis (**Fig. 3**). This concept was elegantly demonstrated in an experimental model in healthy humans who were exposed to inhaled lipopolysaccharide (LPS).[60] BAL and plasma biomarkers for alveolar epithelial-capillary permeability, inflammation, and alveolar endothelial dysfunction were compared between self-reported smokers and nonsmokers. Absolute measurements were consistent with more alveolar permeability to protein and inflammation in smokers, and statistical tests of interaction demonstrated that smoking potentiated these responses to LPS.[60] In mice, cigarette smoke exposure itself does not cause frank lung injury, but mice exposed to cigarette smoke develop worse pulmonary edema, increased vascular permeability, worse histologic injury, and increased biomarker evidence of inflammation after exposure to LPS.[61] A similar pattern was demonstrated in a clinically relevant model of pneumococcal pneumonia after antibiotic treatment,[62] and other animal models have also shown that cigarette smoke increases alveolar epithelial-capillary permeability and susceptibility to lung injury.[63]

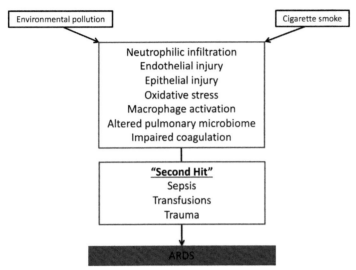

Fig. 3. Pollution and/or cigarette smoke exposure likely predisposes the lung to severe injury in the presence of risk factors for ARDS such as trauma, sepsis, or multiple transfusions.

The relationship between cigarette smoking and COVID-19, which in 2020 was the leading cause of ARDS in the United States,[64] is unclear. There is evidence that the receptor for severe acute respiratory syndrome coronavirus 2 (SARS-CoV-2), angiotensin-converting enzyme 2 (ACE2), is more highly expressed in the lung epithelium of smokers than in nonsmokers.[65,66] It is not obvious from the available data, however, that this leads to an increased risk of SARS-CoV-2 infection or worse outcomes from COVID-19. In fact, smokers are disproportionately underrepresented among patients with COVID-19.[67] It has been proposed that nicotine as an isolated substance may have a protective effect in COVID-19.[68] The relationships among cigarette smoking, ACE2, nicotine, and inflammation are complex, and a full understanding of the implications of smoking on COVID-19 pathogenesis and outcomes requires further study.

E-Cigarettes

E-cigarette use has increased among young people in recent years.[69] Furthermore, using e-cigarettes increases the likelihood of future cigarette smoking among children and adolescents,[70] is associated with increased rates of smoking initiation in adults, and increases the risk of relapse among former cigarette smokers.[71] Therefore, promoting vaping as a harm reduction strategy from traditional cigarettes may be misguided. E-cigarette use likely has negative implications for long-term health based on the cellular and molecular mechanisms it affects,[72,73] although confirming this will require longitudinal studies. In addition, e-cigarettes pose an increased public health risk as a direct cause of ALI.

An outbreak of EVALI, mostly among patients younger than 35 years, emerged in the United States in the spring and summer of 2019. The Centers for Disease Control and Prevention has reported more 2800 cases and 68 deaths.[74] The diagnostic criteria are vaping within the prior 90 days and a new infiltrate on chest imaging in the absence of pulmonary infection.[75] EVALI most commonly presents as acute to subacute constitutional and respiratory symptoms with radiographic findings of bilateral ground glass opacities (**Fig. 4**).[76] In one case series, 26% of patients required mechanical ventilation, and approximately 12% of patients met the Berlin criteria for ARDS by chart review.[77,78]

Vitamin E acetate (VEA) is likely the major causative agent among patients with EVALI. In one case series of patients from 16 different states, VEA was found in 94% of BAL fluid samples from patients with EVALI and in none of the samples from healthy comparators.[79] Most patients report using tetrahydrocannabinol (THC) products, in which VEA is frequently used as a diluent,[80] although some report exclusively using nicotine-based products.[76] The effect of VEA was recently studied in a murine model and in primary alveolar type II (ATII) cell culture.[81] In the mouse model, exposure to aerosolized VEA resulted in significantly increased BAL protein, excess lung water, and BAL biomarkers of alveolar epithelial damage and inflammation when compared with aerosolized tobacco or vegetable glycerin and propylene glycol. Histologic patterns closely mirrored those found in patients with EVALI.[82] VEA was also found to cause direct, dose-dependent ATII toxicity.[81] Because of the many ingredients found in e-cigarettes and the use of unregulated products,[83] however, identifying a single culprit in EVALI is difficult.

It is unknown whether chronic e-cigarette use also increases the risk of developing ARDS from other causes. Studies of cigarette smoke exposure and ARDS using biomarkers for nicotine may have included patients who were using both traditional cigarettes and e-cigarettes, and smoking histories in medical records do not always describe whether patients also vape. E-cigarette vapor both with and without nicotine increases rat endothelial cell permeability in vitro, although the effect is more pronounced with nicotine.[84] Mice chronically exposed to e-cigarette vapor with and without nicotine demonstrate altered lipid homeostasis in alveolar macrophages and changes to ATII lamellar body ultrastructure, which may indicate that e-cigarettes disrupt surfactant production.[85] Chronic e-cigarette exposure also delays the immune response and results in worse lung injury in mice exposed to influenza.[85] Similar changes in humans could plausibly prime the lung for injury as with cigarette use.[60] Further studies should examine whether e-cigarettes increase the risk of developing ARDS from infection, trauma, or other causes.

DIAGNOSIS AND MANAGEMENT IMPLICATIONS

Regardless of the environmental risk factors for ARDS, the cornerstones of diagnosis and management remain the same. None of the aforementioned exposures, including

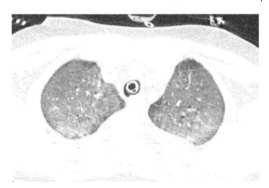

Fig. 4. Computed tomographic scan of a patient with EVALI, demonstrating diffuse bilateral ground glass opacities with characteristic subpleural sparing. (*Courtesy of* Dr. Carolyn Calfee, UCSF.)

e-cigarettes, results in a unique radiographic appearance,[76] and clinicians should use the Berlin criteria for ARDS for diagnosis.[78] Workup should include a thorough investigation of possible pulmonary and extrapulmonary infections, including viral pneumonia, and bronchoscopy may be warranted.[86] Understanding the environmental risk factors for ARDS underscores the importance of an accurate exposure history. For example, patients or surrogates should be asked about both personal use of cigarettes and passive (second-hand) cigarette smoke exposure. A thorough history should also include questions about e-cigarette use (vaping), regardless of whether patients also use combustible cigarettes. Providers should ask about product type; duration and frequency of use; use of nicotine-based products, cannabis products, or both; additives; and where the patient obtains their product.[87] Although corticosteroids are frequently used in EVALI,[76] this treatment has not been assessed in prospective randomized trials. Similarly, there is no pharmacotherapy specific to patients who smoke or who have been exposed to environmental pollutants. Management should therefore be based on the evidence-supported strategies of lung protective ventilation,[88] conservative fluid management,[89] and early prone positioning when Pao_2/ fraction of inspired oxygen is less than 150 mm Hg.[90]

The period during and after critical illness may be a unique opportunity for clinicians to encourage smoking and vaping cessation. Behavioral counseling for hospitalized patients, including critically ill patients, can lead to increased abstinence from smoking.[91] Providers caring for ICU survivors may also have an opportunity to encourage smoking cessation or continued abstinence.[92] Current American Thoracic Society (ATS) guidelines recommend pharmacologic therapy with varenicline and nicotine replacement for smoking cessation in adults.[93] Initiating varenicline therapy in critically ill patients has not been studied, and the role of nicotine replacement therapy in critically ill patients is not well established.[94] Research about pharmacologic therapy for teenagers who use cigarettes or electronic cigarettes is limited. The American Academy of Pediatrics recommends behavioral interventions, adding pharmacologic therapy depending on the severity of tobacco dependence.[95] The best approach for addressing tobacco dependence or e-cigarette use in patients with ARDS requires further investigation. Other exposures such as pollution and wildfire smoke are best addressed by public policy, which also plays a crucial role in smoking and vaping cessation.

PUBLIC HEALTH STRATEGIES AND KNOWLEDGE GAPS

The emerging data about chronic exposures and the risk of ARDS underscores how policy-level interventions impact the practice of critical care. Policy provides opportunities to fill current knowledge gaps through research funding and to limit risks of environmental exposures on a population level. Air quality measures and wildfire mitigation largely depend on public health and policy strategies. Upholding safe air quality standards is necessary to limit population-level exposure, but ambient pollution and the risk of wildfires will continue to increase as climate change progresses. The ATS has made climate change a priority for its public health and research agenda, citing the risk posed to cardiopulmonary health.[96]

Patient-level interventions are important for smoking and vaping cessation, but they should be part of a larger policy agenda (**Table 1**). Declining smoking rates are one of the great public health achievements of the twentieth and twenty-first centuries, and there are still many opportunities for progress such as expanded laws mandating smoke-free public environments, ongoing public awareness campaigns, and widespread adoption of evidence-based treatment of tobacco users.[43] The emergence

Table 1
Individual and policy-level interventions for reducing exposures that increase risk of ARDS

Exposure	Patient-Level Interventions	Policy-Level Interventions
Environmental pollution	Increased awareness of air quality metrics Staying indoors, avoiding strenuous activity when air quality is poor Compliance with evacuation orders during wildfires	Stringent air quality standards Focus on climate and environmental policies to limit impact of climate change
Cigarette smoke	Evidence-based approach to cessation	Expanded public health messaging, including about second-hand smoke Smoke-free public spaces Increased taxation of tobacco products
E-cigarettes	Avoid e-cigarettes as a harm reduction strategy Specific social history questions about e-cigarette use	Strict safety standards and regulation of market, including taxation Reduce availability of products that appeal to young people

of e-cigarettes and other alternative nicotine and cannabis delivery systems require new regulatory efforts. The Food and Drug Administration (FDA) has recently started enforcing regulations of flavored e-cigarette cartridges, for example, but many products still fall outside of this enforcement effort.[97] Illicit products necessarily are not subject to FDA regulations. Rates of EVALI may be higher in regions where cannabis is illegal,[98] and because it remains so on a federal level, there are no federal guidelines for the safe manufacturing or use of cannabis vaping products. There are also federal limitations on cannabis research, which restrict opportunities to study short- and long-term pulmonary effects of THC exposure.

Future research and policy priorities should focus on continuing to limit exposures that increase ARDS risk on both an individual and the population level. Researchers should investigate the optimum timing and method for encouraging smoking cessation after critical illness, including whether it may be appropriate to initiate pharmacologic therapy in the ICU. Priorities for e-cigarettes include strict safety standards, investigating whether e-cigarette exposure increases the risk of ARDS from other causes, and expanding research of potentially harmful electronic marijuana delivery systems. Public messaging about air quality standards should be expanded, and the medical community should continue to raise awareness about the impact of climate change on pollutants that threaten cardiopulmonary health. In summary, the scientific understanding of how environmental exposures increase the risk of ARDS is well established, but there is much to be learned. There are many opportunities to expand our knowledge and implement policy-level changes to continue combat this deadly syndrome.

CLINICS CARE POINTS

- Environmental factors such as cigarette smoking, environmental pollution, and the use of e-cigarettes (vapes) should be recognized as a contributing risk factor for ARDS.
- Evidence-based smoking cessation resources, including pharmacologic aids, should be offered to patients regardless of their stated readiness to quit as per ATS guidelines.

- When patients present with ARDS, clinicians should conduct a detailed exposure history including whether a patient uses combustible cigarettes or e-cigarettes. Vaping history should include frequency, type of product, duration, and source.
- Clinicians should rely on evidence-based cornerstones of ARDS management regardless of exposure history.

DISCLOSURE

K.D. Wick: Grant funding from NIH (5T32GM008440–24). M.A. Matthay: Grant funding from NIH (HL123004, HL134828, and HL140026). Income from Citius Pharmaceuticals and research support from Genentech-Roche for observational studies of ARDS.

REFERENCES

1. Bellani G, Laffey JG, Pham T, et al. Epidemiology, patterns of care, and mortality for patients with acute respiratory distress syndrome in intensive care units in 50 countries. JAMA 2016;315(8):788–800.
2. Lewis SR, Pritchard MW, Thomas CM, et al. Pharmacological agents for adults with acute respiratory distress syndrome. Cochrane Database Syst Rev 2019;7: CD004477.
3. Calfee CS, Delucchi KL, Sinha P, et al. Acute respiratory distress syndrome sub-phenotypes and differential response to simvastatin: secondary analysis of a randomised controlled trial. Lancet Respir Med 2018;6(9):691–8.
4. Matthay MA, McAuley DF, Ware LB. Clinical trials in acute respiratory distress syndrome: challenges and opportunities. Lancet Respir Med 2017;5(6):524–34.
5. World Health Organization. Air pollution: pollutants. Air pollution web site 2020. Available at: https://www.who.int/airpollution/ambient/pollutants/en/. Accessed 26 September, 2020.
6. World Health Organization. Ambient air pollution: a global assessment of exposure and burden of disease. Geneva (Switzerland): World Health Organization; 2016.
7. Clay K, Mullter NZ. Recent increases in air pollution: evidence and implications for mortality. Cambridge (MA): National Bureau of Economic Research Working Paper Series; 2019. p. 1–28. https://doi.org/10.3386/w26381.
8. Yang BY, Qian ZM, Li S, et al. Ambient air pollution in relation to diabetes and glucose-homoeostasis markers in China: a cross-sectional study with findings from the 33 Communities Chinese Health Study. Lancet Planet Health 2018; 2(2):e64–73.
9. Fuks KB, Weinmayr G, Basagana X, et al. Long-term exposure to ambient air pollution and traffic noise and incident hypertension in seven cohorts of the European study of cohorts for air pollution effects (ESCAPE). Eur Heart J 2017; 38(13):983–90.
10. Wang M, Aaron CP, Madrigano J, et al. Association between long-term exposure to ambient air pollution and change in quantitatively assessed emphysema and lung function. JAMA 2019;322(6):546–56.
11. Neupane B, Jerrett M, Burnett RT, et al. Long-term exposure to ambient air pollution and risk of hospitalization with community-acquired pneumonia in older adults. Am J Respir Crit Care Med 2010;181(1):47–53.

12. Dominici F, Peng RD, Bell ML, et al. Fine particulate air pollution and hospital admission for cardiovascular and respiratory diseases. JAMA 2006;295(10): 1127–34.

13. Ware LB, Zhao Z, Koyama T, et al. Long-term ozone exposure increases the risk of developing the acute respiratory distress syndrome. Am J Respir Crit Care Med 2016;193(10):1143–50.

14. Reilly JP, Zhao Z, Shashaty MGS, et al. Low to moderate air pollutant exposure and acute respiratory distress syndrome after severe trauma. Am J Respir Crit Care Med 2019;199(1):62–70.

15. Rhee J, Dominici F, Zanobetti A, et al. Impact of long-term exposures to ambient PM2.5 and ozone on ARDS risk for older adults in the United States. Chest 2019; 156(1):71–9.

16. Rush B, McDermid RC, Celi LA, et al. Association between chronic exposure to air pollution and mortality in the acute respiratory distress syndrome. Environ Pollut 2017;224:352–6.

17. Wu X, Nethery RC, Sabath MB, et al. Air pollution and COVID-19 mortality in the United States: strengths and limitations of an ecological regression analysis. Sci Adv 2020;6(45):eabd4049.

18. Borro M, Di Girolamo P, Gentile G, et al. Evidence-based considerations exploring relations between SARS-CoV-2 pandemic and air pollution: involvement of PM2.5-mediated up-regulation of the viral receptor ACE-2. Int J Environ Res Public Health 2020;17(15):5573.

19. Lin H, Tao J, Kan H, et al. Ambient particulate matter air pollution associated with acute respiratory distress syndrome in Guangzhou, China. J Expo Sci Environ Epidemiol 2018;28(4):392–9.

20. Jahn HJ, Schneider A, Breitner S, et al. Particulate matter pollution in the mega-cities of the Pearl River Delta, China - a systematic literature review and health risk assessment. Int J Hyg Environ Health 2011;214(4):281–95.

21. De Weerdt A, Janssen BG, Cox B, et al. Pre-admission air pollution exposure prolongs the duration of ventilation in intensive care patients. Intensive Care Med 2020;46(6):1204–12.

22. Mudway IS, Kelly FJ. An investigation of inhaled ozone dose and the magnitude of airway inflammation in healthy adults. Am J Respir Crit Care Med 2004; 169(10):1089–95.

23. Williams AE, Chambers RC. The mercurial nature of neutrophils: still an enigma in ARDS? Am J Physiol Lung Cell Mol Physiol 2014;306(3):L217–30.

24. Holter JF, Weiland JE, Pacht ER, et al. Protein permeability in the adult respiratory distress syndrome. Loss of size selectivity of the alveolar epithelium. J Clin Invest 1986;78(6):1513–22.

25. Muller B, Seifart C, Barth PJ. Effect of air pollutants on the pulmonary surfactant system. Eur J Clin Invest 1998;28(9):762–77.

26. Becker S, Fenton MJ, Soukup JM. Involvement of microbial components and toll-like receptors 2 and 4 in cytokine responses to air pollution particles. Am J Respir Cell Mol Biol 2002;27(5):611–8.

27. Chan YL, Wang B, Chen H, et al. Pulmonary inflammation induced by low-dose particulate matter exposure in mice. Am J Physiol Lung Cell Mol Physiol 2019; 317(3):L424–30.

28. Lin CI, Tsai CH, Sun YL, et al. Instillation of particulate matter 2.5 induced acute lung injury and attenuated the injury recovery in ACE2 knockout mice. Int J Biol Sci 2018;14(3):253–65.

29. Pope CA 3rd, Bhatnagar A, McCracken JP, et al. Exposure to fine particulate air pollution is associated with endothelial injury and systemic inflammation. Circ Res 2016;119(11):1204–14.

30. Matthay MA, Zemans RL, Zimmerman GA, et al. Acute respiratory distress syndrome. Nat Rev Dis Primers 2019;5(1):18.

31. Horne BD, Joy EA, Hofmann MG, et al. Short-term elevation of fine particulate matter air pollution and acute lower respiratory infection. Am J Respir Crit Care Med 2018;198(6):759–66.

32. Westerling AL, Hidalgo HG, Cayan DR, et al. Warming and earlier spring increase western U.S. forest wildfire activity. Science 2006;313(5789):940–3.

33. McClure CD, Jaffe DA. US particulate matter air quality improves except in wildfire-prone areas. Proc Natl Acad Sci U S A 2018;115(31):7901–6.

34. Black C, Tesfaigzi Y, Bassein JA, et al. Wildfire smoke exposure and human health: significant gaps in research for a growing public health issue. Environ Toxicol Pharmacol 2017;55:186–95.

35. Pryor WA. Biological effects of cigarette smoke, wood smoke, and the smoke from plastics: the use of electron spin resonance. Free Radic Biol Med 1992;13(6):659–76.

36. Liu JC, Pereira G, Uhl SA, et al. A systematic review of the physical health impacts from non-occupational exposure to wildfire smoke. Environ Res 2015;136:120–32.

37. Enkhbaatar P, Pruitt BA Jr, Suman O, et al. Pathophysiology, research challenges, and clinical management of smoke inhalation injury. Lancet 2016;388(10052):1437–46.

38. Steinvall I, Bak Z, Sjoberg F. Acute respiratory distress syndrome is as important as inhalation injury for the development of respiratory dysfunction in major burns. Burns 2008;34(4):441–51.

39. Zeglinski MR, Turner CT, Zeng R, et al. Soluble wood smoke extract promotes barrier dysfunction in alveolar epithelial cells through a MAPK signaling pathway. Sci Rep 2019;9(1):10027.

40. Liu PL, Chen YL, Chen YH, et al. Wood smoke extract induces oxidative stress-mediated caspase-independent apoptosis in human lung endothelial cells: role of AIF and EndoG. Am J Physiol Lung Cell Mol Physiol 2005;289(5):L739–49.

41. Wegesser TC, Franzi LM, Mitloehner FM, et al. Lung antioxidant and cytokine responses to coarse and fine particulate matter from the great California wildfires of 2008. Inhal Toxicol 2010;22(7):561–70.

42. Ghio AJ, Soukup JM, Case M, et al. Exposure to wood smoke particles produces inflammation in healthy volunteers. Occup Environ Med 2012;69(3):170–5.

43. U.S. Department of Health and Human Services. The health consequences of smoking — 50 years of progress. A report of the surgeon general. Atlanta (GA): US Department of Health and Human Services; 2014.

44. Global Burden of Disease Tobacco Collaborators. Smoking prevalence and attributable disease burden in 195 countries and territories, 1990-2015: a systematic analysis from the Global Burden of Disease Study 2015. Lancet 2017;389(10082):1885–906.

45. Hammond D, Reid JL, Rynard VL, et al. Prevalence of vaping and smoking among adolescents in Canada, England, and the United States: repeat national cross sectional surveys. BMJ 2019;365:l2219.

46. Perrine CG, Pickens CM, Boehmer TK, et al. Characteristics of A Multistate outbreak of lung injury associated with E-cigarette use, or vaping — United States, 2019. MMWR Morb Mortal Wkly Rep 2019;68:860–4.

47. Gajic O, Dabbagh O, Park PK, et al. Early identification of patients at risk of acute lung injury: evaluation of lung injury prediction score in a multicenter cohort study. Am J Respir Crit Care Med 2011;183(4):462–70.

48. Moazed F, Calfee CS. Environmental risk factors for acute respiratory distress syndrome. Clin Chest Med 2014;35(4):625–37.

49. Iribarren C, Jacobs DR Jr, Sidney S, et al. Cigarette smoking, alcohol consumption, and risk of ARDS: a 15-year cohort study in a managed care setting. Chest 2000;117(1):163–8.

50. Hsieh SJ, Zhuo H, Benowitz NL, et al. Prevalence and impact of active and passive cigarette smoking in acute respiratory distress syndrome. Crit Care Med 2014;42(9):2058–68.

51. Hsieh SJ, Ware LB, Eisner MD, et al. Biomarkers increase detection of active smoking and secondhand smoke exposure in critically ill patients. Crit Care Med 2011;39(1):40–5.

52. Toy P, Gajic O, Bacchetti P, et al. Transfusion-related acute lung injury: incidence and risk factors. Blood 2012;119(7):1757–67.

53. Diamond JM, Lee JC, Kawut SM, et al. Clinical risk factors for primary graft dysfunction after lung transplantation. Am J Respir Crit Care Med 2013;187(5):527–34.

54. Bernard GR, Artigas A, Brigham KL, et al. Report of the American-European consensus conference on ARDS: definitions, mechanisms, relevant outcomes and clinical trial coordination. The Consensus Committee. Intensive Care Med 1994;20(3):225–32.

55. Calfee CS, Matthay MA, Eisner MD, et al. Active and passive cigarette smoking and acute lung injury after severe blunt trauma. Am J Respir Crit Care Med 2011;183(12):1660–5.

56. Moazed F, Hendrickson C, Conroy A, et al. Cigarette smoking and ARDS after blunt trauma: the influence of changing smoking patterns and resuscitation practices. Chest 2020;158(4):1490–8.

57. Moazed F, Hendrickson C, Nelson M, et al. Platelet aggregation after blunt trauma is associated with the acute respiratory distress syndrome and altered by cigarette smoke exposure. J Trauma Acute Care Surg 2018;84(2):365–71.

58. Panzer AR, Lynch SV, Langelier C, et al. Lung microbiota is related to smoking status and to development of acute respiratory distress syndrome in critically ill trauma patients. Am J Respir Crit Care Med 2018;197(5):621–31.

59. Calfee CS, Matthay MA, Kangelaris KN, et al. Cigarette smoke exposure and the acute respiratory distress syndrome. Crit Care Med 2015;43(9):1790–7.

60. Moazed F, Burnham EL, Vandivier RW, et al. Cigarette smokers have exaggerated alveolar barrier disruption in response to lipopolysaccharide inhalation. Thorax 2016;71(12):1130–6.

61. Gotts JE, Abbott J, Fang X, et al. Cigarette smoke exposure worsens endotoxin-induced lung injury and pulmonary edema in mice. Nicotine Tob Res 2017;19(9):1033–9.

62. Gotts JE, Chun L, Abbott J, et al. Cigarette smoke exposure worsens acute lung injury in antibiotic-treated bacterial pneumonia in mice. Am J Physiol Lung Cell Mol Physiol 2018;315(1):L25–40.

63. Lu Q, Gottlieb E, Rounds S. Effects of cigarette smoke on pulmonary endothelial cells. Am J Physiol Lung Cell Mol Physiol 2018;314(5):L743–56.

64. Matthay MA, Leligdowicz A, Liu KD. Biological mechanisms of COVID-19 acute respiratory distress syndrome. Am J Respir Crit Care Med 2020;202(11):1489–91.

65. Zhang H, Rostami MR, Leopold PL, et al. Expression of the SARS-CoV-2 ACE2 receptor in the human airway epithelium. Am J Respir Crit Care Med 2020; 202(2):219–29.

66. Smith JC, Sausville EL, Girish V, et al. Cigarette smoke exposure and inflammatory signaling increase the expression of the SARS-CoV-2 receptor ACE2 in the respiratory tract. Dev Cell 2020;53(5):514–29.e3.

67. Farsalinos K, Barbouni A, Niaura R. Systematic review of the prevalence of current smoking among hospitalized COVID-19 patients in China: could nicotine be a therapeutic option? Intern Emerg Med 2020;15(5):845–52.

68. Tindle HA, Newhouse PA, Freiberg MS. Beyond smoking cessation: investigating medicinal nicotine to prevent and treat COVID-19. Nicotine Tob Res 2020;22(9): 1669–70.

69. Cullen KA, Gentzke AS, Sawdey MD, et al. E-cigarette use among youth in the United States, 2019. JAMA 2019;322(21):2095–103.

70. Soneji S, Barrington-Trimis JL, Wills TA, et al. Association between initial use of e-cigarettes and subsequent cigarette smoking among adolescents and young adults: a systematic review and meta-analysis. JAMA Pediatr 2017;171(8): 788–97.

71. McMillen R, Klein JD, Wilson K, et al. E-cigarette use and future cigarette initiation among never smokers and relapse among former smokers in the PATH study. Public Health Rep 2019;134(5):528–36.

72. McAlinden KD, Eapen MS, Lu W, et al. The rise of electronic nicotine delivery systems and the emergence of electronic-cigarette-driven disease. Am J Physiol Lung Cell Mol Physiol 2020;319(4):L585–95.

73. Chun LF, Moazed F, Calfee CS, et al. Pulmonary toxicity of e-cigarettes. Am J Physiol Lung Cell Mol Physiol 2017;313(2):L193–206.

74. Centers for Disease Control and Prevention. Outbreak of lung injury associated with E-cigarette use, or vaping. 2020. Available at: https://www.cdc.gov/tobacco/basic_information/e-cigarettes/severe-lung-disease.html. Accessed October 7, 2020.

75. Centers for Disease Control and Prevention. For state, local, territorial, and tribal health departments: primary case definitions. 2019. Available at: https://www.cdc.gov/tobacco/basic_information/e-cigarettes/severe-lung-disease/health-departments/index.html#primary-case-def. Accessed October 10, 2020.

76. Jonas AM, Raj R. Vaping-related acute parenchymal lung injury: a systematic review. Chest 2020;158(4):1555–65.

77. Layden JE, Ghinai I, Pray I, et al. Pulmonary illness related to E-cigarette use in Illinois and Wisconsin — final report. N Engl J Med 2019;382(10):903–16.

78. ARDS Definition Task Force, Ranieri VM, Rubenfeld GD, et al. Acute respiratory distress syndrome: the Berlin Definition. JAMA 2012;307(23):2526–33.

79. Blount BC, Karwowski MP, Shields PG, et al. Vitamin E acetate in bronchoalveolar-lavage fluid associated with EVALI. N Engl J Med 2019;382(8): 697–705.

80. Duffy B, Li L, Lu S, et al. Analysis of cannabinoid-containing fluids in Illicit vaping cartridges recovered from pulmonary injury patients: identification of vitamin E acetate as a major diluent. Toxics 2020;8(1):8.

81. Matsumoto S, Fang X, Traber MG, et al. Dose-dependent pulmonary toxicity of aerosolized vitamin E acetate. Am J Respir Cell Mol Biol 2020;63(6):748–57.

82. Butt YM, Smith ML, Tazelaar HD, et al. Pathology of vaping-associated lung injury. N Engl J Med 2019;381(18):1780–1.

83. Ghinai I, Pray IW, Navon L, et al. E-cigarette product use, or vaping, among persons with associated lung injury - Illinois and Wisconsin, April-september 2019. MMWR Morb Mortal Wkly Rep 2019;68(39):865–9.

84. Schweitzer KS, Chen SX, Law S, et al. Endothelial disruptive proinflammatory effects of nicotine and e-cigarette vapor exposures. Am J Physiol Lung Cell Mol Physiol 2015;309(2):L175–87.

85. Madison MC, Landers CT, Gu BH, et al. Electronic cigarettes disrupt lung lipid homeostasis and innate immunity independent of nicotine. J Clin Invest 2019; 129(10):4290–304.

86. Papazian L, Calfee CS, Chiumello D, et al. Diagnostic workup for ARDS patients. Intensive Care Med 2016;42(5):674–85.

87. Siegel DA, Jatlaoui TC, Koumans EH, et al. Update: interim guidance for health care providers evaluating and caring for patients with suspected E-cigarette, or vaping, product use associated lung injury - United States, October 2019. MMWR Morb Mortal Wkly Rep 2019;68(41):919–27.

88. Acute Respiratory Distress Syndrome Network, Brower RG, Matthay MA, et al. Ventilation with lower tidal volumes as compared with traditional tidal volumes for acute lung injury and the acute respiratory distress syndrome. N Engl J Med 2000;342(18):1301–8.

89. National Heart L, Blood Institute Acute Respiratory Distress Syndrome Clinical Trials Network, Wiedemann HP, et al. Comparison of two fluid-management strategies in acute lung injury. N Engl J Med 2006;354(24):2564–75.

90. Guerin C, Reignier J, Richard JC, et al. Prone positioning in severe acute respiratory distress syndrome. N Engl J Med 2013;368(23):2159–68.

91. Clark BJ, Moss M. Secondary prevention in the intensive care unit: does intensive care unit admission represent a "teachable moment?". Crit Care Med 2011;39(6): 1500–6.

92. Sevin CM, Bloom SL, Jackson JC, et al. Comprehensive care of ICU survivors: development and implementation of an ICU recovery center. J Crit Care 2018; 46:141–8.

93. Leone FT, Zhang Y, Evers Casey S, et al. Initiating pharmacologic treatment in tobacco-dependent adults. An official American thoracic society clinical practice guideline. Am J Respir Crit Care Med 2020;202(2):e5–31.

94. Wilby KJ, Harder CK. Nicotine replacement therapy in the intensive care unit: a systematic review. J Intensive Care Med 2014;29(1):22–30.

95. Farber HJ, Walley SC, Groner JA, et al. Clinical practice policy to protect children from tobacco, nicotine, and tobacco smoke. Pediatrics 2015;136(5):1008–17.

96. Rice MB, Thurston GD, Balmes JR, et al. Climate change. A global threat to cardiopulmonary health. Am J Respir Crit Care Med 2014;189(5):512–9.

97. Friedman AS, Tam J. E-Cigarettes: matching risks with regulations. Am J Prev Med 2020;60(1):146–50.

98. Smith DM, Goniewicz ML. The role of policy in the EVALI outbreak: solution or contributor? Lancet Respir Med 2020;8(4):343–4.

Toward Optimal Acute Respiratory Distress Syndrome Outcomes
Recognizing the Syndrome and Identifying Its Causes

Maya E. Kotas, MD, PhD[a], B. Taylor Thompson, MD[b],*

KEYWORDS

- Acute respiratory distress syndrome • ARDS • ARDS risk factors
- Lung protective ventilation

KEY POINTS

- Acute respiratory distress syndrome is a heterogeneous clinical syndrome.
- Recognition of the syndrome is essential to use appropriate lung protective ventilation and fluid conservative strategies that reduce morbidity and mortality.
- Recognizing the syndrome is just the start, because many specific causes of acute respiratory distress syndrome require specific therapy.
- Optimal outcomes require both the early recognition of acute respiratory distress syndrome and the identification of the underlying etiology.
- We discuss challenges to recognition of acute respiratory distress syndrome and some specific diseases that may present as acute respiratory distress syndrome, and suggest steps toward diagnosing such diseases.

INTRODUCTION AND IMPORTANCE OF THE PROBLEM

Acute respiratory distress syndrome (ARDS) is an inflammatory lung injury associated with vascular leak, alveolar filling, and hypoxia,[1] and with vast clinical impact. In 2016, an international, multicenter prospective study found that ARDS represented 10.4% of total intensive care unit admissions and 42% of intensive care unit bed occupancy.[2] In the United States, ARDS was estimated to have an age-adjusted incidence of 86.2 per

[a] Division of Pulmonary, Critical Care, Allergy and Sleep Medicine, Department of Medicine, University of California, San Francisco, 505 Parnassus Avenue, Box 0111, San Francisco, CA 94143, USA; [b] Division of Pulmonary and Critical Care Medicine, Department of Medicine, Massachusetts General Hospital, Harvard Medical School, 55 Fruit Street, Boston, MA 02114, USA
* Corresponding author.
E-mail address: tthompson1@mgh.harvard.edu

Crit Care Clin 37 (2021) 733–748
https://doi.org/10.1016/j.ccc.2021.05.011
0749-0704/21/© 2021 Elsevier Inc. All rights reserved.

100,000 person-years, accounting for nearly 200,000 cases per year.[3] Despite the application of supportive standards developed through numerous clinical trials, mortality among patients with ARDS remains in the range of 33% to 45%, depending on the severity of illness.[2] Although such numbers do not account for the fact that patients with ARDS may die of concurrent life-threatening conditions rather than from ARDS per se, they are nevertheless staggering. Further, those who survive may experience long-lasting deficits in physical and psychiatric health.[4] Although a discussion of coronavirus disease 2019 (COVID-19) is beyond the scope of this article, it should be emphasized that the ~600,000 deaths in the United States attributed to COVID-19[5]—a disease whose major mortal complication is ARDS[6]—has greatly magnified the aforementioned incidence and mortality and further underscored the importance of ARDS as a clinical problem.

There are many reasons why it is imperative to define ARDS in clear terms. First, although there is no pharmacologic therapy for ARDS, numerous clinical studies have shown that application of ARDS-specific supportive care can substantially improve clinical outcomes.[7–11] Unfortunately, the diagnosis is often missed, with resulting failure to treat patients according to accepted standards of care.[2] Second, the patients studied in mechanistic and clinical trials must be sufficiently defined and/or homogenous to allow for appropriate power calculations, enrollment, and subgroup analyses that can ultimately identify biomarkers and desperately needed therapies.[12] Third, some patients who have a syndrome that is consistent with or resembles ARDS may benefit from particular medications or interventions—such as the withdrawal of an injurious medication, the addition of antimicrobial agents, or immunosuppression. And finally, because mortality remains high for ARDS, defining the syndrome is important for clinical prognostication. The specificity and sensitivity required to meet each of these objectives is distinct, and may be at odds. For instance, the importance of applying low tidal volume ventilation to all patients who might benefit favors inclusivity, whereas clinical trials of pharmacologic agents typically favor exclusivity.

In this article, we review the historical and current definitions of ARDS and discuss the challenges of diagnosing conditions that present as ARDS but do not fit the conceptual framework of increased lung vascular permeability induced by inflammation (such as disseminated malignancy or alveolar proteinosis), and/or those that are included this framework, but may require specific treatment (such as pneumonia from rare pathogens or drug induced lung injury).

DEFINITIONS AND THEIR LIMITATIONS

Respiratory distress syndrome, which later became known as acute respiratory distress syndrome, was first described by Ashbaugh and colleagues[13] in a case series of 12 patients with severe hypoxemia, decreased lung compliance, and diffuse alveolar infiltrates on chest radiography. Lacking any distinct biomarkers or signs, the syndrome continues to be defined by an overlap of nonspecific radiographic and clinical features. As agreed upon in the Berlin consensus definition, a diagnosis of ARDS requires bilateral opacities on chest imaging, developing within 7 days, incompletely explained by left heart failure, fluid overload, effusions, collapse, or nodules, and resulting in hypoxemia as defined by an arterial partial pressure of oxygen to fraction of inspired oxygen (Pao_2/Fio_2) ratio of 300 mm Hg or less on a minimum positive end-expiratory pressure (PEEP) of 5 cm H_2O^1 (**Box 1**).

The histologic findings from 6 of 7 of Ashbaugh's patients who died were consistent with the stereotyped injury process later called diffuse alveolar damage (DAD),[13,14]

Box 1			
The Berlin definition of ARDS			
Timing	Within 1 wk of a known clinical insult or new/worsening respiratory symptoms		
Chest imaging[a]	Bilateral opacities—not fully explained by effusions, lobar/lung collapse, or nodules		
Origin	Respiratory failure not fully explained by cardiac failure or fluid overload; need objective assessment (eg, echocardiography) to exclude hydrostatic edema if no risk factor present		
	Mild	Moderate	Severe
Oxygenation[b]	$200 < Pao_2:Fio_2 \leq 300$ with PEEP or CPAP ≥ 5 cm H_2O[c]	$100 < Pao_2: \leq 200$ with PEEP ≥ 5 cm H_2O	$Pao_2:Fio_2 \leq 100$ with PEEP ≥ 5 cm H_2O

[a] Chest radiograph or computed tomography scan.
[b] If altitude is higher than 1000 m, correction factor should be made as follows: $Pao_2:Fio_2$ (barometric pressure/760).
[c] This may be delivered noninvasively in the mild ARDS group.

and therefore DAD has historically been considered the pathologic hallmark of ARDS. DAD is characterized by swelling and necrosis of alveolar epithelial cells with resulting hemorrhage and proteinaceous edema, followed days later by hyaline membrane formation, then by type II pneumocyte hyperplasia, fibrosis, and finally resolution.[14] Although the pathophysiologic processes that culminate in DAD and ARDS are incompletely understood, inflammation is almost certainly partially responsible, because the pathology most often follows on the heels of a localized tissue injury such as aspiration, pneumonia, toxic inhalation, sepsis, trauma, fat embolism, pancreatitis, or transfusion. Excellent recent reviews have summarized what is currently known of the pathophysiology that leads to DAD.[5,15,16]

Although ARDS and DAD have often been equated based on Ashbaugh's historical findings, ARDS remains a clinical diagnosis. And although DAD and the aforementioned risk factors remain important aspects of the conceptual framework of ARDS,[1,17] they are excluded from the accepted definitions. DAD is a common pattern of injury and repair that follows diverse tissue insults and is not specific to ARDS.[14] It may be present in patients who do not meet the clinical criteria for ARDS when sufficiently mild and can accompany other dominant histologic patterns. Similarly, the histopathology of ARDS is not limited to DAD. One large study found that, among patients who fit the Berlin criteria, only 45% had histologic evidence of DAD on autopsy, another 49% had findings of multifocal pneumonia, and the remainder was composed of a wide variety of other entities, or no definitive finding at all.[18] Similar findings were observed with the previous widely used American European Consensus definition of ARDS.[19] One interpretation of these discordant findings is that clinical and radiographic criteria are insufficiently specific to define the syndrome. Alternatively, patients with DAD could be considered a subset—or endotype—of ARDS.[20] In favor of the later view, the prevalence of DAD correlates positively with increased severity and duration of illness, but inversely with the application of low tidal volume ventilation.[18,21] All of this could be consistent with a model wherein DAD is a nonspecific pattern that reflects a combination of the initial lung injury and subsequent ventilator-induced lung injury, and upon which a number of pathologies may converge.[20]

In sum, ARDS is a clinical syndrome that results from a wide variety of underlying injuries and is currently defined by the Berlin criteria in deliberately inclusive terms. The current best evidence favors this inclusivity, because patients with diverse risk factors benefit from low tidal volume ventilation and, when severe, ventilation in the prone position.[22] There is no evidence to suggest that patients with different histologic patterns or risk factors should be treated differently.[22] The current definition does not account for the substantial heterogeneity of disease, which remains a challenge to the development and application of specific diagnostics and treatments. Differences in histology, radiographic findings (dense or patchy vs diffuse ground glass), inciting injury, genetics, or biomarkers may ultimately define distinct disease entities best treated in different ways.[23]

RECOGNIZING THE SYNDROME OF ACUTE RESPIRATORY DISTRESS SYNDROME

Despite the relatively simple and inclusive nature of current and past definitions,[24] many practical challenges to diagnosing ARDS persist (**Fig. 1**). For instance, establishing the duration of illness can be challenging if the patient is unable to provide a reliable history or if symptoms attributable to another diagnosis precede the progression to ARDS. Further, the degree of hypoxemia may be challenging to ascertain if arterial blood gas measurements are not easily obtained, as in resource-poor settings, or if the method of supplemental oxygen delivery does not provide PEEP. The Kigali modification, which uses the ratio of oxygen saturation to fraction of inspired oxygen (Fio_2) has been suggested to address the former issue,[25] which seems pragmatic in resource-limited settings. The requirement for PEEP, which was not included in prior definitions of ARDS,[17] presents a progressive challenge because clinicians increasingly use high-flow nasal cannula (HFNC) for patients with acute hypoxemic respiratory failure.[26] This

Recognizing the Syndrome		Identifying the Cause of the Syndrome
Goal:		**Goal:**
Improve outcomes by implementing proper <u>supportive care</u> • Low tidal volume ventilation • Careful fluid management • Prone positioning if severe		Treat the <u>underlying conditions</u> that are causing ARDS
Pitfalls in recognition	**Tips and reminders**	**Classic Causes**
Lack of "classic" radiograph	• Bilateral opacities need not be diffuse; may be very mild, patchy, or asymmetric	• Pneumonia • Sepsis (non pulmonary) • Aspiration • Trauma, toxin/smoke inhalations
Use of HFNC: FiO2 not predictable, PEEP absent	• High risk for ARDS if ≥15L of 100% O2 needed to maintain SpO2 ≥90%–95%	• Pancreatitis
		None likely? Atypical patient features?
		Zebras

Unsure if cardiogenic edema	• Dx not mutually exclusive and often coexist
	• Oxygenation and opacities rapidly improve with treatment of heart failure or volume overload
		• Rare infections
		• Drug induced lung injury
		• Interstitial lung disease:
		    • Acute eosinophilic pneumonia
		    • Cryptogenic organizing pneumonia
		    • NSIP
		    • AE-IPF

Unsure if fully explained by nodules, effusion, or collapse	• Not mutually exclusive, may coexist • Consider CT and/or ultrasound	• Alveolar hemorrhage and/or vasculitis • Malignancy • Pulmonary alveolar proteinosis

Fig. 1. Two key steps in ARDS care: recognizing the syndrome and identifying the cause. When faced with a possible case of ARDS, clinicians should apply Berlin Criteria (see **Box 1**), keeping in mind some classic pitfalls that may lead to missed diagnosis, and initiate appropriate supportive care. Once ARDS has been recognized, clinicians should work to identify the underlying cause to provide targeted treatments. Although the diagnosis of the syndrome is purely clinical, the diagnosis of the underlying condition or disease may require specific imaging or diagnostic testing. AEIPF, Acute exacerbations of idiopathic pulmonary fibrosis; NSIP, nonspecific interstitial pneumonia.

practice shift has become particularly notable during the COVID-19 pandemic.[27,28] Higher HFNC flow rates and Fio_2 deliver correspondingly higher Fio_2 to the trachea (may approach 1.0 at 45 LPM of 100% oxygen), allowing for noninvasive support of patients with severe impairments of gas exchange and accurate assessment of Pao_2/Fio_2, yet are not included in the current definition of ARDS. Because definitions should be adapted to new developments in clinical medicine (as was the case with the Berlin definition in 2012), perhaps an updated definition of ARDS should include spontaneously breathing patients supported with HFNC who have bilateral chest radiographic infiltrates. Although estimates of Fio_2 are notoriously inaccurate at low flow rates, high flow rates allow for accurate estimates of Fio_2 and therefore calculation of Pao_2/Fio_2.[26,29]

Additionally, the interpretation of radiographic findings can be challenging. Plain radiographs may miss qualifying opacities that would be detected on computed tomography (CT) scan (thus, the inclusion of CT scans among imaging modalities in the Berlin definition).[1] Further, although many clinicians consider a diffuse distribution of opacities to be necessary for a diagnosis of ARDS, this classic pattern is not required; although opacities must be bilateral and not fully explained by effusions, lobar/lung collapse, or nodules, they may be very mild, patchy, and asymmetric.[1] Confluent bilateral lobar opacities, for instance, are consistent with ARDS so far as other clinical criteria are met, and examples of such are provided in the Berlin definition supplement.[1] Even in cases where bilateral opacities are evident, interobserver variability results in substantial underdiagnosis,[2,30] likely owing to misconceptions about qualifying opacities, as discussed elsewhere in this article.[16] Furthermore, it may be very difficult to determine that opacities are not fully explained by effusions, lobar/lung collapse, or nodules. Nearly 28% of patients with clinically diagnosed ARDS were found on autopsy to have abscess, emphysema, or no pulmonary abnormality at all,[18] indicating the difficulty of excluding nodules, effusions, and atelectasis.

Finally, the exclusion of cardiogenic pulmonary edema is likely the single most difficult challenge to the diagnosis of ARDS, because differentiating cardiogenic edema from ARDS is rarely possible with chest radiograph alone.[31] Compounding this challenge is that the 2 conditions may coexist.[10] Cardiogenic pulmonary edema refers to the accumulation of fluid within the pulmonary interstitial and/or alveolar spaces as a result of elevated left atrial pressures and that develops through elevated hydrostatic pressure gradients rather than alveolar or vascular barrier disruption.[32] Although the left ventricular dysfunction (either systolic or diastolic) is most often to blame, cardiogenic pulmonary edema can also result from valvular disease, severe systemic hypertension (hypertensive emergency), or systemic volume overload such as in renal or liver disease and over-resuscitation with intravenous fluids. In addition to clinical history, an examination consistent with cardiac dysfunction (gallops, murmurs, displaced point of maximal impulse) or elevated right-sided pressures (elevated jugular venous pressure, peripheral edema), and related radiographic (pulmonary venous congestion, cardiomegaly, pleural effusions), laboratory (elevated B-type natriuretic peptide/N-terminal pro-BNP [BN/NT-proBNP] or troponin) or echographic features (diastolic or systolic dysfunction, valvular disease, a plethoric inferior vena cava), or occasionally right heart catheterization can be used to support the diagnosis of cardiogenic pulmonary edema. When these diagnostic clues are not definitive, a successful trial of diuresis, when not contraindicated owing to competing organ interests, may seal the diagnosis. Reexpansion pulmonary edema, an infrequent iatrogenic complication of thoracostomy or thoracentesis, or negative pressure pulmonary edema[33] are both likely examples of hydrostatic pulmonary edema[34] that may occur in the absence of systemic fluid overload, but are less likely to be confused with ARDS given the specific clinical context in which it occurs.

It is important to note that, although the probability of cardiogenic pulmonary edema is greatly increased if the patient has a history of any cardiac disease or has advanced renal or liver disease, such conditions may also correlate with risk factors for ARDS (such as aspiration or sepsis), and their presence does not exclude a diagnosis of ARDS. In the autopsy study discussed elsewhere in this article, 8% of patients with cardiogenic pulmonary edema also had DAD,[18] whereas a substantial portion of patients with ARDS may have concurrent cardiogenic edema. Conversely, in the FACTT trial, 29% of patients with ARDS also had an elevated pulmonary arterial wedge pressure of greater than 18 mm Hg.[10] Therefore, only when the clinical criteria are resolved by diuresis alone can concurrent ARDS be ruled out.

RECOGNIZING ACUTE RESPIRATORY DISTRESS SYNDROME IS JUST THE START: DIAGNOSING THE CAUSE OF ACUTE RESPIRATORY DISTRESS SYNDROME

Although there is no proven pharmacologic therapy for ARDS per se, a number of conditions that present as ARDS by the Berlin criteria do have specific therapies that should be used alongside ARDS-appropriate supportive care. Such conditions have often been called mimics, but may be better understood as specific pulmonary diagnoses that can cause or present as ARDS. These are in addition to classic extrapulmonary insults (sepsis, trauma, fat embolism, acute pancreatitis), which may also require disorder-specific treatments. Although the number of pulmonary insults leading to hypoxemia and bilateral alveolar infiltrates are too many to exhaustively list in any review, we will briefly summarize some of the entities that frequently meet all Berlin criteria, and may demand specific treatments (see **Fig. 1**).

Infectious Pneumonia

Infectious pneumonia is one of the most common pathologies presenting as ARDS, with studies showing anywhere from 27.0% to 59.4% of patients with ARDS with pre-existing or concurrent diagnosis of pneumonia, and as many of 37% to 65% of ARDS courses complicated by ventilator-associated pneumonia.[35,36] Current numbers are undoubtedly higher in the setting of the current COVID-19 pandemic. Given the very high co-occurrence of pneumonia and/or sepsis with ARDS, it is generally appropriate to treat all patients with ARDS with broad spectrum antibiotics while awaiting culture results. However, a diligent search for the causative organism is indicated to ensure adequate antimicrobial coverage. Typical bacterial organisms, atypical bacterial, viral, fungal, or parasitic infections should all be considered as potential etiologies of ARDS.[5] Patient risk factors such as age, comorbid pulmonary disease, HIV status, other severe immunocompromise, or geographic travel or origins may contribute to diagnostic considerations.[5] In general, we recommend blood, respiratory, and urine cultures and respiratory viral testing by direct fluorescent antibody testing or polymerase chain reaction for all patients with possible ARDS. If all of these cultures are negative, cardiogenic pulmonary edema is unlikely, no other obvious provoking factor for ARDS is present (eg, known gastric aspiration or other etiology of sepsis), and/or the patient is failing to improve on empiric antibiotics, we recommend consideration for further testing in consultation with an infectious disease specialist. Such testing may include bacterial or fungal antigen testing of blood or urine, bronchoalveolar lavage (BAL), serologies, or sequencing/polymerase chain reaction testing depending on the patient characteristics and concurrent symptoms. Again, although a dedicated discussion of COVID-19 is beyond the scope of this article, the proliferation of data supporting the use of steroids[37] and antiviral therapy[38-41] to treat ARDS owing to COVID-19 perfectly underscores the need to diagnose both the syndrome of ARDS and its specific cause to optimize outcomes.

Chemical or Radiation Pneumonitis

Direct or indirect chemical injury to the lung is another common cause of ARDS. Aspiration of gastric contents can present as ARDS and follow a highly variable course, with some patients rapidly improving over 24 to 36 hours and other experiencing a protracted illness lasting days or weeks.[42] A variety of medications, most often antineoplastic therapies (cytotoxic or targeted small molecule), have been associated with pneumonitis that may be severe enough to meet Berlin criteria and can occur anytime from days to weeks after treatment.[43] Cessation of the inciting drug and consideration for steroids may aid in the resolution of ARDS caused by such medications.[43] Similarly, radiation can cause pneumonitis, often but not always localized near the targeted lesion, and usually occurring weeks after the radiation treatment.[44] We suggest consideration of such entities if the patient has recently received antineoplastic therapy, cardiogenic pulmonary edema is ruled out, a microbiologic workup including bronchoscopy is unrevealing, and there are no other obvious potential etiologies of ARDS.

Alveolar Hemorrhage

Diffuse alveolar hemorrhage (DAH) may also present as ARDS. Hemorrhage can be bland (ie, not associated with vascular inflammation) or owing to capillaritis. In bland DAH, hemorrhage can result when elevated cardiac filling pressures (as in cardiogenic pulmonary edema) occur in the setting of coagulopathy or when contusion follows trauma. Alveolar hemorrhage owing to contusion should be considered when alveolar bleeding is coincident with pneumothorax, pneumatoceles, bony fractures, and cutaneous bruising. In contrast, capillaritis can be provoked by a wide range of insults including anti-neutrophil cytoplasmic antibody–associated or other small vessel vasculitides, connective tissue diseases, anti–glomerular basement membrane disease, certain drugs, and infections.[45,46] Hemoptysis is a classic presenting symptom of DAH, although it is absent in at least one-third of patients, and a decrease in hemoglobin may also be observed. DAH is classically diagnosed by BAL showing an increase in red blood cells in serial lavage. Although DAD and DAH may have nearly identical radiologic appearances on the chest radiograph, highly experienced radiologists can sometimes make the diagnosis of DAH based on the differential radiodensity using a CT scan. The identification of DAH does not distinguish between bland hemorrhage and capillaritis, and should be followed by an investigation into the specific cause.

Inflammatory and Autoimmune Causes

There are a number of noninfectious entities, many of which have an inflammatory and/or autoimmune component, that can present as ARDS. Acute eosinophilic pneumonia (AEP), for example, can cause the acute onset of hypoxia and diffuse pulmonary opacities, and typically occurs either after a recent inhalation or without any clear precipitating event in previously healthy young adults. The diagnosis of AEP can be made when the differential on BAL shows more than 25% eosinophils without known causes of eosinophilic pneumonia[47]; this finding is in contrast with other etiologies of ARDS, in which the BAL is more typically neutrophilic. Because eosinophilic pneumonia is exquisitely and rapidly steroid responsive, AEP is a diagnosis not to be missed. Cryptogenic organizing pneumonia can have a similar appearance to AEP, although it is more likely to present with a subacute course. In contrast, acute fibrinous organizing pneumonia, an exceedingly rare entity with an unknown cause, can present with either a subacute or acute course. It is distinguishable only pathologically through the finding of intra-alveolar fibrin balls and organizing pneumonia, and a notable absence of DAD.[48] In those patients who present with an acute course, there is no accepted treatment, and the disease is almost uniformly fatal. Vasculitides, although capable of producing almost any type of pulmonary infiltrate, most often produce an ARDS-like picture if presenting as DAH or AEP, and otherwise are likely to have subacute onset. Finally, although more often chronic or subacute in presentation, interstitial lung diseases in patients with connective tissue disease such as rheumatoid arthritis, Sjogren syndrome, or polymyositis/dermatomyositis can occasionally present with fulminant course and bilateral ground glass opacities, often in the pathologic patterns of nonspecific interstitial pneumonia or organizing pneumonia. Although interstitial lung disease can precede other systemic symptoms, patients with other indicators of connective tissue disease, such as rash, myositis, neuritis, renal impairment, or arthritis, should be considered for these specific diagnoses.

Disseminated Malignancy

Although more commonly presenting with lymphangitic carcinomatosis, in which tumor cells engorge the lymphatic vessels including in the lungs, or as random nodules suggestive of hematogenous spread, aggressive and disseminated cancers can present with almost any radiographic pattern. Although more often subacute in tempo, and usually in patients with a known prior diagnosis of cancer, malignancy occasionally presents acutely and should be considered in the differential diagnosis of ARDS when a signs or history of advanced malignancy are present.

Pulmonary Alveolar Proteinosis

Pulmonary alveolar proteinosis is a rare, pauci-inflammatory condition in which lipoproteinaceous material accumulates in the distal air spaces as a result of impaired granulocyte macrophage colony stimulating factor and/or alveolar macrophage function. In addition to congenital forms, acquired forms may result from autoantibodies that interfere with granulocyte macrophage colony stimulating factor signaling or to inhalations that cause direct macrophage toxicity, such as exposure to some dusts and metals. The onset is more often insidious than acute, but occasionally can present as ARDS, particularly in the case of superinfection (Nocardia being a classic opportunist in this setting, but certainly not the only possibility). The classic crazy-paving pattern of pulmonary alveolar proteinosis is neither sensitive nor specific, and BAL showing copious periodic acid-Schiff–positive material or sometimes biopsy are needed to make the diagnosis. Specific treatment depends on cause of pulmonary alveolar proteinosis, but most commonly includes whole lung lavage and/or granulocyte macrophage colony stimulating factor supplementation.

Acute Exacerbation of Idiopathic Pulmonary Fibrosis

Acute exacerbation of idiopathic pulmonary fibrosis (AEIPF) is a form of acutely exacerbated hypoxemic respiratory failure with unclear provoking factor that occurs in a patient with preexisting IPF, and frequently presents as ARDS.[49] Although a sizable proportion of the available literature suggests usual risk factors for ARDS—such as infection or aspiration—there is often no definitive predisposing event. The prognosis for IPF, which is already poor, is dramatically worsened by the development of AEIPF. On occasion, AEIPF will be the patient's first presentation with IPF. Radiographic findings consistent with usual interstitial pneumonia (reticulations, honeycombing, and traction bronchiectasis) overlaid with the typical ground glass appearance of DAD supports the diagnosis of AEIPF when other causes of ground glass opacities are unlikely or ruled out. Such patients may have stigmata of chronic hypoxemia, such as clubbing or polycythemia. Steroids are typically given in accordance with expert opinion, despite the lack of clinical trials supporting their efficacy, as well other immunosuppressants, such as rituximab.[49]

Other Specific, Nonclassical Causes of Acute Respiratory Distress Syndrome

Neurogenic pulmonary edema is a form of noncardiogenic pulmonary edema that specifically occurs in patients with severe neurologic injury, and is possibly attributable to catecholamine surge.[50] Although the etiology of neurogenic pulmonary edema is hydrostatic in approximately one-half of patients, it is likely owing to increased vascular permeability in the other half.[51]

E-cigarette or vaping product use-associated lung injury is a very recently described inhalation pneumonitis[52] that occurs in patients with history of vaping within the preceding 90 days,[53,54] likely owing to toxicity from vitamin E acetate, a component of e-liquids.[55,56] E-cigarette or vaping product use-associated lung injury should be suspected especially in teenagers or young adults (who are less likely to have other risk factors for ARDS), particularly if accompanied by gastrointestinal symptoms and/or lung function testing abnormalities. Although no clinical trials have yet tested the usefulness of steroids, most cases are so treated based on expert opinion.

Finally, acute interstitial pneumonia, although often listed as a separate entity, is a likely form of idiopathic ARDS with fulminant course and high mortality.[57] Although again lacking evidence to support the approach, high-dose steroids are often attempted.

PRACTICAL SUGGESTIONS FOR IDENTIFYING ACUTE RESPIRATORY DISTRESS SYNDROME AND MAKING THE SPECIFIC DIAGNOSIS

To identify ARDS, we recommend an initial focus on the exclusion of cardiogenic pulmonary edema and inclusion of ARDS based on Berlin criteria. Once the syndrome is recognized and appropriate ARDS-directed supportive therapy initiated, we recommend proceeding to a consideration of the cause of ARDS. To that end, we begin with an investigation of classic etiologies using history, examination, and basic laboratory studies, followed by a consideration of rare causes (zebras) and the performance of further diagnostic maneuvers when an underlying diagnosis is not evident with initial studies (**Fig. 2**). For the purposes of this discussion, we assume that radiographic findings and the degree of hypoxemia are consistent with the Berlin criteria, with one exception. If the patient requires 15 to 20 LPM of 100% O_2 delivered by HFNC or nonrebreather to maintain a hemoglobin saturation of 90% to 95%, we would strongly consider the possibility of ARDS even in the absence of noninvasive or invasive mechanical ventilation with PEEP. Accordingly, careful monitoring of such patients in the intensive care unit for the need for intubation and lung protective ventilation is recommended.

An evaluation for ARDS and its causes should begin with a thorough history and examination. The history should review the duration of illness and precipitating events, as well as the relevant past medical, family, and social history, including substance use, malignancy, and connective tissue disease. A history of cardiac, renal, or liver disease, and/or of substantial volume resuscitation before intensive care unit arrival should increase suspicion for cardiogenic pulmonary edema.

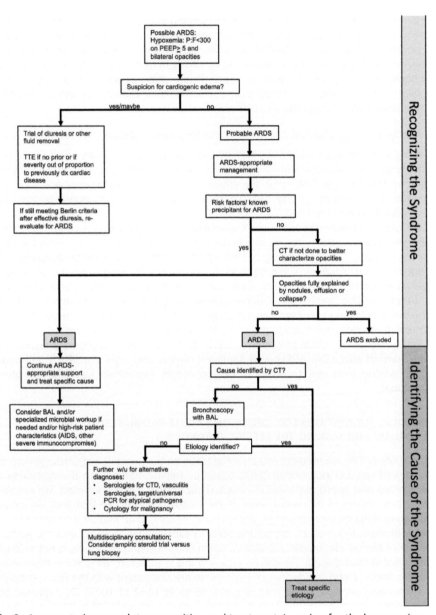

Fig. 2. A suggested approach to recognition and treatment. In caring for the hypoxemic patient with bilateral opacities on either plain radiograph or CT scan, clinicians should determine whether opacities qualify for ARDS and evaluating for cardiogenic pulmonary edema. A workup for specific underlying etiologies should follow and may include advanced imaging, bronchoscopy, specific laboratory testing, biopsy, and/or empiric trials of therapy. A suggested algorithm is presented here with the recognition that clinician preference or resource limitations may require alternative or parallel approaches. BAL, bronchoalveolar lavage; CTD, connective tissue disease; PCR, polymerase chain reaction; TTE, transthoracic echocardiogram.

The examination should start with an evaluation for pulmonary or extrapulmonary infection and a systemic inflammatory response or shock; whereas cardiogenic shock may favor the diagnosis of cardiogenic pulmonary edema, distributive shock would favor sepsis and ARDS. In the absence of shock, the examination should focus first on identifying signs of heart failure or systemic volume overload. Pulmonary examinations are often nonspecific. Rales may or may not be present. Egophany, bronchial breath sounds, or dullness to auscultation/percussion may suggest effusions or atelectasis (which are insufficient to diagnose ARDS and could suggest volume overload), or alternatively, consolidations consistent with ARDS owing to pneumonia. Dental, joint, and skin examinations may reveal potential causes of infection or stigmata of vasculitis, connective tissue disease, or coagulopathy. Point-of-care ultrasound examinations can reasonably be considered an extension of the modern critical care examination[58] and can aid in the qualitative characterization of a decrease in left ventricular ejection fraction, a plethoric inferior vena cava and/or jugular veins, dense pulmonary consolidations, and pericardial, pleural, or intra-abdominal fluid collections.

As a part of the initial workup, we recommend obtaining a complete blood count; basic metabolic panel; coagulation and liver function tests; respiratory, blood, and urine cultures for bacterial pathogens; direct fluorescent antibody testing or polymerase chain reaction panel for common viral and atypical bacterial pathogens; and BNP or NT-proBNP and troponin. Procalcitonin is not required but can be valuable in patients who are suspected to have sepsis without a clear source.

If, after the initial workup as described, the possibility of cardiogenic pulmonary edema remains, we recommend a trial of diuresis when possible (ie, not contraindicated by other organ failure such as distributive shock, and renal function sufficient to achieve diuresis). If this is not possible, or the possibility of cardiogenic pulmonary edema remains even after a reasonable volume of diuresis, we suggest formal transthoracic echocardiography. If none of these evaluations is sufficient to evaluate cardiac function and ensure normal fluid status, right heart catheterization may occasionally be helpful.

In addition to new imaging (chest radiograph or CT scan of the chest), it is imperative that clinicians review any prior imaging, because persistent abnormalities argue for underlying subacute or chronic conditions. Plain radiographs are sufficient to evaluate most cases of ARDS, but CT scanning may be useful if there is no typical risk factor for ARDS, cardiogenic pulmonary edema is unlikely, a disqualifying pulmonary finding (such as nodular or cavitary disease) is suspected, or an atypical cause of ARDS such as hemorrhage or interstitial lung disease is suspected. A CT scan can also be helpful in identifying findings that may be missed on plain radiograph (such as mild ground glass, reticulations, or honeycombing suggestive of interstitial lung disease, or bilateral opacities that were obscured by a diaphragmatic dome or mediastinal structures). Additionally, CT scans may assist with bronchoscopic planning.

When, despite the examinations as described, the underlying etiology of ARDS cannot be identified, bronchoscopy is suggested. In practice, high Fio_2 or PEEP requirements often preclude the ability to perform bronchoscopy. However, when possible, bronchoscopy with BAL can identify aspirated or inhaled material, provide a substrate to test for infectious etiologies, and provide cell counts to evaluate for entities such as eosinophilic pneumonia or DAH. When safe, we recommend bronchoscopy in patients with ARDS in whom a specific underlying etiology has not been identified, including in which an initial infectious workup is negative or the patient is not improving with empiric treatment, and/or when there is high suspicion for DAH based on classic presenting symptoms.

Lung biopsy has no role in confirming the diagnosis of ARDS, because the diagnosis is clinical rather than histologic.[59] However, biopsy may rarely be considered when treatable causes are suspected—for instance, when the patient has no typical risk factors for ARDS, is very young without comorbid disease, there is a high suspicion for a specific diagnosis such as interstitial lung disease—or the patient is worsening rather than improving after several days of appropriate ARDS care without other available explanation.[59] One important exception to this general approach is in suspected AEIPF; in those cases, owing to high associated morbidity, biopsy is usually avoided in favor of empiric therapy.[49] AEIPF aside, case reports and meta-analyses do support the value of biopsy in a very limited set of patients to guide therapy.[60–62] In these studies, however, the majority of cases in which biopsy guided therapy were atypical infections or interstitial processes with possible steroid responsiveness. With the advent of increasingly sensitive diagnostic modalities for atypical infections—such as universal polymerase chain reaction—the relative usefulness of biopsy may decline. Moreover, a significant proportion of patients undergoing biopsy may already be undergoing a therapeutic steroid trial.[61] Because the risk of complications from lung biopsy is significant, the pursuit of biopsy versus a therapeutic trial of steroids when infection is ruled out must be considered on an individual basis, generally in multidisciplinary consultation.[59]

SUMMARY

ARDS is a syndrome, not a disease. To save lives, it is essential to recognize ARDS and provide optimal supportive care with lung protective ventilation[8] and sensible fluid management.[10] ARDS can be the manifestation of myriad underlying conditions, however, and optimal outcomes require identification and treatment of the underlying cause or causes, in addition to recognition of the syndrome itself. An improved understanding of the diverse cellular and molecular processes that lead to ARDS will foster the development of biomarkers and new treatments, and usher in the era of personalized medicine for our patients with this devastating syndrome.

CLINICS CARE POINTS

- The diagnosis of ARDS is based purely on clinical criteria (currently defined by expert consensus according to the Berlin criteria), and does not require any knowledge of the underlying cause or histopathology.
- Clinicians should maintain a high index of suspicion for ARDS in any patient with hypoxia. Although the Berlin criteria require arterial blood gas measurements and PEEP, clinicians may recall that a patient with normal hemoglobin dissociation curve has a Pao_2/Fio_2 ratio of 300 mm Hg or greater if their peripheral saturation is less than 90% on room air. Therefore, the likelihood of hypoxemia qualifying for ARDS further increases with increasing levels of supplemental oxygen needed to maintain a saturation of 90% to 95%.
- Any bilateral airspace opacities that can be captured on plain radiographs or a CT scan qualify if not entirely explained by collapse or effusion. They need not be diffuse, of particular density, or in any specific distribution.
- The overlap between ARDS and DAD is incomplete; neither histology nor a radiographic correlate to DAD are required.
- Although classic causes of ARDS are well-described, almost any pulmonary insult can cause ARDS. Specific diseases that have been called mimics are still consistent with a diagnosis of ARDS if clinical criteria are met.

- Cardiogenic pulmonary edema and ARDS frequently coexist. An index of suspicion for ARDS should remain unless the opacities and hypoxemia that might qualify for ARDS are resolved with treatment of cardiogenic edema alone
- Recognizing ARDS and implementing appropriate supportive care is just the start. Once the syndrome is recognized, clinicians should work to identify and treat the underlying cause using tools such as serology, specialized microbial detection methods, bronchoscopy, radiographic modalities, biopsy, and/or empiric trials of treatment.

DISCLOSURE

The authors gratefully acknowledge the support of the NIH (F32HL140868 and T32HL007185 [M.E.K]; 5R35-HL140026-02 and 5U01HL123009-06 [B.T.T]) and the A.P. Giannini Foundation [M.E.K.].

REFERENCES

1. Force ADT, Ranieri VM, Rubenfeld GD, et al. Acute respiratory distress syndrome: the Berlin Definition. JAMA 2012;307(23):2526–33.
2. Bellani G, Laffey JG, Pham T, et al. Epidemiology, patterns of care, and mortality for patients with acute respiratory distress syndrome in intensive care units in 50 countries. JAMA 2016;315(8).
3. Rubenfeld GD, Caldwell E, Peabody E, et al. Incidence and outcomes of acute lung injury. N Engl J Med 2005;353(16):1685–93.
4. Herridge MS, Tansey CM, Matte A, et al. Functional disability 5 years after acute respiratory distress syndrome. N Engl J Med 2011;364(14):1293–304.
5. Matthay MA, Zemans RL, Zimmerman GA, et al. Acute respiratory distress syndrome. Nat Rev Dis Primers 2019;5(1):18.
6. Tzotzos SJ, Fischer B, Fischer H, et al. Incidence of ARDS and outcomes in hospitalized patients with COVID-19: a global literature survey. Crit Care 2020;24(1):516.
7. Guerin C, Reignier J, Richard JC, et al. Prone positioning in severe acute respiratory distress syndrome. N Engl J Med 2013;368(23):2159–68.
8. Acute Respiratory Distress Syndrome N, Brower RG, Matthay MA, et al. Ventilation with lower tidal volumes as compared with traditional tidal volumes for acute lung injury and the acute respiratory distress syndrome. N Engl J Med 2000; 342(18):1301–8.
9. Petrucci N, De Feo C. Lung protective ventilation strategy for the acute respiratory distress syndrome. Cochrane Database Syst Rev 2013;(2):CD003844.
10. National Heart L, Blood Institute Acute Respiratory Distress Syndrome Clinical Trials N, Wiedemann HP, Wheeler AP, Bernard GR, Thompson BT et al. Comparison of two fluid-management strategies in acute lung injury. N Engl J Med 2006; 354(24):2564–75.
11. Bloomfield R, Noble DW, Sudlow A. Prone position for acute respiratory failure in adults. Cochrane Database Syst Rev 2015;11:CD008095.
12. Ware LB, Matthay MA, Mebazaa A. Designing an ARDS trial for 2020 and beyond: focus on enrichment strategies. Intensive Care Med 2020;46:2153–6.
13. Ashbaugh DG, Bigelow DB, Petty TL, et al. Acute respiratory distress in adults. Lancet 1967;290(7511):319–23.
14. Katzenstein AL, Bloor CM, Leibow AA. Diffuse alveolar damage—the role of oxygen, shock, and related factors. Am J Pathol 1976;85(1):209–28.
15. Ware LB, Matthay MA. The acute respiratory distress syndrome. N Engl J Med 2000;342(18):1334–49.

16. Thompson BT, Chambers RC, Liu KD. Acute respiratory distress syndrome. N Engl J Med 2017;377(6):562–72.

17. Bernard GR, Artigas A, Brigham KL, et al. The American-European Consensus Conference on ARDS. Definitions, mechanisms, relevant outcomes, and clinical trial coordination. Am J Respir Crit Care Med 1994;149(3 Pt 1):818–24.

18. Thille AW, Esteban A, Fernandez-Segoviano P, et al. Comparison of the Berlin definition for acute respiratory distress syndrome with autopsy. Am J Respir Crit Care Med 2013;187(7):761–7.

19. Esteban A, Fernandez-Segoviano P, Frutos-Vivar F, et al. Comparison of clinical criteria for the acute respiratory distress syndrome with autopsy findings. Ann Intern Med 2004;141(6):440–5.

20. Thompson BT, Matthay MA. The Berlin definition of ARDS versus pathological evidence of diffuse alveolar damage. Am J Respir Crit Care Med 2013;187(7): 675–7.

21. Cardinal-Fernandez P, Bajwa EK, Dominguez-Calvo A, et al. The presence of diffuse alveolar damage on open lung biopsy is associated with mortality in patients with acute respiratory distress syndrome: a systematic review and meta-analysis. Chest 2016;149(5):1155–64.

22. Eisner MD, Thompson T, Hudson LD, et al. Efficacy of low tidal volume ventilation in patients with different clinical risk factors for acute lung injury and the acute respiratory distress syndrome. Am J Respir Crit Care Med 2001;164(2):231–6.

23. Reilly JP, Calfee CS, Christie JD. Acute respiratory distress syndrome phenotypes. Semin Respir Crit Care Med 2019;40(1):19–30.

24. Thompson BT, Moss M. A new definition for the acute respiratory distress syndrome. Semin Respir Crit Care Med 2013;34(4):441–7.

25. Riviello ED, Kiviri W, Twagirumugabe T, et al. Hospital incidence and outcomes of the acute respiratory distress syndrome using the Kigali modification of the Berlin definition. Am J Respir Crit Care Med 2016;193(1):52–9.

26. Messika J, Ben Ahmed K, Gaudry S, et al. Use of high-flow nasal cannula oxygen therapy in subjects with ARDS: a 1-year observational study. Respir Care 2015; 60(2):162–9.

27. Yang X, Yu Y, Xu J, et al. Clinical course and outcomes of critically ill patients with SARS-CoV-2 pneumonia in Wuhan, China: a single-centered, retrospective, observational study. Lancet Respir Med 2020;8(5):475–81.

28. Demoule A, Vieillard Baron A, Darmon M, et al. High-flow nasal cannula in critically Ill patients with severe COVID-19. Am J Respir Crit Care Med 2020; 202(7):1039–42.

29. Ritchie JE, Williams AB, Gerard C, et al. Evaluation of a humidified nasal high-flow oxygen system, using oxygraphy, capnography and measurement of upper airway pressures. Anaesth Intensive Care 2011;39(6):1103–10.

30. Rubenfeld GD, Caldwell E, Granton J, et al. Interobserver variability in applying a radiographic definition for ARDS. Chest 1999;116(5):1347–53.

31. Aberle DR, Wiener-Kronish JP, Webb WR, et al. Hydrostatic versus increased permeability pulmonary edema: diagnosis based on radiographic criteria in critically ill patients. Radiology 1988;168(1):73–9.

32. Ware LB, Matthay MA. Clinical practice. Acute pulmonary edema. N Engl J Med 2005;353(26):2788–96.

33. Bhattacharya M, Kallet RH, Ware LB, et al. Negative-pressure pulmonary edema. Chest 2016;150(4):927–33.

34. Sue RD, Matthay MA, Ware LB. Hydrostatic mechanisms may contribute to the pathogenesis of human re-expansion pulmonary edema. Intensive Care Med 2004;30(10):1921–6.
35. Bauer TT, Ewig S, Rodloff AC, et al. Acute respiratory distress syndrome and pneumonia: a comprehensive review of clinical data. Clin Infect Dis 2006;43(6): 748–56.
36. Papazian L, Calfee CS, Chiumello D, et al. Diagnostic workup for ARDS patients. Intensive Care Med 2016;42(5):674–85.
37. Group WHOREAfC-TW, Sterne JAC, Murthy S, et al. Association between administration of systemic corticosteroids and mortality among critically ill patients with COVID-19: a meta-analysis. JAMA 2020;324(13):1330–41.
38. Spinner CD, Gottlieb RL, Criner GJ, et al. Effect of remdesivir vs standard care on clinical status at 11 Days in patients with moderate COVID-19: a randomized clinical trial. JAMA 2020;324(11):1048–57.
39. Goldman JD, Lye DCB, Hui DS, et al. Remdesivir for 5 or 10 Days in patients with severe covid-19. N Engl J Med 2020;383(19):1827–37.
40. Wang Y, Zhang D, Du G, et al. Remdesivir in adults with severe COVID-19: a randomised, double-blind, placebo-controlled, multicentre trial. Lancet 2020; 395(10236):1569–78.
41. Beigel JH, Tomashek KM, Dodd LE, et al. Remdesivir for the treatment of covid-19 - final report. N Engl J Med 2020;383(19):1813–26.
42. Mendelson CL. The aspiration of stomach contents into the lungs during obstetric anesthesia. Am J Obstet Gynecol 1946;52(2):191–205.
43. Skeoch S, Weatherley N, Swift AJ, et al. Drug-induced interstitial lung disease: a systematic review. J Clin Med 2018;7(10).
44. Karpathiou G, Giatromanolaki A, Koukourakis MI, et al. Histological changes after radiation therapy in patients with lung cancer: a prospective study. Anticancer Res 2014;34(6):3119–24.
45. Collard HR, King TE Jr, Schwarz MI. Diffuse alveolar hemorrhage and rare infiltrative disorders of the lung. In: Broaddus VC, Mason RJ, Ernst JD, et al, editors. Murray & Nadel's textbook of respiratory medicine. 6th edition. New York: Elsevier; 2016. p. 1207.
46. Nasser M, Cottin V. Alveolar hemorrhage in vasculitis (primary and secondary). Semin Respir Crit Care Med 2018;39(4):482–93.
47. De Giacomi F, Vassallo R, Yi ES, et al. Acute eosinophilic pneumonia. Causes, diagnosis, and management. Am J Respir Crit Care Med 2018;197(6):728–36.
48. Beasley MB, Franks TJ, Galvin JR, et al. Acute fibrinous and organizing pneumonia: a histological pattern of lung injury and possible variant of diffuse alveolar damage. Arch Pathol Lab Med 2002;126(9):1064–70.
49. Collard HR, Ryerson CJ, Corte TJ, et al. Acute exacerbation of idiopathic pulmonary fibrosis. An international working group report. Am J Respir Crit Care Med 2016;194(3):265–75.
50. Davison DL, Terek M, Chawla LS. Neurogenic pulmonary edema. Crit Care 2012; 16(2):212.
51. Smith WS, Matthay MA. Evidence for a hydrostatic mechanism in human neurogenic pulmonary edema. Chest 1997;111(5):1326–33.
52. Butt YM, Smith ML, Tazelaar HD, et al. Pathology of vaping-associated lung injury. N Engl J Med 2019;381(18):1780–1.
53. Siegel DA, Jatlaoui TC, Koumans EH, et al. Update: interim guidance for health care providers evaluating and caring for patients with suspected E-cigarette,

or vaping, product use associated lung injury - United States, October 2019. MMWR Morb Mortal Wkly Rep 2019;68(41):919–27.

54. Jonas AM, Raj R. Vaping-related acute parenchymal lung injury: a systematic review. Chest 2020;158(4):1555–65.

55. Matsumoto S, Fang X, Traber MG, et al. Dose-dependent pulmonary toxicity of aerosolized vitamin E acetate. Am J Respir Cell Mol Biol 2020;63:748–57.

56. Blount BC, Karwowski MP, Shields PG, et al. Vitamin E acetate in bronchoalveolar-lavage fluid associated with EVALI. N Engl J Med 2020;382(8): 697–705.

57. Travis WD, Costabel U, Hansell DM, et al. An official American Thoracic Society/ European Respiratory Society statement: update of the international multidisciplinary classification of the idiopathic interstitial pneumonias. Am J Respir Crit Care Med 2013;188(6):733–48.

58. Schmidt GA, Koenig S, Mayo PH. Shock: ultrasound to guide diagnosis and therapy. Chest 2012;142(4):1042–8.

59. Palakshappa JA, Meyer NJ. Which patients with ARDS benefit from lung biopsy? Chest 2015;148(4):1073–82.

60. Wong AK, Walkey AJ. Open lung biopsy among critically ill, mechanically ventilated patients. A Metaanalysis. Ann Am Thorac Soc 2015;12(8):1226–30.

61. Donaldson LH, Gill AJ, Hibbert M. Utility of surgical lung biopsy in critically ill patients with diffuse pulmonary infiltrates: a retrospective review. Intern Med J 2016; 46(11):1306–10.

62. Papazian L, Thomas P, Bregeon F, et al. Open-lung biopsy in patients with acute respiratory distress syndrome. Anesthesiology 1998;88(4):935–44.

Pathophysiology of Acute Respiratory Distress Syndrome and COVID-19 Lung Injury

Kai Erik Swenson, MD[a,b],*, Erik Richard Swenson, MD[c,d]

KEYWORDS

- acute respiratory distress syndrome • COVID-19 • pathophysiology

KEY POINTS

- Acute respiratory distress syndrome (ARDS) is a form of noncardiogenic, permeability pulmonary edema associated with systemic inflammatory conditions and marked by diffuse alveolar damage.
- A wide spectrum of ventilation/perfusion defects, including dead space and shunt, is responsible for gas exchange impairments in ARDS.
- Focal parenchymal involvement and derecruitment in ARDS, especially common in posterior and dependent regions, affect ventilation and perfusion heterogeneity and likely contribute to ongoing lung injury due to stress propagation.
- Normal mechanisms for alveolar fluid clearance are impaired in ARDS due to alveolar epithelial injury and inactivation of surfactant.
- Trauma from ventilatory support in ARDS can be roughly divided into 2 categories involving high (barotrauma/volutrauma) and low (atelectrauma) lung volumes; the resulting adverse biologic effects of these traumatic forces on the lung parenchyma and the systemic inflammatory response are broadly termed biotrauma.
- Spontaneous breathing efforts, especially in the presence of ventilator dyssynchrony, may further aggravate lung injury due to the above mechanisms and are broadly termed patient self-inflicted lung injury (P-SILI).
- Some cases of COVID-19-related lung injury may initially present with mild reductions in compliance and less dyspnea in comparison with the degree of worrisome hypoxemia (so-called silent hypoxemia).

Continued

[a] Division of Pulmonary and Critical Care Medicine, Massachusetts General Hospital, 55 Fruit Street, BUL 148, Boston, MA 02114, USA; [b] Division of Pulmonary, Critical Care, and Sleep Medicine, Beth Israel Deaconess Medical Center, Boston, Massachusetts, USA; [c] Department of Medicine, Division of Pulmonary and Critical Care Medicine, University of Washington, Seattle, WA, USA; [d] Medical Service, Veterans Affairs Puget Sound Health Care System, 1660 South Columbian Way, Campus Box 358280 (S-111 Pulm), Seattle, WA 98108, USA
* Corresponding author. Division of Pulmonary and Critical Care Medicine, Massachusetts General Hospital, 55 Fruit Street, BUL 148, Boston, MA 02114.
E-mail address: keswenson@mgh.harvard.edu

Crit Care Clin 37 (2021) 749–776
https://doi.org/10.1016/j.ccc.2021.05.003
0749-0704/21/© 2021 Elsevier Inc. All rights reserved.

criticalcare.theclinics.com

Continued

- However, the overall pathophysiology and clinical course of COVID-19-related lung injury suggests that it is broadly similar to other forms of virally-mediated ARDS.

PATHOPHYSIOLOGY OF ACUTE RESPIRATORY DISTRESS SYNDROME

Acute respiratory distress syndrome (ARDS) is a complex syndrome of acute lung injury leading to noncardiogenic pulmonary edema from many causes that is heterogenous in its clinical presentation and associated with a 40% mortality rate.[1] Extensive work since its initial description in 1967 has elucidated biological pathways causing the many physiologic changes of alveolar collapse/derecruitment, reduced lung compliance, greater pulmonary vascular resistance, and gas exchange impairment that can be compounded by patient's own ventilatory response or assisted ventilatory support, due to regional heterogeneity of the underlying lung injury.

Pathogenesis of Acute Respiratory Distress Syndrome

It is useful to briefly review the pathogenesis of lung injury and repair in ARDS to understand its effects on physiology. Injury begins with activation of alveolar macrophages by microbial or cell injury products,[2] which are locally derived in primary lung injury (pulmonary ARDS) or systemically derived (extrapulmonary ARDS). Cytokine/chemokine release by macrophages recruits and activates circulating neutrophils, which release myriad inflammatory molecules. Although assisting with pathogen killing, they also injure the normally tight alveolar endothelial–epithelial barrier consisting of adherent cell-cell contacts and glycocalyx linings.[3] Alveolar type II pneumocytes secrete surfactant and along with type I pneumocytes reabsorb alveolar fluid by active ion transport back into the interstitium for lymphatic clearance.[4] As a result of loss of the normal low permeability characteristics, the alveolar space fills with an inflammatory cell-rich proteinaceous edema fluid (exudative phase of ARDS), a prime determinant of lung injury severity, alveolar collapse, and derecruitment.[5]

In the proliferative phase of ARDS, with the clearance of pathogens and damaged host cells from the alveolar space, the immune response is recalibrated to prioritize repair and restoration of normal function. This involves neutrophil apoptosis and removal, expansion of resident fibroblasts and interstitial matrix reformation, and regrowth of alveolar epithelium by differentiation of type II alveolar cells into type I cells. If the proliferative phase is impaired or prolonged, ongoing inflammation and fibroblast proliferation impair alveolar clearance and functional recovery.[6] It is likely that uncleared, insoluble proteins in the alveolar space (forming hyaline membranes observed histologically) seed the formation of fibrotic tissue by mesenchymal cells, ultimately leading to the long-term consequence of fibrosing alveolitis (fibrotic phase of ARDS) in some but not all patients.

Gas Exchange Impairment in Acute Respiratory Distress Syndrome

The consequences of the above changes to alveolar structure and histology are gas exchange impairment, increased work breathing, and dyspnea leading to respiratory failure. Alveolar flooding along with pulmonary vascular injury generates the entire spectrum of V_A/Q abnormalities from areas with reduced ventilation-to-perfusion (V_A/Q) ratios and intrapulmonary shunting to high V_A/Q ratios and dead space (**Fig. 1**). Low V_A/Q and shunt are responsible for increased venous admixture and arterial hypoxemia. Given little or no ventilation to these areas, arterial hypoxemia is

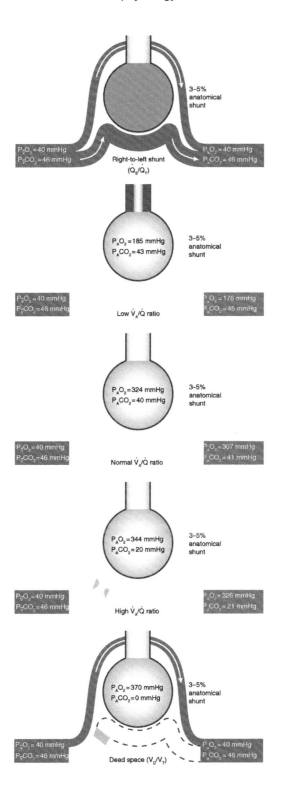

insensitive to global increases in ventilation. Increased F_{io2} can improve oxygenation in low V_A/Q regions, though not in shunts. Although alveolar and interstitial edema widens the alveolar–capillary barrier, the impact of diffusion limitation in causing hypoxemia is dwarfed by contributions of low V_A/Q and shunt[7] as demonstrated by the multiple inert gas elimination technique (MIGET). Increases in alveolar oxygen with higher F_{io2} minimize the impact of any diffusion limitation by increasing the alveolar–capillary oxygen driving gradient. Finally, intracardiac shunting can develop in patients with a preexisting patent foramen ovale, who develop elevated right heart pressures because of increased pulmonary vascular resistance (PVR).

Hypercapnia can also occur but is not incorporated into any ARDS definitions. Several aspects of CO_2 elimination in ARDS merit discussion. As is the case for oxygen uptake, V_A/Q mismatching also impairs CO_2 elimination. Although a diffusion impairment for CO_2 does not occur due to its very high solubility in blood and tissue water and a 20-fold greater diffusivity over oxygen, any failure of alveolar–capillary CO_2 equilibration (widened a-A P_{CO2} gradient) results from rapid capillary transit times and several relatively slower steps in blood CO_2 chemistry including red cell membrane chloride–bicarbonate exchange and the Bohr-Haldane effects.[8] Both high and low V_A/Q regions (including shunt) contribute significantly to hypercapnia, as clarified using MIGET[9] because mixed venous blood flowing through low V_A/Q units enters into the systemic arterial circulation with little or no CO_2 elimination.[10] The use of the Bohr–Enghoff equation to estimate dead space with values as high as 75%[11] overestimates the magnitude of physiologic dead space in ARDS occurring from vascular obstruction and vasoconstriction.[9] Nonetheless, a rising CO_2 dead space may be associated with increased vascular resistance and right heart dysfunction indicative of vascular obstruction.[12] Increases in minute ventilation can effectively improve CO_2 elimination from less injured regions due to the steepness of the blood CO_2 dissociation curve and even cause arterial hypocapnia but become less effective as V_A/Q mismatching worsens and the increased work of breathing generates more CO_2. Ventilation of high V_A/Q regions, especially dead space ($V_A/Q > 100$), wastes respiratory effort without contributing to CO_2 elimination.[13]

Hypercapnia with protective lung ventilation is better accepted since the landmark ARDSNet study showing mortality reduction with this strategy.[14] However, whether this permissive hypercapnia itself might have benefits remains uncertain. It may have both positive and deleterious effects on the ongoing process of lung injury, such as the attenuation of lung inflammation, but results in reduced alveolar fluid clearance.[15,16]

Fig. 1. Spectrum of V_A/Q abnormalities in ARDS. The spectrum of V_A/Q abnormalities in ARDS (from top to bottom) ranging from shunt ($V_A/Q = 0$), low ventilation-to-perfusion ratio ($V_A/Q = 0.2$–0.01), normal ratio ($V_A/Q = 0.2$–5), high ventilation-to-perfusion ratio ($V_A/Q = 5$–100) to dead space ($V_A/Q = $ infinity). Typical mixed venous, alveolar (A), and arterial (A), and mixed venous (mv) P_{O2} and P_{CO2} values are shown. Values are those at a fractional inspired O_2 concentration of 0.5 at a hemoglobin of 15 g/dL and a respiratory exchange ratio of 0.8. (*From* Radermacher P, Maggiore SM, Mercat A. Fifty years of research in ARDS. Gas exchange in acute respiratory distress syndrome. Am J Respir Crit Care Med. 2017; 196(8): 964-84.; with permission.)

Regional Differences in Lung Density, Ventilation, and Blood Flow in Acute Respiratory Distress Syndrome

ARDS does not affect the lung uniformly, as shown by CT imaging (**Fig. 2**). The greatest degree of edema, parenchymal densities, consolidation, and shunting are often in the dorsal and basilar regions of the lung, particularly in the supine position, the position in which most patients are maintained while on mechanical ventilation or during hemodynamic instability. However, this heterogeneity can be altered with position changes, such as with turning to the prone position.[17] Quantification of heterogeneity in lung units using MIGET demonstrates a wide range of VA/Q lung units indirectly, with a bimodal distribution of considerable shunt and elevated alveolar dead space,[18] but it provides no regional information. Advanced imaging techniques, including radiolabeled inert gas inhalation/infusion, can provide spatial resolution for the physiologic heterogeneity seen with MIGET in ARDS.[19] Areas of lowest ventilation and lowest VA/Q (areas of CT densities) are found in gravitationally dependent regions; regional ventilation heterogeneity is greater in the supine than in the prone position (**Fig. 3**), likely a consequence of the more compressive effect of lung and soft tissue weight (cardiac and abdominal) on basilar lung regions and higher regional pleural pressure differences in the supine position.[20] Oxygenation in ARDS improves in most patients with prone positioning resulting from the reduction in regional VA/Q heterogeneity.

Pulmonary blood flow, on the other hand, is less affected by gravitational forces and positioning,[21] as regional blood vessel density and local vascular tone are the primary

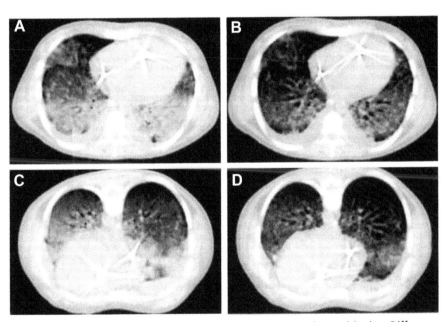

Fig. 2. Differences in lung density by CT imaging in prone vs. supine positioning. Differences in lung density by CT scanning in ARDS, taken in the supine position at end exhalation (*A*), end inspiration (*B*), and in the prone position at end exhalation (*C*) and at end inspiration (*D*). The improvement in aeration in the prone images is consistent with the more uniform VA/Q matching and improved oxygenation with prone positioning. (*From* Kallet RH. A Comprehensive Review of Prone Position in ARDS. Respir Care. 2015; 60(11): 1660-87; with permission.)

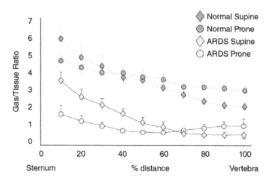

Fig. 3. Changes in lung tissue heterogeneity over the anterior-posterior plane. The gas/tissue ratios reflect the degree of uniformity of ventilated lung as a function of the distance between the sternum and the vertebrae. In the supine position, the gas/tissue ratio sharply decreases from the sternum to the vertebrae suggesting that both in normal and in patients with ARDS distending forces are about 3 times higher closer to the sternum than to the vertebrae. In prone position, the gas/tissue ratio is far more homogeneous, indicating a more even distribution of forces and more uniform ventilation throughout the lung. (*From* Guérin C, Albert RK, Beitler J, et al. Prone position in ARDS patients: why, when, how and for whom. Intensive Care Med. 2020;46(12):2385-2396. doi:10.1007/s00134-020-06306-w; with permission.)

determinants of regional perfusion. Perfusion is higher in posterior and caudal lung regions, and therefore, prone positioning (which improves ventilation in these areas) is associated with significant gas exchange improvement in most patients with ARDS. Pulmonary vascular tone is presumed to be mediated most directly by hypoxic pulmonary vasoconstriction (HPV) and hypercapnic pulmonary vasoconstriction that redirect perfusion to greater ventilated and oxygenated lung units to optimize V_A/Q matching. The only direct evidence that HPV is operative and contributes significantly to regional vascular tone in ARDS because it has never been tested formally by hypoxic gas inspiration,[22] comes from patients receiving extracorporeal membrane oxygenation in whom mean PA pressure decreased, and PVR fell 25% when the mixed venous P_{O_2} was raised from 47 to 84 mm Hg by increasing extracorporeal blood flow.[23] HPV augmentation with pulmonary vasoconstrictors (almitrine) and inhalation of pulmonary vasodilators (such as nitric oxide) to vasodilate ventilated areas are both associated with reductions in hypoxemia; the latter treatment, however, only exerts effects on ventilated lung units to which it can be delivered.[24]

Respiratory Mechanics in Acute Respiratory Distress Syndrome

Lung parenchyma is formed from millions of interdependent alveoli, which share the alveolar volume throughout the lung, preventing overdistension during inspiration and collapse during expiration.[25] This allows for parenchymal stress during inspiration to be somewhat homogenized, despite variability in alveolar size and location. In ARDS, increased permeability and loss of surfactant cause some alveoli to become flooded and unrecruitable or poorly recruitable. As a result, lung volume remaining for gas exchange shrinks, and lung compliance is reduced, though it varies widely based on disease severity from 5 to 40 mL/cmH$_2$0,[26,27] and functional residual capacity is decreased by 20% to 30% compared with normal.[28] The volume of derecruited lung appears to roughly correlate with the degree of pulmonary shunt and gas exchange abnormalities.[29]

It has been long recognized that alveolar edema and derecruitment occur in a heterogeneous regional fashion, with dependent regions most affected.[30,31] Focal and nonfocal patterns of lung involvement in ARDS respond differently to recruitment maneuvers such as positive end-expiratory pressure (PEEP) or position change.[32] These radiographic findings reinforce the idea that the lung in ARDS can be conceptually divided into nonaerated diseased regions and aerated healthy regions. The diminished size of normal aerated lung tissue in relation to overall lung mass has been termed the "baby lung in an adult body."[26] As is clear from the radiographic studies above, the "baby lung" need not be a distinct anatomic but rather a physiologic entity, and its area can shift dramatically depending on body position.[30]

Global measurements of compliance and airway, plateau, and transpulmonary pressures may not adequately account for such regional variation in physiology. For example, there may be significant variations in pleural pressure in ARDS, especially between dependent and nondependent regions, that are not captured by a point estimate of pleural pressure via esophageal balloon and can be as high as 10 cmH$_2$0 in cadaveric studies.[33] Additionally, airway pressure measurements may not accurately estimate local stresses in regions with airway closure, particularly in obese patients.[32]

These regional variations in compliance can lead to heterogeneous injury risk. In a process called stress concentration, local alveolar derecruitment causes inhomogeneity in distending pressures, with surrounding alveoli bearing the greatest stress. In effect, this creates a penumbra of at-risk lung units (**Fig. 4**) surrounding an area of injury that may propagate.[34,35] These areas have been termed "stress raisers" and may involve up to a quarter of the parenchyma as visualized by dynamic CT imaging. Mechano-transduction associated with shear stresses caused by cyclic atelectasis in these regions may contribute to cleavage of cell-cell adhesion molecules, further disrupting membranes and preventing alveolar clearance of edema.[36] Despite retaining grossly normal mechanical properties,[37] PET imaging demonstrates that well-aerated lung regions have abnormal permeability and higher metabolic rate, suggesting ongoing and worsening inflammation even with lung-protective ventilation.[38,39]

Though ARDS is predominantly a restrictive disorder, airway obstruction can also occur from edematous distal airways and increased lung weight causing small airway narrowing/closure, with total airway resistance elevated roughly 2-fold.[40] Expiratory flow limitation does appear to exist in ARDS and improves with PEEP though not with bronchodilators.[41] Although rapid flows and rapid changes in pressure likely exert some degree of additional stress to the lung parenchyma given its viscoelastic nature, the clinical importance of this stress is not fully known.

Alveolar and Lymphatic Fluid Clearance in Acute Respiratory Distress Syndrome

The ability of the lung to maintain a highly compliant and dry alveolar air space for efficient gas exchange at a low work of breathing cost depends upon a number of factors, including surfactant production and active vectorial alveolar epithelial sodium and water transport from the alveolar space into the interstitium for reuptake into the blood or lymphatic transport. In ARDS, the surfactant is inactivated, and alveolar epithelial injury leads to loss of fluid reabsorption (**Fig. 5**). Type I and II alveolar epithelial cells actively reabsorb sodium and fluid from the airspace via apical membrane sodium entry through epithelial sodium channels (ENaCs) driven by the concentration gradient established by sodium pumping into the interstitium by basolateral membrane energy-consuming Na$^+$/K$^+$ ATPase.[42] Chloride follows paracellularly and via cystic fibrosis transmembrane conductance regulator (CFTR)-mediated transcellular uptake[43] and water by paracellular movement and by aquaporin-5 mediated transcellular movement.[44] Fluid reabsorption rates in the isolated human lung average about 12%

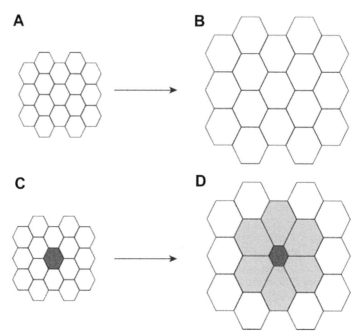

Fig. 4. Local ventilatory inhomogeneity as a stress raiser. A stress raiser is a region of early injury that leads to inhomogeneous tissue forces that apply stress and strain to surrounding neighbor regions. An equal volume of gas is introduced into an area of normal lung (*A*) and into one with a stress raiser (either a collapsed or non-air-filled region-the dark region in (*C*). In a normal lung, the introduced air with inflation is evenly distributed and leads to uniform inflation at minimal stress (*B*). In contrast, the lung with a stress raiser, when further inflated (*D*), subjects the immediate neighboring regions (colored gray) to greater stress (and potential injury) as they are inflated, but the collapsed or fluid-filled region itself is not inflated. (*From* Henderson WR, Chen L, Amato MB, Brochard LJ. Fifty years of research in ARDS. Respiratory mechanics in acute respiratory distress syndrome. Am J Respir Crit Care Med. 2017; 196(7): 822-33; with permission.)

per hour[45] but likely are higher in vivo. Reabsorption can be stimulated several-fold by beta-2 adrenergic agonist- and corticosteroid-mediated upregulation of ENaCs and Na^+/K^+ ATPase membrane expression and activity.[42,45] Fluid clearance from the lung interstitium by lung lymphatics is mediated passively by ventilatory efforts and by active, spontaneous contractions that can be stimulated by beta-2 adrenergic drugs[46] that may enhance lymph drainage from the lung.

In conditions wherein the alveolar epithelium is not injured, such as cardiogenic pulmonary edema, beta-2 adrenergic agonists increase fluid reabsorption, but the hope that this might be realized in ARDS could not be demonstrated in 2 large clinical trials involving systemic[47] and inhaled[48] drug administration. The success in heart failure and lack of efficacy in ARDS is likely explained by a functioning intact alveolar epithelium in cardiogenic pulmonary edema and injury and denudation of the epithelium in acute lung injury, either unable to reabsorb sodium at all or keep pace with ongoing rates of microvascular leakage. The increase in alveolar surface tension with cessation of production and inactivation of surfactant in ARDS leads to a lower interstitial pressure that increases the microvascular transmural pressure gradient. This favors greater extravascular fluid accumulation for the same microvascular pressure.[49]

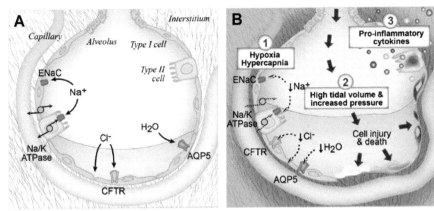

Fig. 5. Alveolar fluid clearance in uninjured lung vs. ARDS. Alveolar fluid clearance pathways in edematous uninjured lungs (*A*) and in ARDS (*B*). Both types I and II alveolar epithelial cells absorb sodium, chloride, and water, respectively, via epithelial sodium channels (ENaCs), cystic fibrosis transmembrane conductance regulator (CFTR), and aquaporin-5 (AQ-5) channels. Energy-dependent Na^+/K^+ ATPase activity on the basolateral membrane of epithelial cells establishes an osmotic driving gradient for movement of sodium from the alveolar space into the interstitium for removal by capillary blood or lymphatic clearance. Chloride follows passively either by CFTR or paracellularly with water moving transcellularly via AQ-5 or paracellularly. Other cation channels not illustrated are also involved. These pathways along with surfactant maintain a dry and compliant alveolar space for efficient gas exchange. With injury to the lung (*B*) and loss of the normal tight alveolar–capillary barrier such as in ARDS, fluid moves into the lungs and is less readily reabsorbed. Hypoxia and hypercapnia cause downregulation and loss of the ion and water channels as well as Na^+/K^+ ATPase activity. This may be compounded by various proinflammatory cytokines and mechanical ventilator-induced lung injury involving high distending volumes and pressures. (*From* Huppert LA, Matthay MA, Ware LB. Pathogenesis of Acute Respiratory Distress Syndrome. Semin Respir Crit Care Med. 2019 Feb; 40(1):31-39; with permission.)

Pathophysiology of Lung Injury from Ventilatory Support in Acute Respiratory Distress Syndrome

An understanding of ARDS physiology, whose key features include gas exchange abnormalities often requiring ventilatory support and atelectasis/decreased compliance with significant regional heterogeneity, has implications for ventilatory support strategies. The role of lung injury while on positive pressure ventilation is the best studied. Positive pressure ventilation along with PEEP reduces the work of breathing and prevents atelectasis of nearly collapsed lung units to improve gas exchange. Furthermore, positive airway pressure helps reduce further edema formation in many edematous states, including the increased alveolar permeability of ARDS.[50] However, as long known, mechanical ventilation also exacerbates the ongoing processes of lung injury and even injury to other critical organs beyond the lung (**Fig. 6**), broadly termed ventilator-induced lung injury (VILI). VILI is often differentiated at the extremes of lung volume[51]; injury at high lung volumes is due to alveolar overdistension (barotrauma/volutrauma), whereas injury at low lung volumes is due to cyclical opening and closing of distal airways and alveoli (atelectrauma). High respiratory rate and inspiratory flow theoretically would increase total stress at both high and low lung volumes, although the effect of these variables within normal clinical ranges on the progression of injury remains uncertain.[52] Other etiologies of VILI include patient self-inflicted lung

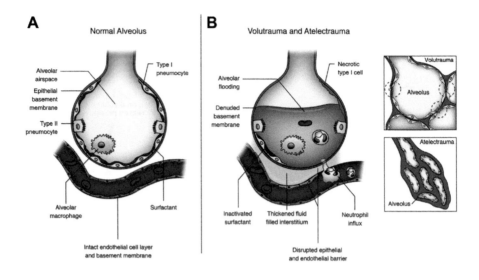

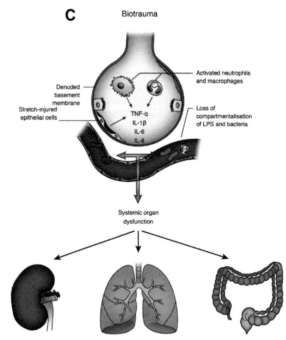

Fig. 6. Events and forms of ventilator-induced lung injury (VILI). The normal alveolus (*A*) is contrasted with the alveolus (*B*) injured by mechanical ventilation by volutrauma and atelectrauma causing endothelial and epithelial injury, greater alveolar–capillary permeability, proteinaceous alveolar edema, and recruitment of inflammatory cells. Activation of resident and recruited cells results in biotrauma (*C*) with the production of proinflammatory mediators that propagate the injury and spillover into the circulation to cause systemic organ damage and dysfunction (*D*). (*From* Curley GF, Laffey JG, Zhang H, Slutsky AS. Biotrauma and Ventilator-Induced Lung Injury: Clinical Implications. Chest. 2016; 150(5): 1109-17; with permission.)

injury (P-SILI) described below, and biotrauma, the downstream local and systemic biological effects of all ventilation-related injury.

Volutrauma, Barotrauma, Atelectrauma, and Biotrauma

Volutrauma and barotrauma represent 2 depictions of the same process, in which excessive mechanical power causes alveolar overdistension and repetitive strain[53] and has been well-described for decades.[54] Clinical strategies to avoid volutrauma and barotrauma, termed lung-protective ventilation, are strongly associated with improved mortality in ARDS.[14] These include targeted tidal volumes of 6 mL/kg ideal body weight, plateau pressures less than 30 cmH$_2$0, driving pressures (plateau pressure − PEEP) < 16 cmH$_2$O, and judicious PEEP; however, even these goals may not be adequately protective. None allow for delivered tidal volumes to scale with the fraction of nonaerated lung; a more individualized approach would incorporate some measurement of aerated lung volume, such as with nitrogen wash-in/wash-out or helium dilution techniques, or CT quantitation of aerated lung volume.[55]

It is important to note that plateau pressure decreases as the duration of time spent at end-inspiratory occlusion lengthens, likely due to delayed recruitment of additional lung volume via surfactant spread and alveolar pendelluft. Thus, a shorter end-inspiratory occlusion plateau pressure is recommended as a marker of lung injury.[27] Additionally, plateau pressures may not correlate well with transpulmonary pressure, especially if there is significant extrathoracic restriction, such as with severe obesity, ascites, advanced pregnancy, or extensive thoracic burns.[56] Lastly, regional heterogeneity of lung compliance can lead to local overdistension, as visualized on CT, despite global lung-protective ventilation[57]; this likely occurs predominantly in areas of stress concentration. Various bedside techniques, especially electrical impedance tomography (EIT) to noninvasively monitor changes in regional lung ventilation across the transverse plane of the chest, may help tailor ventilatory support to avoid such injury.[58] Gross overdistension and rupture of alveoli can also lead to pneumothorax, pneumomediastinum, and air embolism in ARDS, though this is rare in the age of lung-protective ventilation.

Injury at low lung volumes due to stresses from cyclical opening and closing of alveoli and distal airways, associated with parenchymal shear injury, is collectively termed atelectrauma. Animal models of ARDS demonstrate that cyclical opening and closing of alveolar ducts and even bronchioles (depending on the level of PEEP) leads to site-specific lung injury,[59] which correlates with findings in human lungs on autopsy series.[60] Pressures required to maintain open airways vary depending on patient and lung region but globally can be as high as 13 cmH$_2$0 when monitoring the lower inflection point of the pressure/volume curve.[61] Thus, injury from cyclical atelectasis may be prevented with the application of higher PEEP.[62] Although large trials of high versus low PEEP in ARDS have shown no mortality reduction,[63,64] there are likely patient subsets who might benefit from higher or lower PEEP. Notably, decremental PEEP trials to identify the pressure–volume curve associated with the best dynamic compliance ("open lung strategy") may reduce mortality in ARDS.[65,66] PEEP titration targeting a transpulmonary pressure of 0 to 10 cmH$_2$O at end expiration using esophageal balloon pressure measurement for estimation of pleural pressure is also promising for optimizing respiratory parameters and reducing overall lung injury.[67] Evaluation of regional recruitability continues to be an active area of investigation; emerging bedside techniques include the multiple pressure–volume curves method[68] and EIT.[58]

The genetic, molecular, and cell biological events of parenchymal stress and strain in all types of VILI are termed biotrauma. It is the cellular response to alveolar and small airway cellular injury with gene transcription and elaboration of numerous proinflammatory mediators that drive ongoing lung injury and cause systemic organ damage and dysfunction.[52] These processes, mediators, and their effects are more fully presented by other articles in this series.

Patient Self-Inflicted Lung Injury

Afferent signaling to the CNS of impaired gas exchange, lung irritant and stretch receptor activation, and the work of breathing can lead to vigorous injurious respiratory efforts to both diseased and at-risk lung regions even when tidal volumes and plateau pressures are limited.[69] Convincing data come from animal models, in which neurologically-stimulated hyperventilation itself directly induces acute lung injury.[70] It is likely that the effects of P-SILI are most profound on basilar lung units where swings in local intrapleural negative pressure caused by the proximity of the diaphragm are greatest.[71–73]

Most clinical data suggesting P-SILI derive from studies correlating spontaneous breathing efforts during mechanical ventilation with increased mortality. Despite similar tidal volumes and plateau pressures, assisted breaths can lead to worsened lung injury in early ARDS compared to controlled breaths, offering supportive evidence for neuromuscular blockade, especially in the presence of significant patient-ventilator dyssynchrony,[73] but controlled trials have not convincingly demonstrated a mortality benefit.[74] The dangers of spontaneous ventilation on the progression of lung injury must be weighed carefully alongside its beneficial effects in preventing respiratory muscle atrophy and the risks with additional sedation or neuromuscular blockade to abrogate spontaneous efforts.[75]

PATHOPHYSIOLOGY OF COVID-19 LUNG INJURY

The SARS-CoV-2 pandemic beginning in early 2020 has caused millions of deaths from severe COVID-19 lung injury and respiratory failure, often complicated by multi-system injury. While infection can present in myriad ways, SARS-CoV-2 is largely transmitted by aerosolization and typically causes symptoms of fatigue, malaise, fever, cough, sore throat, and dyspnea from pneumonitis, hypoxemia, and respiratory failure. People of all ages and backgrounds are afflicted. Risk factors for poorer outcomes include older age, obesity, male sex, diabetes, hypertension, cardiovascular disease, smoking, cancer, autoimmune disorders, and other chronic diseases. Those with limited reserve, particularly in lung function, have the worst prognosis. While COVID-19 has been described as an atypical form of ARDS, the issue remains highly controversial, as pathophysiologic similarities with ARDS from other causes outnumber any differences (**Table 1**). In many ways, the advent of COVID-19 as a trigger for ARDS has reopened many questions on the pathophysiology of ARDS itself.

Pathogenesis of COVID-19 Lung Injury

The pathogenesis of COVID-19 lung injury involves direct viral damage and a host defense response with thrombotic and inflammatory reactions in the lung and elsewhere.[76] The alveolar epithelium and vascular endothelium express angiotensin-converting enzyme 2 (ACE-2), to which the virus attaches and then is internalized along with the membrane-bound ACE-2. Consequently, cellular damage ensues and evolves to interstitial edema and alveolar fluid filling, similar to the process of alveolar flooding in ARDS. Autopsy data, reflecting advanced disease, reveal typical ARDS features, including exudative proliferative and fibrotic phases of diffuse alveolar damage, hyaline membranes, alveolar and interstitial edema, atypical pneumocyte hyperplasia, alveolar hemorrhage, infarction, endothelial cell injury, and capillary congestion with microthrombosis and dilation.[77,78] Notably, there is greater vasculopathy,

Table 1
Comparisons between pathophysiology of COVID-19 lung injury and acute respiratory distress syndrome

	COVID-19 Lung Injury	Acute Respiratory Distress Syndrome
Onset	8–12 d	< 7 d (Berlin definition)
Cause	SARS-CoV-2 (agent of COVID-19) via direct viral and immune response-mediated-injury	Multiple pulmonary and nonpulmonary (systemic) causes, both infectious and noninfectious
Histologic features	• DAD • Organizing pneumonia • More severe vasculopathy - Thromboembolism - In situ microthrombi - Capillary dilatations - Endothelial damage	• DAD - Exudative phase - Proliferative phase - Fibrotic phase • Vascular changes - Thromboembolism - In situ microthrombi - Capillary dilatations - Endothelial damage
Imaging	• Peripheral and basilar ground-glass opacities in early disease • Progression to typical consolidation as in ARDS	• Consolidations, often patchy and dependent
Respiratory mechanics	• C_{ST} range: 20–90 mL/cmH$_2$O • Compliance and oxygenation often improved with increased PEEP or prone positioning	• C_{ST} range: 10–78 mL/cmH$_2$O • Compliance and oxygenation often improved with increased PEEP or prone positioning
Pulmonary vasculature	• Mild-moderate pulmonary hypertension • Unknown whether HPV intact or impaired • Vasculature responsive to almitrine and inhaled NO	• Mild-moderate pulmonary hypertension • HPV intact • Vasculature responsive to almitrine, calcium channel blockers, nitrates, PDE-5 inhibitors, and inhaled NO
Gas exchange	V_A/Q mismatching: • Hypoxemia due to low V_A/Q and shunt • No evidence for diffusion limitation • Hypercapnia due to permissive hypoventilation, and all forms of V_A/Q mismatch	V_A/Q mismatching: • Hypoxemia due to low VA/Q and shunt • No evidence for diffusion limitation • Hypercapnia due to permissive hypoventilation, and all forms of V_A/Q mismatch
Alveolar epithelial fluid clearance	Likely reduced due to alveolar type I and II cell damage, but not formally tested	Reduced due to alveolar type I and II cell damage; unresponsive to beta-adrenergic therapy

Abbreviations: ARDS, acute respiratory distress syndrome; C $_{ST}$, static compliance; COVID-19, coronavirus disease-2019; HPV, hypoxic pulmonary vasoconstriction; NO, nitric oxide; PDE-5, phosphodiesterase-5; PEEP, positive end-expiratory pressure; V$_A$/Q, alveolar ventilation–perfusion ratio.

including macro- and microthrombosis, endothelial cell injury, vascular dilation, and aberrant angiogenesis[77,79] in COVID-19 and the earlier SARS injury than with H1N1 influenza and ARDS.[80] However, lung biopsies in early COVID-19[81–83] do not show the marked vascular pathology noted at autopsy. Limited bronchoalveolar lavage data demonstrate a more monocytic and lymphocytic predominance in the airspace typical of viral pneumonias[84] compared with the dominantly neutrophilic cell population in ARDS.[85] Understanding the respiratory pathophysiology of COVID-19 lung injury and ARDS is fundamental to better clinical care and support.

Lung Compliance and Respiratory Mechanics

A possible unique ARDS presentation was reported by Gattinoni and colleagues (2020) and followed up with a larger study of 32 patients[86] with potential implications for physiologic support.[87] In these studies, a small fraction (<20%) had "near normal" static total respiratory system compliance (C_{ST}) of 70 to 90 mL/cmH$_2$O with an average of 50 (**Fig. 7**) compared with an average of 40 in series of ARDS patients.[88] On the basis of a slightly higher average C_{ST} observed in earlier ARDS patients, they proposed a controversial high compliance L phenotype (L for low elastance, low PEEP recruitability, and more dominant low V_A/Q gas exchange abnormality than shunt) combined with vasoplegia and loss of HPV. Nonetheless, many patients continue to worsen, suggesting only a temporal sequence of early disease evolving to more classic ARDS pathophysiology. A small fraction of patients with higher compliance of the L phenotype has been described in equal proportions in subsequent series.[89–93] This is neither unique to COVID-19, as shown in ARDS before the pandemic,[93–95] nor to patients with other influenza pneumonias requiring mechanical ventilation.[96]

Several explanations for better compliance early in COVID-19 lung injury and even in ARDS are possible. The first is the predominantly peripheral and basilar ground-glass opacities (GGO) very prevalent on CT imaging (**Fig. 8**) early in the course of the disease.[97,98] While never directly studied, GGOs, by virtue of their lesser CT density than consolidations, could be more compliant. This is suggested indirectly in patients when dynamic (but not static) compliance was measured and surprisingly correlated with the volume of CT-defined GGO, in contrast to a negative correlation with

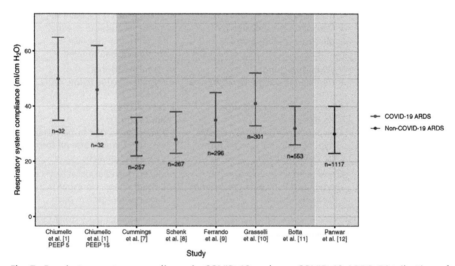

Fig. 7. Respiratory system compliance in COVID-19 and non-COVID-19 ARDS. Distribution of respiratory system compliance (C_{ST}) values in various studies of patients with COVID-19 lung injury and compared with patients with ARDS. Most studies find no significant differences between the 2 forms of lung injury. (*From* Goligher EC, Ranieri VM, Slutsky AS. Is severe COVID-19 pneumonia a typical or atypical form of ARDS? And does it matter? Intensive Care Med. 2021;47(1):83-85. doi:10.1007/s00134-020-06320-y; with permission.)

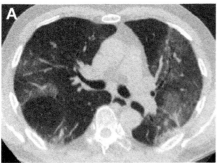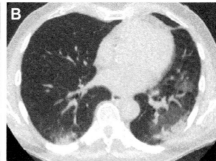

Fig. 8. Representative CT imaging of early COVID-19 lung injury. Two axial slices of a patient with COVID-19 lung injury at presentation to the emergency department after several days of fever, mild dyspnea, cough, and malaise. The images show multiple areas of typical ground-glass opacities and some early consolidation (A, B). (From Schalekamp S, Bleeker-Rovers CP, Beenen LFM, Quarles van Ufford HME, Gietema HA, Stöger JL, Harris V, Reijers MHE, Rahamat-Langendoen J, Korevaar DA, Smits LP, Korteweg C, van Rees Vellinga T, Vermaat M, Stassen PM, Scheper H, Wijnakker R, Borm FJ, Dofferhoff ASM, Prokop WM. Chest CT in the Emergency Department for Diagnosis of COVID-19 Pneumonia: Dutch Experience. Radiology. 2020: 203465; with permission.)

consolidated lung.[99] Surfactant producing AE type II cells express ACE-2 and contain almost 50% of total lung surfactant.[100] With injury and release of these stores, the compliance decline expected with microvascular leakage might be buffered, but only temporarily before surfactant inactivation occurs and production ceases. Hyaluronan, also produced by AE type II cells[101] as part of the alveolar glycocalyx, enhances surfactant function and reduces fluid accumulation;[102] in early injury before excessive accumulation occurs, it may limit surfactant inactivation.[103,104]

Several other aspects of compliance in ARDS and COVID-19 lung injury warrant discussion. The idea that a more vascular type injury may lead to better-than-expected compliance[99] runs counter to the fact that poorly perfused or nonperfused lung regions become stiffer by hypocapnic pneumoconstriction and then by cessation of surfactant production.[105] This normal V_A/Q matching mechanism based on responses to changes in local blood-borne CO_2 delivery redirects ventilation from poorly perfused regions to those with greater blood flow. Several studies have in fact found no correlation between the amount of affected lung by CT imaging and C_{ST}.[106–108] It should also be pointed out that initial higher compliance is a poor predictor of risk and progression to severe lung injury in ARDS.[109]

Pulmonary Hemodynamics and Vascular Regulation

One proposed aspect of COVID-19 lung injury is vasoplegia and loss of HPV that may even result in paradoxic hyperperfusion. CT imaging of the vasculature shows large and small vessel dilations in areas of affected lung and dual-energy CT perfusion imaging (Fig. 9) reveals greater perfusion, particularly in GGO areas, supporting the possible idea of vasoplegia and dysregulated perfusion.[99,110] Estimated PA pressures by transesophageal echocardiography in severe COVID-19 lung injury show only modest elevations[111,112] as in ARDS.[113,114] This has now been corroborated with right heart catheterization data in 21 mechanically ventilated patients, showing mild pulmonary hypertension (mean PAP—27 mm Hg, PVR—1.6 Woods units, and cardiac output—7.3 L/min).[115] These data do not rule out pulmonary hypertension (PH) in some with COVID-19 lung injury as there are case reports of right heart dysfunction

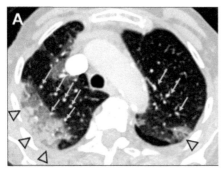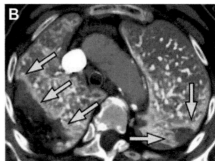

Fig. 9. Changes in pulmonary vascular anatomy in focal COVID-19 lung disease. Conventional (*A*) and dual-energy CT (*B*) in a patient with COVID-19 pneumonia without evidence of pulmonary emboli. (*A*) There is a large area of peripheral ground-glass opacity and consolidation within the right upper lobe and smaller ground-glass opacity in the posterior left upper lobe (green *arrowheads*), which are accompanied by dilated subsegmental vessels proximal to, and within, the opacities (green *arrows*). (*B*) The accompanying image of pulmonary blood volume shows corresponding wedge-shaped areas of decreased perfusion within the upper lobes, with a peripheral halo of higher perfusion (green *arrows*). (*From* Lang M, Som A, Mendoza DP, et al. Hypoxaemia related to COVID-19: vascular and perfusion abnormalities on dual-energy CT. Lancet Infect Dis. 2020;20(12):1365-1366. doi:10.1016/ S1473-3099(20)30367-4; Reprinted with permission from Elsevier.)

and cor pulmonale consistent with either PH or viral myocardial injury.[116] At this time, all analyses of pulmonary hemodynamics are complicated by the likelihood of wide regional PVR differences such that vascular beds with low resistance and possible lack of HPV are counterbalanced by other areas of higher resistance due to obstruction from pulmonary embolism and/or in situ thrombosis, as observed in over 30% of patients despite anticoagulant prophylaxis.[117] Loss of ACE-2 activity from internalization with the virus will result in less breakdown of vasoconstricting angiotensin II to its vasodilating and antiinflammatory metabolite Ang1-7.[118] In addition, bradykinin and some of its active edema-promoting metabolites are elevated in COVID-19, several of which are metabolized by ACE-2.[119]

If HPV is blunted or absent, multiple mechanisms may be responsible. Reductions in alveolar P_{CO_2} will blunt HPV.[22] Another possibility is that SARS-CoV-2 may cause changes in proteins involved in vascular O_2 sensing.[120] Finally, viral-mediated alveolar–capillary endothelial cell injury[77,79,121,122] may impair alveolar hypoxia sensing and transduction to the vascular smooth muscle.[123] Another explanation, unrelated to the above possible viral-mediated effects, is that those with hypoxemia out of proportion to the extent of lung involvement may have intrinsically blunted HPV at the low end of the wide 5-fold variation in this response among healthy persons.[22] It remains unknown whether HPV is altered in COVID-19 lung injury because to do so would require brief testing with inspired hypoxic gas. As in ARDS, almitrine improves gas exchange in patients with COVID-19 lung injury,[124] as does inhaled nitric oxide.[125] However, because these drugs also alter PVR in normoxia,[126–128] they are not wholly ideal to evaluate HPV and thus do not clearly establish an alteration in HPV in patients with COVID-19 lung injury.

Causes of Hypoxemia, Hypercapnia, and Dyspnea in COVID-19 Lung Injury

There have been alarming reports of what has been termed silent hypoxemia or happy hypoxia, denoting marked arterial hypoxemia despite an apparent lack of dyspnea in otherwise conscious and spontaneously breathing patients. Delirium associated with the infection may increase the presentation of silent hypoxemia.[129] The diagnosis of possible silent hypoxemia varies from a small minority of patients to as many as one-third when assessed simply as the absence of dyspnea.[89,90,130–132] The hypoxemia can be profound, with values of SpO_2 and Pao_2 as low as 70% and 40 mm Hg,[133] yet surprisingly in the half-century since the description of ARDS, silent hypoxemia has never been reported before. In reviews of ARDS, a few patients have presented without dyspnea, but no percentages are given and none in relation to the degree of severe hypoxemia.[85] In severe viral-induced ARDS, including SARS-CoV-1 and H1N1 influenza infection, those requiring oxygen without dyspnea ranged from 0% to 27%,[109,134–136] suggesting this phenomenon is virally-mediated. In a recent analysis of prehospitalized patients, the average SpO_2 divided by respiratory rate was 5.0 in March 2020, compared with 3.2 to 3.5 in March of the preceding 3 years, suggestive of more silent hypoxemia and less tachypnea in the COVID-19 era.[137]

Hypoxemia in COVID-19 as described in ARDS is caused by low ventilation-to-perfusion (V_A/Q) mismatching and shunt. In ARDS, there is no evidence for diffusion limitation, but this has not yet been studied in COVID-19 lung injury using MIGET. Recently, detection of small bubbles with intravenous injection by transcranial Doppler correlated with hypoxemia and reduced compliance in patients with COVID-19 lung injury and was attributed to diffusion limitation due to microvascular dilations noted at autopsy.[138] However, normally occurring intrapulmonary arteriovenous anastomoses of similar diameters causing equal bubble scores in healthy people do not cause hypoxemia.[139] Modeling of early COVID-19 lung injury is conflicting. One study suggests the reported hypoxemia severity in early disease can be reasonably explained by a combination of pulmonary embolism, V_A/Q mismatching in noninjured lung regions from redirection of blood flow from obstructed regions, and normal perfusion of the relatively small fraction of injured lung and does not require the loss of HPV, hypoxic vasodilation, or diffusion limitation.[140] Another finds that the L-type phenotype can only be explained by hyperperfusion of collapsed lung regions, loss of HPV, extensive microvascular obstruction, and diffusion limitation in affected areas.[141] Hypercapnia also develops in very severe COVID-19 lung injury for the same reasons as described earlier in the section on ARDS. As in ARDS, the entire spectrum of V_A/Q mismatching contributes to the CO_2 dead space calculation. Reported values of dead space as high as 75% in COVID-19 lung injury[142] due largely to vascular obstruction would be inconsistent with the mild PH and preserved cardiac output in most patients as noted above.

The absence of respiratory distress in some patients with COVID-19 lung injury include better-than-expected lung compliance (discussed above) with arterial hypocapnia in those that can increase ventilation sufficiently to partially blunt dyspnea arising from hypoxemia and other stimuli from the injured lung and elsewhere in the body. Furthermore, there is speculation that neural infection by SARS-CoV-2 (given the presence of ACE-2 in the carotid body[143] and elsewhere in the CNS[144]) leads to a loss of normal perception of increased breathing from hypoxemia, lung irritant and stretch receptor activity, respiratory muscle effort, fever, anxiety, sympathetic nervous system activation, increased metabolism, and metabolic acidosis. Other coronaviruses infect the brainstem via viral transmission along afferent nerves arising in the lung, nasopharynx, and other peripheral mechanoreceptors and chemoreceptors.[145] Regarding the respiratory muscles, they express ACE-2 and can develop myopathic changes with infection that might lessen afferent signaling of their effort.[146]

Control of ventilation and dyspnea perception is complex.[147] Afferent signals to the brain regarding breathing and its perception (**Fig. 10**) include (a) chemoreception by

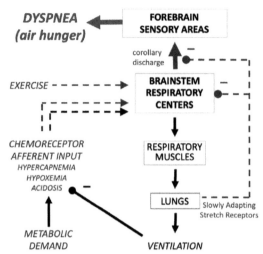

Fig. 10. Signaling pathways in the control of ventilation. Schematic representation of the multiple afferent signaling pathways to the brainstem respiratory centers that control ventilation from mechano-stretch receptors in muscles and joints, irritant and stretch receptor in the lungs, arterial Po_2 and Pco_2 (from peripheral chemoreceptors in the carotid body, arterial pH and Pco_2 (from central chemoreceptors in the brainstem), fear, and emotional and pain stimuli from the hypothalamus. Signals from the brainstem are also conveyed (corollary projection) to the conscious regions of the brain (amygdala and insular cortex) that perceive dyspnea, work of breathing, and respiratory distress. In COVID-19, it is proposed that some of this signaling and cortical perception may be impaired by direct viral injury to these pathways. (*From* Simonson T, Baker T, Banzett R, et al. Silent hypoxaemia in COVID-19 patients. J Physiol 2021;599(4):1057-1065. doi:10.1113/jp280769; with permission.)

peripheral and central chemoreceptors of arterial Po_2, pH, and Pco_2 and (b) signaling from the lungs, respiratory muscles, and chest wall to the brainstem respiratory control center and its "corollary projection" to higher cortical centers in the anterior insular cortex and amygdala, where the conscious sensation of breathing resides.[148] Signaling from peripheral and central chemoreceptors in response to arterial Pco_2 and Po_2 changes, like that of HPV,[22] varies 5-fold to 10-fold among individuals[149,150] and is lower in older and patients with diabetes.[133] In addition to interindividual variability of hypoxic ventilatory response (HVR), a similar high variability exists with the symptomatic dyspnea threshold onset during hypoxemia, with an observed threshold range of end-tidal Po_2 from 35 to 60 mm Hg in healthy subjects maintained eucapnic at a fixed ventilation that likely correlates with HVR.[151]

Whatever the pathophysiologic underpinnings of silent hypoxemia, it represents a significant threat for patients sent home with mild COVID-19 and told to seek care only when they become dyspneic or sicker. The fate of many with silent hypoxemia is one of eventual deterioration and death. It can be reasonably argued that many hours and days of severe unrecognized hypoxemia exact a multi-organ toll that if prevented sooner might improve outcomes because severe hypoxemia itself, in conjunction with systemic inflammation in COVID-19, contributes to further lung damage via exacerbation of local inflammatory injury.[152] Additionally, hypoxemia may contribute to hypercoagulability and thrombosis in the lung and other organs.[153] Hypoxia-inducible factor-1 is increased in response to hypoxemia and in an animal model of herpes virus infection was shown to increase viral replication.[154]

Treatment Strategies for COVID-19 Lung Injury

As already discussed, the numerous published large series of patients with COVID-19 lung injury and respiratory failure find little difference in many of the usual respiratory parameters of compliance, driving pressure, PEEP, V_A/Q mismatching, and shunt seen in ARDS. Accordingly, most physicians have employed low tidal volume ventilation with permissive hypercapnia, prone positioning, intermediate levels of PEEP, neuromuscular blockade, and conservative fluid therapy, in addition to pharmacologic therapies specific for COVID-19 as supportive data emerged. The concern raised for patients with the L type phenotype being harmed by smaller tidal volumes and higher PEEP has never been subjected to rigorous clinical trial, and the improving survival rates of patients with severe COVID-19 to that with standard ARDS support suggests that harms of greater PEEP with overdistension and injury of more compliant lung (VILI) and hemodynamic compromise have not been realized.

Nonetheless, some aspects of COVID-19 have stimulated considerations of therapies either tried and found unsuccessful in ARDS or novel possibilities based on the pathophysiology of the injured lung in COVID-19. These include inhaled nitric oxide to improve V_A/Q matching and reduce shunt by pulmonary vasodilation only in ventilated areas as well as possible direct viral killing and antiinflammatory effects. Other forms of inhaled vasodilators including prostacyclin and its analogs are being used. Enhancement of HPV with almitrine in affected areas in the few countries where this is available has had success in improving oxygenation. The recent success with dexamethasone and in ARDS[155] may be multifactorial beyond suppression of inflammation to include stimulation of fluid absorption, surfactant secretion, and reduction in HPV.[156] Studies are underway to test whether the prominent hypercoagulopathy of COVID-19 may require higher dosing of standard prophylactic anticoagulants. The critical role of ACE-2 and its role in setting the balance of the renin–angiotensin system offers the possibility of using Ang1-7 to reduce inflammation and reduce vasoconstriction.[157]

SUMMARY

The pathophysiology of ARDS and COVID-19 lung injury share many of the same aspects of reduced lung parenchymal compliance, vasculopathy, alveolar flooding, and gas exchange impairment arising from direct infectious causes and noninfectious injuries. Exuberant host defense inflammatory responses lead to endothelial and epithelial cell damage and loss of the normally tight alveolar–capillary barrier and its ability to maintain a dry alveolar space for efficient gas exchange. The heterogenous regional extent of injury creates stress factors on surrounding lung that can further propagate injury with mechanical ventilation and possibly with vigorous spontaneous breathing efforts. While there may be some differences between ARDS and COVID-19 lung injury in aspects of lung compliance, pulmonary vascular responses, and hypoxia sensing and responses that underlie the phenomenon of silent hypoxemia, there remains considerable dispute as to whether they really are distinguishing and important enough to warrant different strategies of care. The pathophysiologic features of both lung injuries have important ramifications for life-sustaining supportive care, and it is hoped that pharmacologic therapies may reduce mortality and enhance functional outcomes.

CLINICS CARE POINTS

- COVID-19-related lung injury should be managed using the same principles of lung-protective ventilation proven efficacious in classic ARDS.

- The degree of heterogeneity seen in parenchymal injury in both classic ARDS and COVID-19-related lung injury supports the use of early proning in severe or rapidly-deteriorating patients to limit ongoing stress concentration and propagation.
- Treatments that improve hypoxemia via ventilation–perfusion matching without addressing ongoing mechanical stresses on lung parenchyma, such as inhaled vasodilators, may temporize refractory hypoxemia but are unlikely to alter the course of disease in ARDS.
- Avoidance of significant patient-ventilator dyssynchrony during the progression of lung injury may limit further injury from P-SILI.
- Hypoxemia and pulmonary infiltrates in the absence of respiratory distress or impaired compliance appear to be common in early COVID-19-related lung injury and do not preclude the development of progressive respiratory failure seen in classic ARDS.

REFERENCES

1. Villar J, Blanco J, Kacmarek RM. Current incidence and outcome of the acute respiratory distress syndrome. Curr Opin Crit Care 2016;22(1):1–6.
2. Taylor PR, Martinez-Pomares L, Stacey M, et al. Macrophage receptors and immune recognition. Annu Rev Immunol 2005;23:901–44.
3. Wiener-Kronish J, Albertine K, Matthay M. Differential responses of the endothelial and epithelial barriers of the lung in sheep to Escherichia coli endotoxin. J Clin Invest 1991;88(3):864–75.
4. Matthay MA, Folkesson HG, Verkman A. Salt and water transport across alveolar and distal airway epithelia in the adult lung. Am J Physiol 1996;270(4): L487–503.
5. Ware LB, Matthay MA. Alveolar fluid clearance is impaired in the majority of patients with acute lung injury and the acute respiratory distress syndrome. Am J Respir Crit Care Med 2001;163(6):1376–83.
6. Pugin J, Verghese G, Widmer M-C, et al. The alveolar space is the site of intense inflammatory and profibrotic reactions in the early phase of acute respiratory distress syndrome. Crit Care Med 1999;27(2):304–12.
7. Dantzker DR, Brook CJ, Dehart P, et al. Ventilation-perfusion distributions in the adult respiratory distress syndrome. Am Rev Resp Dis 1979;120(5):1039–52.
8. Klocke RA. Velocity of CO2 exchange in blood. Annu Rev Physiol 1988;50(1): 625–37.
9. Robertson HT, Swenson ER. What do dead-space measurements tell us about the lung with acute respiratory distress syndrome? Respir Care 2004;49(9): 1006–7.
10. Wagner PD. Causes of a high physiological dead space in critically ill patients. Crit Care 2008;12(3):148.
11. Nuckton TJ, Alonso JA, Kallet RH, et al. Pulmonary dead-space fraction as a risk factor for death in the acute respiratory distress syndrome. N Eng J Med 2002; 346(17):1281–6.
12. Papolos AI, Schiller NB, Belzer A, et al. Pulmonary dead space monitoring: Identifying subjects with ARDS at risk of developing right ventricular dysfunction. Respir Care 2019;64(9):1101–8.
13. Radermacher P, Maggiore SM, Mercat A. Fifty years of research in ARDS. Gas exchange in acute respiratory distress syndrome. Am J Respir Crit Care Med 2017;196(8):964–84.

14. ARDS Network. Ventilation with lower tidal volumes as compared with traditional tidal volumes for acute lung injury and the acute respiratory distress syndrome. N Eng J Med 2000;342(18):1301–8.

15. Swenson ER, Robertson HT, Hlastala MP. Effects of inspired carbon dioxide on ventilation-perfusion matching in normoxia, hypoxia, and hyperoxia. Am J Respir Crit Care Med 1994;149(6):1563–9.

16. Briva A, Vadász I, Lecuona E, et al. High CO_2 levels impair alveolar epithelial function independently of pH. PLoS One 2007;2(11):e1238.

17. Kallet RH, Kallet RH. A comprehensive review of prone position in ARDS. Respir Care 2015;60(11):1660–87.

18. Radermacher P, Santak B, Wüst HJ, et al. Prostacyclin for the treatment of pulmonary hypertension in the adult respiratory distress syndrome: effects on pulmonary capillary pressure and ventilation—perfusion distributions. Anesthesiology 1990;72(2):238–44.

19. Kaushik SS, Freeman MS, Cleveland ZI, et al. Probing the regional distribution of pulmonary gas exchange through single-breath gas-and dissolved-phase 129Xe MR imaging. J Appl Physiol 2013;115(6):850–60.

20. Guérin C, Albert RK, Beitler J, et al. Prone position in ARDS patients: why, when, how and for whom. Intensive Care Med 2020;46(12):2385–96.

21. Glenny RW, Bernard S, Robertson HT, et al. Gravity is an important but secondary determinant of regional pulmonary blood flow in upright primates. J Appl Physiol 1999;86(2):623–32.

22. Swenson ER. Hypoxic pulmonary vasoconstriction. High Alt Med Biol 2013; 14(2):101–10.

23. Benzing A, Mols G, Brieschal T, et al. Hypoxic pulmonary vasoconstriction in nonventilated lung areas contributes to differences in hemodynamic and gas exchange responses to inhalation of nitric oxide. Anesthesiology 1997;86(6): 1254–61.

24. Payen D, Muret J, Beloucif S, et al. Inhaled nitric oxide, almitrine infusion, or their coadministration as a treatment of severe hypoxemic focal lung lesions. Anesthesiology 1998;89(5):1157–65.

25. Mead J, Takishima T, Leith D. Stress distribution in lungs: a model of pulmonary elasticity. J Appl Physiol 1970;28(5):596–608.

26. Gattinoni L, Pesenti A. The concept of "baby lung". Appl Physiol Intensive Care Med 2006;303–11.

27. Henderson WR, Chen L, Amato MB, et al. Fifty years of research in ARDS. Respiratory mechanics in acute respiratory distress syndrome. Am J Respir Crit Care Med 2017;196(7):822–33.

28. Heinze H, Eichler W. Measurements of functional residual capacity during intensive care treatment: the technical aspects and its possible clinical applications. Acta Anaesthesiol Scand 2009;53(9):1121–30.

29. Reske AW, Costa EL, Reske AP, et al. Bedside estimation of nonaerated lung tissue using blood gas analysis. Crit Care Med 2013;41(3):732–43.

30. Maunder RJ, Shuman WP, McHugh JW, et al. Preservation of normal lung regions in the adult respiratory distress syndrome: analysis by computed tomography. JAMA 1986;255(18):2463–5.

31. Pelosi P, D'Andrea L, Vitale G, et al. Vertical gradient of regional lung inflation in adult respiratory distress syndrome. Am J Respir Crit Care Med 1994; 149(1):8–13.

32. Behazin N, Jones SB, Cohen RI, et al. Respiratory restriction and elevated pleural and esophageal pressures in morbid obesity. J Appl Physiol 2010; 108(1):212–8.

33. Yoshida T, Amato MB, Grieco DL, et al. Esophageal manometry and regional transpulmonary pressure in lung injury. Am J Respir Crit Care Med 2018; 197(8):1018–26.

34. Cressoni M, Chiurazzi C, Gotti M, et al. Lung inhomogeneities and time course of ventilator-induced mechanical injuries. Anesthesiology 2015;123(3):618–27.

35. Gaver DP III, Nieman GF, Gatto LA, et al. The poor get POORer: a hypothesis for the pathogenesis of ventilator-induced lung injury. Am J Respir Crit Care Med 2020;202(8):1081–7.

36. Villar J, Zhang H, Slutsky AS. Lung repair and regeneration in ARDS: role of PE-CAM1 and Wnt signaling. Chest 2019;155(3):587–94.

37. Gattinoni L, Pesenti A, Avalli L, et al. Pressure-volume curve of total respiratory system in acute respiratory failure: computed tomographic scan study. Am Rev Resp Dis 1987;136(3):730–6.

38. Cressoni M, Chiumello D, Chiurazzi C, et al. Lung inhomogeneities, inflation and [18F] 2-fluoro-2-deoxy-D-glucose uptake rate in acute respiratory distress syndrome. Eur Respir J 2016;47(1):233–42.

39. Bellani G, Messa C, Guerra L, et al. Lungs of patients with acute respiratory distress syndrome show diffuse inflammation in normally aerated regions: a [18F]-fluoro-2-deoxy-D-glucose PET/CT study. Crit Care Med 2009;37(7): 2216–22.

40. Eissa N, Ranieri VM, Corbeil C, et al. Analysis of behavior of the respiratory system in ARDS patients: effects of flow, volume, and time. J Appl Physiol 1991; 70(6):2719–29.

41. Kondili E, Prinianakis G, Athanasakis H, et al. Lung emptying in patients with acute respiratory distress syndrome: effects of positive end-expiratory pressure. Eur Respir J 2002;19(5):811–9.

42. Huppert LA, Matthay MA, Ware LB. Pathogenesis of acute respiratory distress syndrome. Semin Respir Crit Care Med 2019;40(1):31–9.

43. Fang X, Fukuda N, Barbry P, et al. Novel role for CFTR in fluid absorption from the distal airspaces of the lung. J Gen Physiol 2002;119(2):199–208.

44. Verkman A, Mitra AK. Structure and function of aquaporin water channels. Am J Physiol 2000;278(1):F13–28.

45. Sakuma T, Gu X, Wang Z, et al. Stimulation of alveolar epithelial fluid clearance in human lungs by exogenous epinephrine. Crit Care Med 2006;34(3):676.

46. Takahashi N, Kawai Y, Ohhashi T. Effects of vasoconstrictive and vasodilative agents on lymphatic smooth muscles in isolated canine thoracic ducts. J Pharmacol Exp Ther 1990;254(1):165–70.

47. Smith FG, Perkins GD, Gates S, et al. Effect of intravenous β-2 agonist treatment on clinical outcomes in acute respiratory distress syndrome (Balti-2): a multicentre, randomised controlled trial. Lancet 2012;379(9812):229–35.

48. National Heart, Lung, and Blood Institute Acute Respiratory Distress Syndrome (ARDS) Clinical Trials Network, Matthay MA, Brower RG, et al. Randomized, placebo-controlled clinical trial of an aerosolized β2-agonist for treatment of acute lung injury. Am J Respir Crit Care Med 2011;184(5):561–8.

49. Albert RK, Lakshminarayan S, Hildebrandt J, et al. Increased surface tension favors pulmonary edema formation in anesthetized dogs' lungs. The J Clin Invest 1979;63(5):1015–8.

50. Nieman GF, Gatto LA, Habashi NM. Impact of mechanical ventilation on the pathophysiology of progressive acute lung injury. J Appl Physiol 2015; 119(11):1245–61.
51. Slutsky AS, Ranieri VM. Ventilator-induced lung injury. N Eng J Med 2013; 369(22):2126–36.
52. Curley GF, Laffey JG, Zhang H, et al. Biotrauma and ventilator-induced lung injury: clinical implications. Chest 2016;150(5):1109–17.
53. Gattinoni L, Tonetti T, Cressoni M, et al. Ventilator-related causes of lung injury: the mechanical power. Intensive Care Med 2016;42(10):1567–75.
54. Webb HH, Tierney DF. Experimental pulmonary edema due to intermittent positive pressure ventilation with high inflation pressures. Protection by positive end-expiratory pressure. Am Rev Resp Dis 1974;110(5):556–65.
55. Chiumello D, Cressoni M, Chierichetti M, et al. Nitrogen washout/washin, helium dilution and computed tomography in the assessment of end expiratory lung volume. Crit Care 2008;12(6):R150.
56. Grasso S, Terragni P, Birocco A, et al. ECMO criteria for influenza A (H1N1)-associated ARDS: role of transpulmonary pressure. Intensive Care Med 2012; 38(3):395–403.
57. Terragni PP, Rosboch G, Tealdi A, et al. Tidal hyperinflation during low tidal volume ventilation in acute respiratory distress syndrome. Am J Respir Crit Care Med 2007;175(2):160–6.
58. Bachmann MC, Morais C, Bugedo G, et al. Electrical impedance tomography in acute respiratory distress syndrome. Crit Care 2018;22(1):1–11.
59. Muscedere J, Mullen J, Gan K, et al. Tidal ventilation at low airway pressures can augment lung injury. Am J Respir Crit Care Med 1994;149(5):1327–34.
60. Rouby J, Lherm T, De Lassale EM, et al. Histologic aspects of pulmonary barotrauma in critically ill patients with acute respiratory failure. Intensive Care Med 1993;19(7):383–9.
61. Chen L, Del Sorbo L, Grieco DL, et al. Airway closure in acute respiratory distress syndrome: an underestimated and misinterpreted phenomenon. Am J Respir Crit Care Med 2018;197(1):132–6.
62. Dreyfuss D, Saumon G. Ventilator-induced lung injury: lessons from experimental studies. Am J Respir Crit Care Med 1998;157(1):294–323.
63. Mercat A, Richard J-CM, Vielle B, et al. Positive end-expiratory pressure setting in adults with acute lung injury and acute respiratory distress syndrome: a randomized controlled trial. JAMA 2008;299(6):646–55.
64. Meade MO, Cook DJ, Guyatt GH, et al. Ventilation strategy using low tidal volumes, recruitment maneuvers, and high positive end-expiratory pressure for acute lung injury and acute respiratory distress syndrome: a randomized controlled trial. JAMA 2008;299(6):637–45.
65. Kacmarek RM, Villar J, Sulemanji D, et al. Open lung approach for the acute respiratory distress syndrome: a pilot, randomized controlled trial. Crit Care Med 2016;44(1):32–42.
66. Lu J, Wang X, Chen M, et al. An open lung strategy in the management of acute respiratory distress syndrome: a systematic review and meta-analysis. Shock 2017;48(1):43–53.
67. Talmor D, Sarge T, Malhotra A, et al. Mechanical ventilation guided by esophageal pressure in acute lung injury. N Eng J Med 2008;359(20):2095–104.
68. Chen L, Chen G-Q, Shore K, et al. Implementing a bedside assessment of respiratory mechanics in patients with acute respiratory distress syndrome. Crit Care 2017;21(1):84.

69. Yoshida T, Uchiyama A, Matsuura N, et al. Spontaneous breathing during lung-protective ventilation in an experimental acute lung injury model: high transpulmonary pressure associated with strong spontaneous breathing effort may worsen lung injury. Crit Care Med 2012;40(5):1578–85.
70. Mascheroni D, Kolobow T, Fumagalli R, et al. Acute respiratory failure following pharmacologically induced hyperventilation: an experimental animal study. Intensive Care Med 1988;15(1):8–14.
71. Kallet RH, Alonso JA, Luce JM, et al. Exacerbation of acute pulmonary edema during assisted mechanical ventilation using a low-tidal volume, lung-protective ventilator strategy. Chest 1999;116(6):1826–32.
72. Kiss T, Bluth T, Braune A, et al. Effects of positive end-expiratory pressure and spontaneous breathing activity on regional lung inflammation in experimental acute respiratory distress syndrome. Crit Care Med 2019;47(4):e358–65.
73. Yoshida T, Fujino Y, Amato MB, et al. Fifty years of research in ARDS. Spontaneous breathing during mechanical ventilation. Risks, mechanisms, and management. Am J Respir Crit Care Med 2017;195(8):985–92.
74. National Heart L, Network BIPCT. Early neuromuscular blockade in the acute respiratory distress syndrome. N Engl J Med 2019;380(21):1997–2008.
75. Putensen C, Zech S, Wrigge H, et al. Long-term effects of spontaneous breathing during ventilatory support in patients with acute lung injury. Am J Respir Crit Care Med 2001;164(1):43–9.
76. Dorward DA, Russell CD, Um IH, et al. Tissue-specific immunopathology in fatal COVID-19. Am J Respir Crit Care Med 2020;203(2):192–201.
77. Carsana L, Sonzogni A, Nasr A, et al. Pulmonary post-mortem findings in a series of COVID-19 cases from northern Italy: a two-centre descriptive study. Lancet Infect Dis 2020;20(10):1135–40.
78. Tomashefski J Jr, Davies P, Boggis C, et al. The pulmonary vascular lesions of the adult respiratory distress syndrome. Am J Pathol 1983;112(1):112.
79. Ackermann M, Verleden SE, Kuehnel M, et al. Pulmonary vascular endothelialitis, thrombosis, and angiogenesis in Covid-19. N Eng J Med 2020;383(2):120–8.
80. Hariri LP, North CM, Shih AR, et al. Lung histopathology in coronavirus disease 2019 as compared with severe acute respiratory sydrome and H1N1 influenza: a systematic review. Chest 2021;159(1):73–84.
81. Tian S, Hu W, Niu L, et al. Pulmonary pathology of early phase 2019 novel coronavirus (COVID-19) pneumonia in two patients with lung cancer. J Thorac Oncol 2020;15(5):700–4.
82. Pogatchnik BP, Swenson KE, Sharifi H, et al. Radiology-pathology correlation in recovered COVID-19, demonstrating organizing pneumonia. Am J Respir Crit Care Med 2020;202(4):598–9.
83. Pernazza A, Mancini M, Rullo E, et al. Early histologic findings of pulmonary SARS-CoV-2 infection detected in a surgical specimen. Virchows Archiv 2020; 477:743–8.
84. Liao M, Liu Y, Yuan J, et al. Single-cell landscape of bronchoalveolar immune cells in patients with COVID-19. Nat Med 2020;26:842–4.
85. Matthay MA, Zemans RL, Zimmerman GA, et al. Acute respiratory distress syndrome. Nat Rev Dis Primers 2019;5(1):1–22.
86. Chiumello D, Busana M, Coppola S, et al. Physiological and quantitative CT-scan characterization of COVID-19 and typical ARDS: a matched cohort study. Intensive Care Med 2020;46(12):2187–96.
87. Marini JJ, Gattinoni L. Management of COVID-19 respiratory distress. JAMA 2020;323(22):2329–30.

88. Goligher EC, Ranieri VM, Slutsky AS. Is severe COVID-19 pneumonia a typical or atypical form of ARDS? And does it matter? Intensive Care Med 2021; 47:83–5.

89. Ziehr DR, Alladina J, Petri CR, et al. Respiratory pathophysiology of mechanically ventilated patients with COVID-19: a cohort study. Am J Respir Crit Care Med 2020;201(12):1560–4.

90. Bhatraju PK, Ghassemieh BJ, Nichols M, et al. Covid-19 in critically ill patients in the Seattle region—case series. N Eng J Med 2020;382(21):2012–22.

91. Pan C, Chen L, Lu C, et al. Lung recruitability in COVID-19–associated acute respiratory distress syndrome: a single-center observational study. Am J Respir Crit Care Med 2020;201(10):1294–7.

92. Botta M, Tsonas AM, Pillay J, et al. Ventilation management and clinical outcomes in invasively ventilated patients with COVID-19 (PRoVENT-COVID): a national, multicentre, observational cohort study. Lancet Respir Med 2020. https:// doi.org/10.1016/S2213-2600(20)30459-8. in press.

93. Grieco DL, Bongiovanni F, Chen L, et al. Respiratory physiology of COVID-19-induced respiratory failure compared to ARDS of other etiologies. Crit Care 2020;24(1):1–11.

94. Guérin C, Reignier J, Richard JC, et al. Prone positioning in severe acute respiratory distress syndrome. N Eng J Med 2013;368(23):2159–68.

95. Panwar R, Madotto F, Laffey JG, et al. Compliance phenotypes in early ARDS before the COVID-19 pandemic. Am J Respir Crit Care Med 2020;202(9): 1244–52.

96. Cobb NL, Sathe NA, Duan KI, et al. Comparison of clinical features and outcomes in critically ill patients hospitalized with COVID-19 versus influenza. Ann Am Thorac Soc 2020. https://doi.org/10.1513/AnnalsATS.202007-805OC. in press.

97. Schalekamp S, Bleeker-Rovers CP, Beenen LFM, et al. Chest CT in the emergency department for diagnosis of COVID-19 pneumonia: Dutch experience. Radiology 2020;203465.

98. Rousan LA, Elobeid E, Karrar M, et al. Chest x-ray findings and temporal lung changes in patients with COVID-19 pneumonia. BMC Pulm Med 2020; 20(1):245.

99. Patel BV, Arachchillage DJ, Ridge CA, et al. Pulmonary angiopathy in severe COVID-19: physiologic, imaging and hematologic observations. Am J Respir Crit Care Med 2020;202(5):690–9.

100. Jobe AH, Ikegami M. Biology of surfactant. Clin Perinatol 2001;28(3):655–69, vii-viii.

101. Sahu SC, Tanswell AK, Lynn WS. Isolation and characterization of glycosaminoglycans secreted by human foetal lung type II pneumocytes in culture. J Cell Sci 1980;42:183–8.

102. Ochs M, Hegermann J, Lopez-Rodriguez E, et al. On top of the alveolar epithelium: surfactant and the glycocalyx. Int J Mol Sci 2020;21(9):3075.

103. Hellman U, Karlsson MG, Engström-Laurent A, et al. Presence of hyaluronan in lung alveoli in severe Covid-19: an opening for new treatment options? J Biol Chem 2020;295(45):15418–22.

104. Lu KW, Taeusch HW, Clements JA. Hyaluronan with dextran added to therapeutic lung surfactants improves effectiveness in vitro and in vivo. Exp Lung Res 2013;39(4–5):191–200.

105. Swenson ER. The unappreciated role of carbon dioxide in ventilation/perfusion matching. Anesthesiology 2019;131(2):226–8.

106. Bos L, Paulus F, Vlaar A, et al. Subphenotyping ARDS in COVID-19 patients: consequences for ventilator management. Ann Am Thorac Soc 2020;17(9): 1161–3.

107. Haudebourg A-F, Perier F, Tuffet S, et al. Respiratory mechanics of COVID-19 vs. Non-COVID-19 associated acute respiratory distress syndrome. Am J Respir Crit Care Med 2020;202(2):287–90.

108. Beloncle FM, Pavlovsky B, Desprez C, et al. Recruitability and effect of PEEP in SARS-Cov-2-associated acute respiratory distress syndrome. Ann Intensive Care 2020;10:1–9.

109. Sheng W-H, Chiang B-L, Chang S-C, et al. Clinical manifestations and inflammatory cytokine responses in patients with severe acute respiratory syndrome. J Formos Med Assoc 2005;104(10):715–23.

110. Lang M, Som A, Carey D, et al. Pulmonary vascular manifestations of COVID-19 pneumonia. Radiol Cardiothorac Imaging 2020;2(3):e200–77.

111. Evrard B, Goudelin M, Montmagnon N, et al. Cardiovascular phenotypes in ventilated patients with COVID-19 acute respiratory distress syndrome. Crit Care 2020;24(1):1–5.

112. Pagnesi M, Baldetti L, Beneduce A, et al. Pulmonary hypertension and right ventricular involvement in hospitalised patients with COVID-19. Heart 2020;106(17): 1324–31.

113. Squara P, Dhainaut J-F, Artigas A, et al. Hemodynamic profile in severe ARDS: results of the European Collaborative ARDS Study. Intensive Care Med 1998; 24(10):1018–28.

114. Bull T, Clark B, McFann K, et al. National Institutes of Health/National Heart, Lung, and Blood Institute ARDS Network. Pulmonary vascular dysfunction is associated with poor outcomes in patients with acute lung injury. Am J Respir Crit Care Med 2010;182(9):1123–8.

115. Caravita S, Baratto C, Di Marco F, et al. Haemodynamic characteristics of COVID-19 patients with acute respiratory distress syndrome requiring mechanical ventilation. An invasive assessment using right heart catheterization. Eur J Heart Fail 2020. https://doi.org/10.1002/ejhf.2058. in press.

116. Potus F, Mai V, Lebret M, et al. Novel insights on the pulmonary vascular consequences of COVID-19. Am J Physiol 2020;319(2):L277–88.

117. Klok F, Kruip M, Van der Meer N, et al. Incidence of thrombotic complications in critically ill ICU patients with COVID-19. Thromb Res 2020;191:145–7.

118. Vaduganathan M, Vardeny O, Michel T, et al. Renin–angiotensin–aldosterone system inhibitors in patients with Covid-19. N Eng J Med 2020;382(17):1653–9.

119. de Maat S, de Mast Q, Danser AHJ, et al. Impaired breakdown of bradykinin and its metabolites as a possible cause for pulmonary edema in COVID-19 infection. Semin Thromb Hemost 2020;46(7):835–7.

120. Archer SL, Sharp WW, Weir EK. Differentiating COVID-19 pneumonia from acute respiratory distress syndrome (ARDS) and high altitude pulmonary edema (HAPE): therapeutic implications. Circulation 2020;142:101–4.

121. Menter T, Haslbauer J, Nienhold R, et al. Post-mortem examination of COVID19 patients reveals diffuse alveolar damage with severe capillary congestion and variegated findings of lungs and other organs suggesting vascular dysfunction. Histopathology 2020. https://doi.org/10.1111/his.14134.

122. Ranucci M, Ballotta A, Di Dedda U, et al. The procoagulant pattern of patients with COVID-19 acute respiratory distress syndrome. J Thromb Haemost 2020; 18(7):1747–51.

123. Grimmer B, Kuebler WM. The endothelium in hypoxic pulmonary vasoconstriction. J Appl Physiol 2017;123(6):1635–46.
124. Bendjelid K, Giraud R, Von Düring S. Treating hypoxemic COVID-19 "ARDS" patients with almitrine: the earlier the better? Anaesth Crit Care Pain Med 2020; 39(4):451–2.
125. Parikh R, Wilson C, Weinberg J, et al. Inhaled nitric oxide treatment in spontaneously breathing COVID-19 patients. Ther Adv Respir Dis 2020. https://doi.org/ 10.1177/1753466620933510.
126. Mélot C, Dechamps P, Hallemans R, et al. Enhancement of hypoxic pulmonary vasoconstriction by low dose almitrine bismesylate in normal humans. Am Rev Resp Dis 1989;139(1):111–9.
127. Watt M, Peacock A, Newell J, et al. The effect of amlodipine on respiratory and pulmonary vascular responses to hypoxia in mountaineers. Eur Respir J 2000; 15(3):459–63.
128. Pavelescu A, Naeije R. Effects of epoprostenol and sildenafil on right ventricular function in hypoxic volunteers: a tissue Doppler imaging study. Eur J Appl Physiol 2012;112(4):1285–94.
129. Kennedy M, Helfand BK, Gou RY, et al. Delirium in older patients with COVID-19 presenting to the emergency department. JAMA Netw Open 2020;3(11). e2029540-e.
130. Chen G, Wu D, Guo W, et al. Clinical and immunological features of severe and moderate coronavirus disease 2019. J Clin Invest 2020;130(5).
131. Yang X, Yu Y, Xu J, et al. Clinical course and outcomes of critically ill patients with SARS-CoV-2 pneumonia in Wuhan, China: a single-centered, retrospective, observational study. Lancet Respir Med 2020;8(5):475–81.
132. Guan W-j, Liang W-h, Zhao Y, et al. Comorbidity and its impact on 1590 patients with Covid-19 in China: a Nationwide analysis. Eur Respir J 2020;55(5).
133. Tobin MJ, Laghi F, Jubran A. Why COVID-19 silent hypoxemia is baffling to physicians. Am J Respir Crit Care Med 2020;202(3):356–60.
134. Xiao Z, Li Y, Chen R, et al. A retrospective study of 78 patients with severe acute respiratory syndrome. Chin Med J 2003;116(6):805–10.
135. Chen C-Y, Lee C-H, Liu C-Y, et al. Clinical features and outcomes of severe acute respiratory syndrome and predictive factors for acute respiratory distress syndrome. J Chin Med Assoc 2005;68(1):4–10.
136. Siau C, Law J, Tee A, et al. Severe refractory hypoxaemia in H1N1 (2009) intensive care patients: initial experience in an Asian regional hospital. Singapore Med J 2010;51(6):490–5.
137. Jouffroy R, Jost D, Prunet B. Prehospital pulse oximetry: a red flag for early detection of silent hypoxemia in COVID-19 patients. Crit Care 2020;24(1):1–2.
138. Reynolds AS, Lee AG, Renz J, et al. Pulmonary vascular dilatation detected by automated transcranial Doppler in COVID-19 pneumonia. Am J Respir Crit Care Med 2020;202(7):1037–9.
139. Swenson ER, Hopkins SR, Stickland MK. Positive bubble study in severe COVID-19: bubbles may be unrelated to gas exchange impairment. Am J Respir Crit Care Med 2020. https://doi.org/10.1164/rccm.202010-3800LE. in press.
140. Herrmann J, Mori V, Bates JHT, et al. Modeling lung perfusion abnormalities to explain early COVID-19 hypoxemia. Nat Commun 2020;11(1):4883.
141. Das A, Saffaran S, Chikhani M, et al. In Silico modeling of coronavirus disease 2019 acute respiratory distress syndrome: pathophysiologic insights and potential management implications. Crit Care Explor 2020;2(9):e0202.

142. Diehl JL, Peron N, Chocron R, et al. Respiratory mechanics and gas exchanges in the early course of COVID-19 ARDS: a hypothesis-generating study. Ann Intensive Care 2020;10(1):95.

143. Fung ML. The role of local renin-angiotensin system in arterial chemoreceptors in sleep-breathing disorders. Front Physiol 2014;5:336.

144. Kabbani N, Olds JL. Does COVID19 infect the brain? If so, smokers might be at a higher risk. Mol Pharmacol 2020;97(5):351–3.

145. Li YC, Bai WZ, Hashikawa T. The neuroinvasive potential of SARS-CoV2 may play a role in the respiratory failure of COVID-19 patients. J Med Virol 2020; 92(6):552–5.

146. Shi Z, de Vries HJ, Vlaar APJ, et al. Diaphragm pathology in critically ill patients with COVID-19 and postmortem findings from 3 medical centers. JAMA Intern Med 2021;181(1):122–4.

147. Parshall M, Schwartzstein R, Adams L, et al. American Thoracic Society Committee on Dyspnea. An official American Thoracic Society statement: update on the mechanisms, assessment, and management of dyspnea. Am J Respir Crit Care Med 2012;185(4):435–52.

148. Simonson T, Baker T, Banzett R, et al. COVID-19 respiratory distress: not so much 'happy hypoxia' as 'silent hypoxemia'. J Physiol 2020. https://doi.org/10.1113/JP280769. in press.

149. Swenson ER, Duncan TB, Goldberg SV, et al. Diuretic effect of acute hypoxia in humans: relationship to hypoxic ventilatory responsiveness and renal hormones. J Appl Physiol 1995;78(2):377–83.

150. McGurk S, Blanksby B, Anderson M. The relationship of hypercapnic ventilatory responses to age, gender and athleticism. Sports Med 1995;19(3):173–83.

151. Moosavi SH, Golestanian E, Binks AP, et al. Hypoxic and hypercapnic drives to breathe generate equivalent levels of air hunger in humans. J Appl Physiol 2003; 94(1):141–54.

152. Eltzschig HK, Carmeliet P. Hypoxia and inflammation. N Eng J Med 2011;364(7):656–65.

153. Su H, Yang M, Wan C, et al. Renal histopathological analysis of 26 postmortem findings of patients with COVID-19 in China. Kidney Int 2020;98(1):219–27.

154. López-Rodríguez DM, Kirillov V, Krug LT, et al. A role of hypoxia-inducible factor 1 alpha in Mouse Gammaherpesvirus 68 (MHV68) lytic replication and reactivation from latency. PLoS Pathog 2019;15(12):e1008192.

155. Villar J, Ferrando C, Martínez D, et al. Dexamethasone treatment for the acute respiratory distress syndrome: a multicentre, randomised controlled trial. Lancet Respir Med 2020;8(3):267–76.

156. Bärtsch P, Swenson ER. Clinical practice: acute high-altitude illnesses. N Engl J Med 2013;368(24):2294–302.

157. Jia H, Neptune E, Cui H. Targeting ACE2 for COVID-19 therapy: opportunities and challenges. Am J Respir Cell Mol Biol 2020. https://doi.org/10.1165/rcmb.2020-0322PS. in press.

COVID-19–Associated Acute Respiratory Distress Syndrome: Lessons from Tissues and Cells

Elizabeth A. Middleton, MD, Guy A. Zimmerman, MD*

KEYWORDS

- COVID-19 • SARS-CoV-2 • ARDS • Acute lung injury • Histopathology
- Vasculopathy

KEY POINTS

- Specific histologic patterns with pathogenetic implications are emerging from clinical and experimental studies of coronavirus disease 2019 (COVID-19) acute lung injury.
- Physiologic variables and clinical outcomes in COVID-19–associated acute respiratory distress syndrome linked to histopathologic patterns may be identified.
- These studies may provide a rationale for targeted interventions based on specific cellular events and temporal phases of COVID-19 acute lung injury.

INTRODUCTION

Patients with coronavirus disease 2019 (COVID-19) induced by severe acute respiratory syndrome coronavirus 2 (SARS-CoV-2) frequently develop acute, precipitous respiratory failure with features of the acute respiratory distress syndrome (ARDS).[1] Understanding the biology, mechanisms of acute lung injury, and pathophysiology of COVID-19–associated ARDS is essential for its rational management,[1,2] but these elements are largely uncharacterized. ARDS is a common, complex, and lethal syndrome that is caused by a spectrum of infectious and noninfectious insults.[3,4] COVID-19–associated ARDS may be, in large part, similar to ARDS of other causes.[5,6] Alternatively, it may have novel features and it is possible, and perhaps likely, that COVID-19–associated ARDS represents a unique phenotype.[7,8] It is also possible that there is biological and physiologic heterogeneity and that there are subphenotypes of COVID-19–associated ARDS, as there are in classic ARDS (a term that is used here to indicate ARDS unrelated to COVID-19).[2,4,7]

Division of Pulmonary and Critical Care Medicine, Department of Internal Medicine, Program in Molecular Medicine, University of Utah School of Medicine, Eccles Institute of Human Genetics, 15 North 2030 East, Room #4220, Salt Lake City, UT 84112, USA
* Corresponding author.
E-mail address: guy.zimmerman@u2m2.utah.edu

Crit Care Clin 37 (2021) 777–793
https://doi.org/10.1016/j.ccc.2021.05.004
0749-0704/21/© 2021 Elsevier Inc. All rights reserved.

Histopathology and clinical cell biology are fundamental to understanding human diseases and for elucidation of their mechanisms and physiologic consequences, and may be critical for precise characterization of new or emerging syndromes. For clinicians, description of the anatomy of the disorder provides correlates for interpretation of imaging and other diagnostic measures, understanding pathophysiology, and formulating therapeutic strategies; for translational investigators, human histopathology is a basis for devising reduced experimental models and for evaluating outcomes in surrogate in vivo experiments; for medical scientists new to a field, histopathology can provide an unbiased sense of complexity of a disease and insights regarding the cellular and molecular issues that underpin it. Linking pathologic patterns to clinical variables can be particularly informative.[9] This article profiles available information on the pathology of SARS-CoV-2 pneumonia, focusing on histology and cellular characterization and lessons and questions that these studies provide regarding COVID-19–associated ARDS.

OVERVIEW OF THE PATHOLOGY OF SEVERE ACUTE RESPIRATORY SYNDROME CORONAVIRUS-2 PNEUMONIA

Current synthesis of the pathology of SARS-CoV-2 pneumonia is based on reports of autopsies, more limited postmortem sampling, surgically excised lung tissue, and cytologic analysis. Multiple studies of documented SARS-CoV-2 infection from Asia, Europe, and the United States have appeared. Early cases and case series are summarized in reviews.[10–13] This article also discusses findings reported in selected early and more recent primary reports.

Macroscopic features of the lung in COVID-19 are nonspecific and include edema, hemorrhage, and thrombosis.[12] Lung weights are substantially increased. In an international report of 68 autopsies, the combined lung weight was greater than 1300 g (normal average 840 g) in 92% of cases.[14] In a smaller series, the mean weight of lungs from subjects with COVID-19 (1681 $\pm$ 49 g) was greater than that of uninfected control lungs (1045 $\pm$ 91 g) but lower than that of patients dying of influenza-associated ARDS (2404 $\pm$ 560 g).[15] Macroscopic involvement is frequently patchy but there can be extensive consolidation, corresponding with a spectrum of patterns on diagnostic imaging.[11,12,16]

In early case reports and series, the most commonly reported histologic finding, by far, was diffuse alveolar damage (DAD),[10–13] including cellular features of the acute, exudative, and proliferative, or organizing, phases (**Box 1, Fig. 1**). More recent autopsy series, some multicenter involving large numbers of patients, extend early findings and frequently also emphasize pulmonary vascular involvement and apparent temporal evolution of acute lung injury.[14,15,22–32] Tracheobronchial injury and inflammation, independent of intubation and mechanical ventilation, have been documented in addition to alveolar involvement.[14,30] The conclusion is that SARS-CoV-2 pneumonia is a complex respiratory disorder involving the tracheobronchial, alveolar, and vascular compartments.[11,12,14]

Evidence for viral infection of tracheobronchial and alveolar epithelial cells (AECs) by ultrastructure, immunohistochemistry, or in situ hybridization has been a consistent finding in COVID-19; detection of viral particles or markers in endothelial and immune cells has been reported in some, but not all, studies.[11–15,22,23,28,30,32–35] Angiotensin-converting enzyme 2 (ACE2), a requisite component of the molecular system by which SARS-CoV-2 enters host cells, was detected on alveolar epithelial and endothelial cells.[15] Persistent viral infection may drive ongoing focal alveolar injury and clinical manifestations[14,23] but is absent in the organizing phase of DAD in some patients.[32]

Box 1
Diffuse alveolar damage is the characteristic histologic pattern of classic acute respiratory distress syndrome

DAD was originally characterized as a nonspecific response to acute or subacute alveolar injury incited by a variety of insults, alone or in combination. Specific histologic features identifying early exudative and later proliferative phases, often progressing to extensive interstitial fibrosis, were described[17] (see **Fig. 1**). Ultrastructural analysis confirmed and extended observations by light microscopy.[18,19] Hyaline membranes, alveolar epithelial cell (AEC) type I (pneumocyte) injury and loss, interstitial and alveolar edema, and interstitial and alveolar inflammatory infiltrates are key histologic features of the acute exudative phase. The inflammatory infiltrate was originally described to be mononuclear,[17] but neutrophils are prominent in classic DAD of many causes.[4,20] Fibrin thrombi are common in alveolar capillaries and pulmonary arterioles. Platelets are frequently detected in microvascular thrombi, especially when specific markers are used.[17–19,21] Intra-alveolar fibrin, hemorrhage, and cellular debris are variably seen. Ultrastructural studies reveal denuded alveolar epithelial basement membrane and cellular details of epithelial and endothelial injury.[18,19] The organizing, proliferative phase is indicated by AEC II (type II pneumocyte) hyperplasia and by interstitial fibrosis that can be severe.[17–19] At present, hyaline membranes are considered the required feature for pathologic diagnosis of DAD in classic ARDS, and the other elements of the histologic pattern are used to establish its evolutionary stage.[21]

Histologic patterns that vary from the dominant DAD phenotype have been reported,[10,11,14,22,25,33–35] including acute fibrinous and organizing pneumonia.[10,36] They may be sentinel subsets that indicate biological heterogeneity, potentially underlying clinical heterogeneity.[2]

In addition to the respiratory system, multiple studies have examined other organs and tissues. Although this article does not review extrapulmonary features of SARS-CoV-2 infection, they indicate, along with clinical manifestations and circulating biomarkers, that SARS-CoV-2 infection is frequently a systemic syndrome.[1,10–13,16]

There are several caveats regarding current reports of the pathology of COVID-19. The lung tissue examined to date has largely been from elderly patients, frequently with a variety of comorbidities, consistent with the well-known susceptibility to severe SARS-CoV-2 infection and increased mortality in this population. Common features of the lung pathology could therefore partly be caused by responses of the aged, multiply compromised lung. Nevertheless, observations in nonhuman primates indicate that DAD occurs across the age spectrum and in otherwise healthy lungs in response to SARS-CoV-2 infection (discussed later). A second issue is that most of the lung tissue from patients with COVID-19 examined so far is from patients that expired well after onset of the clinical illness, often after days or weeks of medical intervention and intensive care unit support. Thus, the early patterns of lung involvement in SARS-CoV-2 infection in humans are not known. Tissue from patients undergoing lung resection while in the undiagnosed, apparently early, phase of COVID-19 infection provides useful but limited information.[37–39] Experimental animal models[40] will likely be essential in addressing this unknown feature. Experimental animal studies will also likely be the only avenue immediately available for determining patterns of histologic and cellular evolution in SARS-CoV-2–induced acute lung injury, although molecular imaging or histology-specific biomarkers[21,31] may be informative in humans in the future. In addition, virtually no patients in reports of COVID-19 lung histopathology have been ascertained to have ARDS according to the Berlin definition[3,4,9] or other consensus criteria, although relevant clinical and physiologic data are available for some. Therefore, it is currently necessary to extrapolate existing histopathologic findings to COVID-19–associated ARDS.

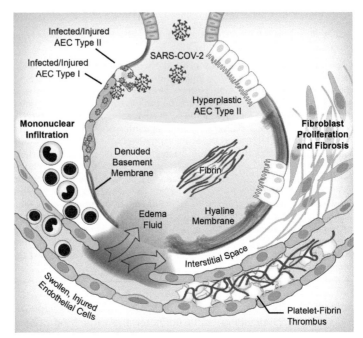

Fig. 1. DAD is the histologic signature of COVID-19 acute lung injury. The pattern and cardinal features of DAD (see **Box 1**) have been consistently observed in the lungs of patients with documented SARS-CoV-2 infection, including in autopsies of critically ill subjects described to have COVID-19–associated ARDS. Frequently hyaline membranes and alveolar epithelial cell (AEC) type II hyperplasia occur in the same foci of affected lung, indicating temporal overlap and potentially evolution of acute lung injury. Other histologic features besides the cardinal criteria of DAD, including squamous metaplasia, AEC atypia, and intense scarring with obliteration of alveolar spaces, have been variably reported. Variations in the cellular makeup of the inflammatory infiltrate, including the specific pattern of acute neutrophilic bronchopneumonia together with DAD and additional variant histologic patterns, have also been reported. See text for details. DAD was noted to be caused by viral pneumonias in the classic description (Katzenstein and colleagues[17]) and is the characteristic histologic pattern in the lungs in SARS, Middle East respiratory syndrome, and pandemic influenza.

DIFFUSE ALVEOLAR DAMAGE: THE SIGNATURE BUT NONSPECIFIC HISTOLOGIC PATTERN OF CLASSIC ACUTE RESPIRATORY DISTRESS SYNDROME AND CORONAVIRUS DISEASE 2019 LUNG INJURY

DAD is a specific constellation of histologic features that defines a characteristic but nonspecific pattern of response to acute or subacute lung injury[17] (see **Box 1**, **Fig. 1**). It is the signature pathologic lesion and is central in current concepts of ARDS, although not all patients with classic ARDS have DAD on autopsy or diagnostic lung biopsy examination and the physiologic syndrome of ARDS can be associated with other histologic patterns.[3,4,9,21] The presence of hyaline membranes is a requisite criterion for DAD diagnosis, and other histologic features are used to determine evolutionary stages of the response.[21]

As noted previously, DAD is a consistent, almost ubiquitous, finding when lungs from decedents with COVID-19 are examined.[10–15,22–32,35] DAD is also a key component of the acute lung injury induced by coronaviruses in Middle East respiratory syndrome (MERS-CoV) and severe acute respiratory syndrome (SARS-CoV) infection.[11,12,24]

DAD in lungs of patients infected with SARS-CoV-2 could not be differentiated from DAD in acute lung injury induced by other insults when early case reports and case series were reviewed.[12] A focused study concluded that DAD in COVID-19 infection is morphologically indistinguishable from DAD of other causes.[29] This determination was based on consensus blinded analysis of histopathology of lungs from hospitalized patients with SARS-CoV-2 infection, patients infected with SARS-CoV-2 who died in the community, and historical hospitalized and outpatient controls previously determined to have DAD induced by sepsis, lung infection, or other conditions, including hospitalized controls assessed to have clinical ARDS. The findings were interpreted as indicating that DAD (without distinctive histologic features that differentiate it from DAD of other causes) is the primary manifestation of COVID-19–associated lung injury in patients who die in the hospital or in the community. A corollary was that mechanical ventilation and high inspired oxygen concentration are not primary drivers of the histologic changes.[29] Both supportive interventions induce the DAD phenotype.[3,17]

Correlation of the histologic pattern of DAD with physiologic data and clinical variables in classic ARDS has been informative.[9,21,41,42] Evolution of histologic features of DAD in patients with classic ARDS suggests a time-dependent set of biological events that alter physiologic variables and might be modified by time-sensitive interventions.[41] Cellular features indicating evolution of acute lung injury seem to also correlate with duration of disease in COVID-19.[14,22,28,32] A recent histologic and transcriptomic analysis extending findings in one of the early major COVID-19 autopsy series suggests distinct phases of immune disorder, varying in interferon-stimulated genes, cytokines, viral load, and cellular injury, and natural progression culminating in DAD.[31] If verified, this may provide a basis for timing of administration of targeted therapeutics in clinical trials and, ultimately, in practice. Evaluation of the impact of DAD on physiologic variables and response to supportive measures in COVID-19–associated ARDS[5,6] requires future study.

Examination of the complex relationship between DAD and classic ARDS indicates that the presence of DAD influences clinical outcomes.[21] ARDS with DAD detected by open lung biopsy is associated with higher mortality than is ARDS in the absence of DAD.[43] This finding may also be true of COVID-19–associated ARDS, but it is unclear whether lung biopsy will be widely used in COVID-19 because of risk of viral dissemination and other concerns, underscoring the potential benefits of biomarkers and molecular imaging techniques that reflect this histologic pattern.[21,31]

Although DAD in COVID-19 and DAD in acute lung injury of other causes are indistinguishable by light microscopy,[12,29] they may be different at the molecular level. Future analysis of clinical lung tissue and bronchoalveolar lavage (BAL) samples, and samples from in vivo and in vitro experimental models, may reveal unique biochemical and cellular features that influence evolution of the alveolar injury or its resolution and repair.[4]

ALVEOLAR IMMUNE EFFECTOR CELLS IN CORONAVIRUS DISEASE 2019–ASSOCIATED LUNG INJURY

Leukocytes are a common feature of DAD (see **Box 1**), classically as a prominent interstitial infiltrate.[17] Inflammatory cells also concentrate in microvessels in numbers greater than those seen in the normal lung, suggesting intravascular activation and sequestration, and accumulate in the alveolar spaces in some cases.[4,18,19]

In COVID-19–associated DAD, perivascular and interstitial mononuclear cell infiltrates of variable intensity composed primarily of cluster of differentiation (CD) 4+ and CD8+ lymphocytes were commonly reported in early studies and were assessed to be consistent with viral infection.[10–13] Macrophages may have particular activities that drive acute lung injury early in the evolution of SARS-CoV-2 infection.[31,37–39,44,45] Limited early reports of BAL sampling also indicated predominant lymphocytic and mononuclear cell inflammation, including plasma cells and macrophages.[46–48] Although characteristic of viral infection, mononuclear leukocyte infiltrates are also found in acute lung injury of other causes, including oxygen toxicity[17] and malaria-associated ARDS.[49]

Angiocentric accumulation of lymphocytes in the alveolar perivascular interstitium and microvessels was observed in lung tissue from patients with COVID-19[15] and SARS-CoV-2–infected primates.[45] CD68+ macrophages and an activated T-cell signature correlated with DAD in a detailed study of lungs from COVID-19 decedents involving histology, immunophenotyping, and transcriptomics.[31] The activities and mechanisms of accumulation of alveolar lymphocytes in COVID-19 are unknown; they are suggested to contribute to both viral clearance and acute lung injury based on histologic and blood analysis.[31,50] In influenza infection, signaling interplay between lymphocyte subsets, injured alveolar cells, and fibroblasts influences immune cell accumulation and lung dysfunction, suggesting that similar events may occur in COVID-19.[51] Circulating platelet-lymphocyte and platelet-monocyte aggregates were increased in the blood of patients with COVID-19 compared with samples from control patients,[52,53] indicating one potential mechanism of lung accumulation of mononuclear leukocytes and showing interaction of key immune effector cells.[54]

Myeloid leukocyte subsets may also have critical effector activities in COVID-19 pneumonia.[44,47,55] Neutrophils (polymorphonuclear leukocytes) are hallmarks of classic ARDS induced by a variety of common infectious and noninfectious triggers,[20] but their involvement in SARS-CoV-2 lung infection is unclear. Neutrophils were infrequently identified in early COVID-19 autopsies, surgical cases, and BAL samples.[12,38,39,46,48] They were much less frequently detected by quantitative scoring in alveoli of patients with COVID-19 than in the lungs of patients dying of influenza.[15] Nevertheless, neutrophils were present in lung tissue from some patients with COVID-19.[10,12,14,22,33–37,56] One possibility is that neutrophils in these samples were indicators of superimposed bacterial pneumonia, and it was suggested that they are not effector cells in the primary inflammatory response to SARS-CoV-2 because they are not typically found in the lung in uncomplicated viral infection.[12] Autopsy evidence shows that bacterial pneumonia occurs in COVID-19 infection (discussed later), supporting this possibility.

Alternative possibilities are that neutrophils are transient cellular components or are a subpopulation of effector cells in SARS-CoV-2 lung infection, or that DAD with neutrophilic inflammation is a distinct phenotypic response to SARS-CoV-2. Observations in nonhuman primates suggest that SARS-CoV-2 has the biological potential to directly or indirectly trigger early alveolar accumulation of neutrophils in combination with mononuclear leukocytes. Neutrophils were present in cellular infiltrates together with lymphocytes and macrophages in foci of inflammation localized with AEC type I and AEC II positive for SARS-CoV-2 antigen in necropsy samples collected 4 days after infection of cynomolgus macaques.[57] Neutrophils were also identified together with mononuclear leukocytes in focal areas in lungs of rhesus macaques sacrificed 2 to 4 days after infection with SARS-CoV-2.[58,59] These models further showed key features of DAD at these early time points after infection. Nevertheless, evolution and changes in the immune effector cell populations and, specifically, persistence of neutrophils were not determined, which is an issue for future investigation.

One potential consequence of neutrophil accumulation in inflammatory syndromes is generation of neutrophil extracellular traps (NETs). NETs have both defensive and injurious activities, are triggered by viral and nonviral pathogens, and are generated in ARDS.[49,60] Neutrophil accumulation in capillaries, alveoli, and airways of 3 patients dying of COVID-19 suggested that NETs contribute to the pathobiology of SARS-CoV-2 infection.[60] Neutrophils in the process of NET formation (NETosis) and extracellular NET lattices were subsequently shown in autopsy sections of lung tissue from decedents COVID-19, 1 of whom expired after 5 days of intensive care treatment of ARDS (with concomitant empiric treatment of community-acquired pneumonia) and 2 others who died shortly after emergency room admission.[61] Plugs composed of neutrophils alone, and neutrophils interpreted to be undergoing NETosis based on swollen nuclei that stained positively for citrullinated histone H_3, on a background of DAD with interstitial T-lymphocyte infiltrates, were observed in lungs of a subset of a second series of patients dying of COVID-19; 9 out of 21 subjects (43%) had fungal or bacterial superinfections in this report.[35]

In correlative studies, myeloperoxidase/DNA complexes, a plasma marker of NETs, were increased in blood samples from hospitalized patients with COVID-19, including subjects with ARDS.[61] The levels were directly correlated with severity of illness and inversely correlated with oxygenation indexed by the Pao_2/fraction of inspired oxygen ratio. In parallel, neutrophils from patients with COVID-19 underwent unstimulated NETosis in vitro and plasma from patients with COVID-19 triggered NET formation by control neutrophils, a process that could be blocked by a novel inhibitor.[61] In a different analysis of circulating blood cells and postmortem lung tissue, aberrant patterns of neutrophil and platelet activation and plateletneutrophil aggregate formation were related to severity of COVID-19 pneumonia, providing evidence for immunothrombosis involving platelets, neutrophils, and fibrin.[62] Increased platelet-neutrophil aggregates were also detected in investigations of the platelet transcriptome in COVID-19.[53] These studies[35,53,61,62] suggest that neutrophils, platelets, and NETs may contribute to inflammatory lung injury and systemic thromboinflammation in COVID-19–associated ARDS.[60] Nevertheless, participation and contributions of neutrophils to COVID-19 and its complications remain to be defined.

VASCULOPATHY AND THROMBOINFLAMMATION ARE COMMON IN CLASSIC ACUTE RESPIRATORY DISTRESS SYNDROME AND CORONAVIRUS DISEASE 2019 LUNG INFECTION

Vasculopathy is a central component of DAD in acute lung injury and classic ARDS of diverse causes.[4,17–19,21] Endothelial dysfunction, with endothelial cells injured but largely intact by ultrastructural examination, contributes to increased alveolar-capillary permeability to protein and interstitial and alveolar edema in the exudative phase of DAD; alterations in the endothelial network can be dramatic in the later proliferative phase.[18,19] Thrombosis of pulmonary vessels is a common feature of both the exudative and proliferative phases. In systematic studies of lung vessels by postmortem angiography and histology correlated with antemortem balloon arteriography, vascular occlusion was detected in as many as 95% of cases. By microscopic examination, platelet-fibrin thrombi were commonly observed in alveolar capillaries and arterioles in acute ARDS, and platelet-fibrin thrombi in microvessels and laminated fibrin clots in pre-acinar and intra-acinar arteries were detected across the time line spectrum. The pulmonary vascular bed was found to be extensively remodeled in later proliferative and fibrotic phases of ARDS in lungs from some patients.[19]

Vasculopathy is also a component of acute lung injury in COVID-19, and it is suggested that SARS-CoV-2 induces a distinct vascular endotype of ARDS.[8] Pulmonary vascular injury was identified in 16 out of 23 early reports of acute lung injury in COVID-19.[11] In a quantitative histologic study that also used micro–computed tomography, ultrastructural analysis, and molecular assays, lungs from decedents with COVID-19 respiratory failure or ARDS secondary to H1N1 influenza were equally likely to have thrombi in precapillary pulmonary arteries, but alveolar-capillary microthrombi were 9 times more prevalent in patients with COVID-19. Structurally deformed capillaries with evidence for intussusceptive angiogenesis were also significantly more frequent in the lungs of subjects with COVID-19 compared with those with influenza, although the number of patients in each group was small.[15] In a different analysis, platelet and/or fibrin microthrombi were identified in lungs from 84% of 68 patients with COVID-19, several whom had large vessel pulmonary thrombi and extrapulmonary thrombotic involvement.[14] Macrovascular and microvascular thrombi have been reported in multiple additional studies of COVID-19 lungs.[10,12,23–27,29,32,61–63]

Endotheliitis (also termed endothelialitis) has been identified in lungs from patients with COVID-19[15,33] and SARS-CoV-2–infected rhesus macaques.[45] The term implies endothelial injury and dysfunction with a component of perivascular inflammation, but there is not yet a consensus definition or rigorous determination of whether it is commonly present in COVID-19 pneumonia or represents a unique histologic subphenotype. Endothelial damage, swelling, and vacuolization shown by light and electron microscopy have been attributed to endothelial cell infection by SARS-CoV-2 via ACE2, but, in some studies, viral particles or antigen were detected in AECs but not in capillary endothelium.[11,15,22,24,32,33,36,56] Perivascular leukocyte involvement has been reported as lymphocytic angiocentric inflammation[15,45] and lymphocytic and myeloid cell accumulation in different patients,[33] intravascular fibrin deposition with septal accumulation of neutrophils,[34] and neutrophilic capillaritis.[22,60] In 1 report, focal microthrombi were found, but no histologic evidence of endotheliitis.[56] Perivascular inflammation did not reliably separate COVID-19 from other causes of DAD in a comparative analysis.[29] Thus, there are many questions related to pulmonary endotheliitis in COVID-19 to be resolved. In addition, there are multiple fundamental issues to be explored. For example, it may be critical to know whether SARS-CoV-2–induced acute lung injury differentially affects recently described alveolar endothelial cell subtypes.[64] Direct contributions of injured endothelial cells to other facets of alveolar damage and inflammation (see **Fig. 1**), and to viral containment versus spread, are also yet to be examined.

Thrombocytopenia, which is common and often profound in critically ill patients with classic ARDS,[49] is generally mild in COVID-19, although it can be progressive in nonsurvivors.[65] Platelets have dual roles as hemostatic and immune effector cells in the lung and other tissues,[54] and can have thromboinflammatory activities in ARDS.[49] Aggregates of platelets and platelet-fibrin thrombi have been commonly observed in microvessels in SARS-CoV-2–infected lungs,[10,14,24–26,62,63] and molecular signatures associated with platelet activation, aggregation, and adhesion were detected in infected macaques.[45] Altered platelet reactivity was detected in mild and severe COVID-19 infection.[52,53,62] Platelet-neutrophil aggregates, a marker of platelet activation,[54] were observed in COVID-19 lungs and blood.[35,53,62] Platelets trigger NETosis, are effectors of pathologic clotting,[49,60,65] and may contribute to NET formation and immunothrombosis in COVID-19[61,62,66] (discussed earlier).

Megakaryocytes, the precursors of platelets, are present in normal and injured lungs and generate platelets in the pulmonary compartment (reviewed by Middleton and colleagues[49]). Megakaryocytes, including cells actively producing platelets, were detected in lung microvessels of decedents of COVID-19.[10,26] Two autopsy series that included patients dying of COVID-19 or of classic ARDS found increased numbers of megakaryocytes in the pulmonary vasculature of subjects with COVID-19 infection, although only 1 comparison reached statistical significance.[63,67] Megakaryocyte transcript signatures were increased in blood from patients[68] and macaques[45] infected with SARS-CoV-2. It is unknown whether megakaryocytes in the lungs of patients with COVID-19 have anti–SARS-CoV-2 activities that may influence COVID-19 infection, as with other viruses.[69] In contrast, novel functions of megakaryocytes may contribute to acute lung injury or repair in COVID-19.[49] Circulating megakaryocytes with a strong interferon-associated molecular signature were one of 3 cell types reported to be hallmarks of severe COVID-19 and were linked to inflammatory markers in plasma.[68]

Dysregulated systemic hemostasis may contribute to pulmonary vasculopathy in COVID-19.[65] As markers, increase of plasma D-dimer concentration has been widely reported, and increased thrombin generation and relative impairment in fibrinolysis have been shown in severe COVID-19.[6,65,70,71] Increased circulating platelet-monocyte aggregates were found in blood samples from patients with severe COVID-19 pneumonia, particularly those requiring mechanical ventilation. Platelets from these patients induced tissue factor expression by monocytes in vitro,[52] suggesting a mechanism for pulmonary and systemic thromboinflammation.[54]

The causal links between deranged coagulation and macrothrombosis and microthrombosis in COVID-19 have not been elucidated,[65] establishing key priorities for basic and clinical investigation. As an example, altered complement activation may link dysregulated inflammation and coagulation in COVID-19, including in patients with respiratory failure and systemic complications.[34,65,66,72,73] The SARS-CoV-2 spike protein activates the alternate pathway of complement,[74] suggesting a possible mechanism. SARS-CoV-2 also induces complement and coagulation pathways in macaques.[45] Lung and systemic manifestations were mitigated in C3-deficient mice infected with SARS-CoV-2.[73]

PULMONARY COINFECTION IN CORONAVIRUS DISEASE 2019 PNEUMONIA: A COMMON PHENOTYPE

Microbial coinfection is common in COVID-19–induced acute lung injury, based on autopsy series in which the frequency of suspected or documented bacterial or fungal coinfection, usually termed superimposed bronchopneumonia or superinfection, was 13% to 79%.[11,14,23–25,27,30,32,35,63] The histologic pattern has been described as dense accumulations of neutrophils in alveoli and airways, alveolar hemorrhage, and vascular congestion on a background of DAD with lymphocytic interstitial infiltrates.[27] Special stains, microbial cultures, and molecular techniques have been used to confirm histologic findings and identify a variety of non–COVID-19 pathogens,[14,27,30] although in some reports the diagnosis was made exclusively on the pattern of neutrophilic bronchopneumonia with DAD and, in others, coinfection was not detected.[26] Frequent coinfection was also reported in a recent study of blood and airway myeloid leukocyte subsets in patients with severe COVID-19 lung involvement.[55] For comparison, coinfection was present in 26% of 100 fatal cases of pandemic influenza A; DAD was a ubiquitous underlying histologic pattern.[75] In contrast, coinfection was not frequently reported in the SARS and MERS pandemics.[30]

In classic ARDS, DAD, acute neutrophilic pneumonia caused by bacterial or fungal pathogens, and DAD together with acute neutrophilic pneumonia are each distinct histologic phenotypes that carry physiologic significance and have different clinical outcomes.[21] This finding may also be true for COVID-19–associated ARDS, an issue that should be addressed in future clinical and experimental investigations. Application of metagenomic techniques will also be revealing.

ANIMAL MODELS: EXPERIMENTAL CORRELATES AND CONSISTENT HISTOPATHOLOGY

Specific findings in primate models of SARS-CoV-2 lung infection were mentioned earlier. Although overt clinical signs do not develop short term, histopathology in cynomolgus macaques is consistent with that in human COVID-19 pneumonia (see **Fig. 1**). Foci of pulmonary consolidation were found in 2 of 4 animals (young and aged) 4 days after infection with SARS-CoV-2 isolated from a human patient.[57] The major histologic changes included areas of acute lung injury with features of exudative and proliferative DAD, indicating that this pattern of response is a facet of the biology of SARS-CoV-2 lung infection that can develop rapidly and supporting the conclusion that DAD is not exclusively secondary to respiratory therapy measures.[29] DAD histopathology was also observed in animals infected in parallel with MERS-CoV for comparison. SARS-CoV-2 antigen was detected in AEC I and AEC II in areas of DAD, a proximity that suggested that SARS-CoV-2 infection drives evolution of the DAD histologic pattern.[57] Similarly, SARS-CoV-2 antigen and viral RNA were detected in focal areas of DAD in human COVID-19 pneumonia.[14,32]

Histologic changes of DAD also occur in rhesus macaques infected with SARS-CoV-2. Hyaline membranes, alveolar edema, fibrin deposition, interstitial infiltrates, and AEC II hyperplasia were observed in multifocal areas of involvement 3 days after infection.[59] In a second study, hyaline membranes were present together with interstitial and alveolar inflammatory infiltrates and edema 2 days after infection.[58] In a study to examine age as a variable, histologic findings were generally similar but the specific components of interstitial inflammation and edema were more severe in aged rhesus macaques than in younger animals 7 days after SARS-CoV-2 infection.[76] In cynomolgus macaques, age did not affect the histologic pattern at an early time point, but aged animals shed SARS-CoV-2 longer after infection.[57]

Additional animal models of COVID-19 have been developed, including experimental infection of rodents.[40] Severe disease has been reported in some, depending on the animal species, genetic background, and conditions of viral challenge.[40,77–79] To date, studies of mice have largely described alveolar interstitial infiltrates and edema, recapitulating some but not all of the histologic determinants of DAD (see **Fig. 1**). Acute lung injury with hyaline membranes and other DAD features were reported in 2 recently described murine models.[77,79]

Although the rapidly expanding repertoire of primate and small animal models will provide correlates of human COVID-19 and experimental infrastructure for mechanistic studies and for evaluation of therapeutics and vaccines, none yet developed is a faithful surrogate for human COVID-19–associated ARDS.[40] As existing models are further refined and others developed for this purpose, lung histology will be a critical variable, as it has been in experimental acute lung injury of other causes.[80] A recently reported model in standard laboratory mouse strains infected with a murine-adapted SARS-CoV-2 was interpreted to have features of ARDS based on assessment of acute lung injury and DAD by histologic scoring,[77] although oxygenation and other key determinants of ARDS[3,4,80] were not examined. The severity of injury was greater in BALB/c than in C57/BL6 mice.

SUMMARY

In January of 2020, nothing was known of the anatomic basis for respiratory failure caused by the novel SARS-CoV-2 virus. Since that time, examination of lung tissue from patients with COVID-19 has yielded a body of information with clinical and basic relevance, showing the unique value of analysis of pathologic anatomy in emerging and reemerging infectious diseases.[11] The findings provide an initial foundation for understanding pathophysiologic features of COVID-19–associated ARDS[1,2,5,6,16] and priorities for future investigations.

It is clear that SARS-CoV-2 infection can cause injury from the tracheobronchial epithelium to the pleura.[10–13] Injury to the alveoli characterized by DAD is central to COVID-19 respiratory failure, consistent with the histopathology of severe infections caused by other respiratory viruses, including SARS-CoV, MERS-CoV, and influenza.[11,12,17,75] Features of DAD were also prominent in lungs of patients reported in the original description of ARDS, several of whom were thought to have fatal viral pneumonia.[81] Pulmonary vascular and microvascular involvement is common in COVID-19 pneumonia and may have unique features. DAD and its microvascular component are histologic counterparts for altered compliance, dead space, and oxygenation and for perfusion and other imaging abnormalities in patients with COVID-19–associated ARDS.[6] Further study may provide additional useful insights, as it has in classic ARDS.[19,21,41,42] Although the common histopathologic and cellular features of established COVID-19 acute lung injury are becoming clear, the early events in alveolar damage, the temporal progression to DAD, and the cellular and molecular mechanisms involved are obscure. Further definition of these features may have therapeutic significance. Current anatomic findings with clinical correlates suggest that pathways inherent to both the pathogen and the host contribute to COVID-19–associated ARDS.[12,15,31,82,83]

Findings from examination of COVID-19 lung tissue raise many additional questions and priorities for investigation, some of which are identified in this article, and potential controversies. The frequency, mechanisms, and physiologic significance of histologic patterns that vary from established DAD[10,11,14,22,25,27,33–36] are open questions that need to be resolved. The specific issue of endotheliitis, which is currently based on a small number of diverse observations, needs further definition. The extent to which alveolar microvascular involvement is greater, or not different, compared with that of classic ARDS,[15,29] potential SARS-CoV-2–specific mechanisms of alveolar vasculopathy,[15,45,79] and whether COVID-19–associated ARDS is a distinct vascular endotype of ARDS[8] each merit additional examination. Similarly, the specific contributions of neutrophils, NETs, platelets, and megakaryocytes to the pathogenesis of SARS-CoV-2 pneumonia and COVID-19–associated ARDS, in the broader context of activities of key immune effector cells, are unresolved issues with possible therapeutic relevance. Histopathologic analysis amplified by the tools of modern biology and molecular immunology,[15,31] in parallel with rigorous animal models[40] and reduced experimental approaches including isolated cell-based assays and organoid preparations, has the potential to provide needed answers and contribute to vetting of emerging hypotheses.[84] Such insights may then refine understanding of the place of COVID-19 acute lung injury in the broader spectrum of ARDS.[2–4,7–9]

CLINICS CARE POINTS

- DAD has been consistently identified as the key histologic pattern of acute lung injury in SARS-CoV-2–associated pneumonia and ARDS.
- The histologic pattern of DAD in SARS-CoV-2–associated lung injury is not different from DAD in classic ARDS not associated with SARS-CoV-2 infection and COVID-19 pneumonia.
- Biological activities of injured alveolar cells and immune effector cells recruited to the alveoli in SARS-CoV-2–associated pneumonia and ARDS may contribute to unique physiologic responses and to outcomes in these syndromes.

- Additional histologic patterns besides DAD have been identified in SARS-CoV-2–associated acute lung injury and may be the basis for heterogeneity and subphenotypes in COVID-19–associated ARDS.
- COVID-19–associated ARDS is histologically similar to ARDS of other causes in the presence of DAD and perivascular inflammation; however, there is evidence of direct viral infection in the tracheobronchial epithelium and AECs.
- Deranged coagulation and presence of immunothrombi is a notable finding in COVID-19–associated ARDS and has many potential drivers, including the presences of NETs, complement activation and increased platelet activation/aggregation, and increased monocyte tissue factor levels induced by platelet-monocyte aggregates.
- Lung tissue examined is largely from elderly patients who succumbed to the disease; therefore, distinguishing direct disease from SARS-CoV-2 infection or complex comorbid disease is challenging.
- Secondary bacterial and fungal pneumonias commonly occur in COVID-19–associated ARDS, although the clinical outcomes driven by the physiologic consequences of coinfection are not yet clear.

ACKNOWLEDGMENTS

The authors greatly appreciate the efforts and creative contributions of Kendra Richardson and Diana Lim in preparation of the article and figure. E.A. Middleton is supported by a research career development award (1 KO8 HL153953-02) from the National Heart, Lung, and Blood Institute and an award from the University of Utah Immunology, Inflammation, and Infectious Disease Program. G.A. Zimmerman was supported by awards from the National Institutes of Health (R37 HL044525, HL077671, HL130541, HD093826) while the work cited was done.

DISCLOSURE

The authors have nothing to disclose.

REFERENCES

1. Berlin DA, Gulik RM, Martinez FJ. Severe COVID-19. N Engl J Med 2020. https://doi.org/10.1056/NEJMcp2009575.
2. Ware LB. Physiological and biological heterogeneity in COVID-19-associated acute respiratory distress syndrome. Lancet Respir Med 2020. https://doi.org/10.1016/S2213-2600(20)30369-6. S2213-2600(20)30369-6.
3. Thompson BT, Chambers RC, Liu KD. Acute respiratory distress syndrome. N Engl J Med 2017;377:562–72.
4. Matthay MA, Zemans RL, Zimmerman GA, et al. Acute respiratory distress syndrome. Nat Rev 2019;5:18.
5. Ferrando C, Suarez-Sipmann F, Mellado-Artigas R, et al. Clinical features, ventilatory management, and outcome of ARDS caused by COVID-19 are similar to other causes of ARDS. Intensive Care Med 2020. https://doi.org/10.1007/s00134-020-06192-2.
6. Grasselli G, Tonetti T, Protti A, et al. Pathophysiology of COVID-19-associated acute respiratory distress syndrome: a multicentre prospective observational study. Lancet Respir Med 2020;8(12):1201–8.
7. Sinha P, Calfee CS, Cherian S, et al. Prevalence of phenotypes of acute respiratory distress syndrome in critically ill patients with COVID-19: a prospective

observational study. Lancet Respir Med 2020. https://doi.org/10.1016/S2213-2600(20)30366-0. S2213-2600(20)30366-0.

8. Mangalmurti NS, Reilly JP, Cines DB, et al. COVID-19-associated acute respiratory distress syndrome clarified: a vascular endotype? Am J Respir Crit Care Med 2020;202(5):750–3.

9. Thompson BT, Matthay MA. The Berlin Definition of ARDS versus pathological evidence of diffuse alveolar damage. Am J Respir Crit Care Med 2013;187(7):675–7.

10. Buja LM, Wolf DA, Zhao B, et al. The emerging spectrum of cardiopulmonary pathology of the coronavirus disease 2019 (COVID-19): report of 3 autopsies from Houston, Texas, and review of autopsy findings from other United States cities. Cardiovasc Pathol 2020;48:107233.

11. Calabrese F, Pezzuto F, Fortarezza F, et al. Pulmonary pathology and COVID-19: lessons from autopsy. The experience of European Pulmonary Pathologists. Virchows Arch 2020;477(3):359–72.

12. Mohanty SK, Satapathy A, Naidu MM, et al. Severe acute respiratory syndrome coronavirus-2 (SARS-CoV-2) and coronavirus disease 19 (COVID-19) – anatomic pathology perspective on current knowledge. Diagn Pathol 2020;15:103.

13. Vasquez-Bonilla W, Orozco R, Argueta V, et al. A review of the main histopathological findings in coronavirus disease 2019. Hum Pathol 2020;105:74–83.

14. Borczuk AC, Salvatore SP, Seshan SV, et al. COVID-19 pulmonary pathology: a multi-institutional autopsy cohort from Italy and New York City. Mod Pathol 2020;33(11):2156–68.

15. Ackermann M, Verleden SE, Kuehnel M, et al. Pulmonary vascular endothelialitis, thrombosis, and angiogenesis in COVID-19. N Engl J Med 2020;383:120–8.

16. Wiersinga WJ, Rhodes A, Cheng AC, et al. Pathophysiology, transmission, diagnosis, and treatment of Coronavirus disease 2019 (COVID-19). JAMA 2020;324(8):782–93.

17. Katzenstein AL, Bloor CM, Leibow AA. Diffuse alveolar damage–the role of oxygen, shock, and related factors. A review. Am J Pathol 1976;85(1):209–28.

18. Bachofen M, Weibel ER. Structural alterations of lung parenchyma in the adult respiratory distress syndrome. Clin Chest Med 1982;3(1):35–56.

19. Tomashefski JF Jr. Pulmonary pathology of acute respiratory distress syndrome. Clin Chest Med 2000;21(3):435–66.

20. Zemans RL, Matthay MA. What drives neutrophils to the alveoli in ARDS? Thorax 2017;72(1):1–3.

21. Cardinal-Fernández P, Lorente JA, Ballén-Barragán A, et al. Acute respiratory distress syndrome and diffuse alveolar damage. New insights on a complex relationship. Ann Am Thorac Soc 2017;14(6):844–50.

22. Bössmüller H, Traxier S, Bitzer M, et al. The evolution of pulmonary pathology in fatal COVID-19 disease: an autopsy study with clinical correlation. Virchows Arch 2020;477(3):349–57.

23. Bussani R, Schneider E, Zentilin L, et al. Persistence of viral RNA, pneumocyte syncytia and thrombosis are hallmarks of advanced COVID-19 pathology. EBioMedicine 2020;61:103104.

24. Carsana L, Sonzogni A, Nasr A, et al. Pulmonary post-mortem findings in a series of COVID-19 cases from northern Italy: a two-centre descriptive study. Lancet Infect Dis 2020;20(10):1135–40.

25. De Michele S, Sun Y, Yilaz MM, et al. Forty postmortem examinations in COVID-19 patients. Am J Clin Pathol 2020;154(6):748–60.

26. Fox SE, Akmatbekov A, Harbert JL, et al. Pulmonary and cardiac pathology in African American patients with COVID-19: an autopsy series from New Orleans. Lancet Respir Med 2020;8(7):681–6.

27. Grosse C, Grosse A, Salzer HJF, et al. Analysis of cardiopulmonary findings in COVID-19 fatalities: high incidence of pulmonary artery thrombi and acute suppurative bronchopneumonia. Cardiovasc Pathol 2020;49:107263.

28. Hanley B, Naresh KN, Roufosse C, et al. Histopathological findings and viral tropism in UK patients with severe fatal COVID-19: a post-mortem study. Lancet Microbe 2020;1(6):e245–53.

29. Konopka KE, Nguyen T, Jentzen JM, et al. Diffuse alveolar damage (DAD) resulting from coronavirus disease 2019 infection is morphologically indistinguishable from other causes of DAD. Histopathology 2020;77(4):570–8.

30. Martines RB, Ritter JM, Matkovic E, et al. Pathology and pathogenesis of SARS-CoV-2 associated with fatal Coronavirus Disease, United States. Emerg Infect Dis 2020;26(9):2005–15.

31. Nienhold R, Ciani Y, Koelzer VH, et al. Two distinct immunopathological profiles in autopsy lungs of COVID-19. Nat Commun 2020;11(1):5086.

32. Schaefer IM, Padera RF, Solomon IH, et al. In situ detection of SARS-CoV-2 in lungs and airways of patients with COVID-19. Mod Pathol 2020;1–11. https://doi.org/10.1038/s41379-020-0595-z.

33. Varga Z, Flammer AJ, Steiger P, et al. Endothelial cell infection and endotheliitis in COVID-19. Lancet 2020;395(10234):1417–8.

34. Magro C, Mulvey JJ, Berlin D, et al. Complement associated microvascular injury and thrombosis in the pathogenesis of severe COVID-19 infection: a report of five cases. Transl Res 2020;220:1–13.

35. Schurink B, Roos E, Radonic T, et al. Viral presence and immunopathology in patients with lethal COVID-19: a prospective autopsy cohort study. Lancet Microbe 2020;1(7):e290–9.

36. Copin MC, Parmentier E, Duburcq T, et al. Time to consider histologic pattern of lung injury to treat critically ill patients with COVID-19 infection. Intensive Care Med 2020;46(6):1124–6.

37. Pernazza A, Mancini M, Rullo E, et al. Early histologic findings of pulmonary SARS-CoV-2 infection detected in a surgical specimen. Virchows Arch 2020; 477(5):743–8.

38. Tian S, Hu W, Niu L, et al. Pulmonary pathology of early-phase 2019 novel Coronavirus (COVID-19) pneumonia in two patients with lung cancer. J Thorac Oncol 2020;15(5):700–4.

39. Zeng Z, Xu L, Xie XY, et al. Pulmonary pathology of early-phase COVID-19 pneumonia in a patient with a benign lung lesion. Histopathology 2020;77(5):823–31.

40. Muñoz-Fontela C, Dowling WE, Funnell SGP, et al. Animal models for COVID-19. Nature 2020;586(7830):509–15.

41. Thille AW, Esteban A, Fernández-Segoviano P, et al. Chronology of histological lesions in acute respiratory distress syndrome with diffuse alveolar damage: a prospective cohort study of clinical autopsies. Lancet Respir Med 2013;1(5): 395–401.

42. Thille AW, Esteban A, Fernández-Segoviano P, et al. Comparison of the Berlin definition for acute respiratory distress syndrome with autopsy. Am J Respir Crit Care Med 2013;187(7):761–7.

43. Cardinal-Fernández P, Bajwa EK, Dominguez-Calvo A, et al. The presence of diffuse alveolar damage on open lung biopsy is associated with mortality in

patients with acute respiratory distress syndrome: a systematic review and meta-analysis. Chest 2016;149(5):1155–64.

44. Merad M, Martin JC. Pathological inflammation in patients with COVID-19: a key role for monocytes and macrophages. Nat Rev Immunol 2020;1–8. https://doi.org/10.1038/s41577-020-0331-4.

45. Aid M, Busman-Sahay K, Vidal SJ, et al. Vascular disease and thrombosis in SARS-CoV-2-infected rhesus macaques. Cell 2020;183(5):1354–66.

46. Giani M, Seminati D, Lucchini A, et al. Exuberant plasmocytosis in bronchoalveolar lavage specimen of the first patient requiring extracorporeal membrane oxygenation for SARS-CoV-2 in Europe. J Thorac Oncol 2020;15(5):e65–6.

47. Liao M, Liu Y, Yuan J, et al. Single-cell landscape of bronchoalveolar immune cells in patients with COVID-19. Nat Med 2020;26(6):842–4.

48. Voiriot G, Fajac A, Lopinto J, et al. Bronchoalveolar lavage findings in severe COVID-19 pneumonia. Intern Emerg Med 2020;15(7):1333–4.

49. Middleton EA, Rondina MT, Schwertz HJ, et al. Amicus or adversary revisited: platelets in acute lung injury and acute respiratory distress syndrome. Am J Respir Cell Mol Biol 2018;59(1):18–35.

50. Song JW, Zhang C, Fan X, et al. Immunological and inflammatory profiles in mild and severe cases of COVID-19. Nat Commun 2020;11(1):3410.

51. Boyd DF, Allen EK, Randolph AG, et al. Exuberant fibroblast activity compromises lung function via ADAMTS4. Nature 2020;587:466–71.

52. Hottz ED, Azevedo-Quintanilha IG, Palhinha L, et al. Platelet activation and platelet-monocyte aggregate formation trigger tissue factor expression in patients with severe COVID-19. Blood 2020;136(11):1330–41.

53. Manne BK, Denorme F, Middleton EA, et al. Platelet gene expression and function in patients with COVID-19. Blood 2020;136:1317–29.

54. Middleton EA, Weyrich AS, Zimmerman GA. Platelets in pulmonary immune responses and inflammatory lung diseases. Physiol Rev 2016;96(4):1211–59.

55. Sanchez-Cerrillo I, Landete P, Aldave B, et al. COVID-19 severity associates with pulmonary redistribution of $CD_{1C}+$ DCs and inflammatory transitional and nonclassical monocytes. J Clin Invest 2020;130(12):6290–300.

56. Bradley BT, Maioli H, Johnston R, et al. Histopathology and ultrastructural findings of fatal COVID-19 infections in Washington State: a case series. Lancet 2020;396(10247):320–32.

57. Rockx B, Kuiken T, Herfst S, et al. Comparative pathogenesis of COVID-19, MERS, and SARS in a nonhuman primate model. Science 2020;368(6494):1012–5.

58. Chandrashekar A, Liu J, Martinot AJ, et al. SARS-CoV-2 infection protects against rechallenge in rhesus macaques. Science 2020;369(6505):812–7.

59. Munster VJ, Feldmann F, Williamson BN. Respiratory disease in rhesus macaques inoculated with SARS-CoV-2. Nature 2020;585(7824):268–72.

60. Barnes BJ, Adrover JM, Baxter-Stoltzfus A, et al. Targeting potential drivers of COVID-19: neutrophil extracellular traps. J Exp Med 2020;217(6):e20200652.

61. Middleton EA, He XY, Denorme F, et al. Neutrophil extracellular traps contribute to immunothrombosis in COVID-19 acute respiratory distress syndrome. Blood 2020;136(10):1169–79.

62. Nicolai L, Leunig A, Brambs S, et al. Immunothrombotic dysregulation in COVID-19 pneumonia is associated with respiratory failure and coagulopathy. Circulation 2020;142(12):1176–89.

63. Rapkiewicz AV, Mai X, Carsons SE, et al. Megakaryocytes and platelet-fibrin thrombi characterize multi-organ thrombosis at autopsy in COVID-19: a case series. EClinicalMedicine 2020;24:100434.

64. Gillich A, Zhang F, Farmer CG, et al. Capillary cell-type specialization in the alveolus. Nature 2020;586(7831):785–9.

65. Mackman N, Antoniak S, Wolberg AS, et al. Coagulation abnormalities and thrombosis in patients infected with SARS-CoV-2 and other pandemic viruses. Arterioscler Thromb Vasc Biol 2020;40(9):2033–44.

66. Skendros P, Mitsios A, Chrysanthopoulou A, et al. Complement and tissue factor-enriched neutrophil extracellular traps are key drivers in COVID-19 immunothrombosis. J Clin Invest 2020;130(11):6151–7.

67. Valdivia-Mazeyra M, Salas C, Nieves-Alonso J, et al. Increased number of pulmonary megakaryocytes in COVID-19 patients with diffuse alveolar damage: an autopsy study with clinical correlation and review of the literature. Virchows Arch 2020;1–10. https://doi.org/10.1007/s00428-020-02926-1.

68. Bernardes JP, Mishra N, Tran F, et al. Longitudinal multi-omics analyses identify responses of megakaryocytes, erythroid cell, and plasmablasts as hallmarks of severe COVID-19. Immunity 2020;53(6):1296–314.

69. Campbell RA, Schwertz H, Hottz ED, et al. Human megakaryocytes possess intrinsic antiviral immunity through regulated induction of IFITM3. Blood 2019; 133(19):2013–26.

70. Bouck EG, Denorme F, Holle LA, et al. COVID-19 and sepsis are associated with different abnormalities in plasma procoagulant and fibrinolytic activity. Arterioscler Thromb Vasc Biol 2020;41(1):401–14.

71. Ranucci M, Sitzia C, Baryshnikova E, et al. COVID-19-associated coagulopathy: biomarkers of thrombin generation and fibrinolysis leading the outcome. J Clin Med 2020;9(11):3487.

72. Cugno M, Meroni PL, Gualtierotti R, et al. Complement activation in patients with COVID-19: a novel therapeutic target. J Allergy Clin Immunol 2020;146(1):215–7.

73. Gralinski LE, Sheahan TP, Morrison TE, et al. Complement activation contributes to severe acute respiratory syndrome coronavirus pathogenesis. mBio 2018;9(5): e01753-18.

74. Yu J, Yuan X, Chen H, et al. Direct activation of the alternative complement pathway by SARS-CoV-2 spike proteins is blocked by factor D inhibition. Blood 2020;136(18):2080–9.

75. Shieh WJ, Blau DM, Denison AM, et al. 2009 pandemic influenza A (H1N1): pathology and pathogenesis of 100 fatal cases in the United States. Am J Pathol 2010;177(1):166–75.

76. Yu P, Qi F, Xu Y, et al. Age-related rhesus macaque models of COVID-19. Anim Model Exp Med 2020;3(1):93–7.

77. Leist SR, Dinnon KH 3rd, Schäfer A, et al. A mouse-adapted SARS-CoV-2 induces acute lung injury and mortality in standard laboratory mice. Cell 2020; 183(4):1070–85.e12.

78. Tostanoski LH, Wegmann F, Martinot AJ, et al. Ad26 vaccine protects against SARS-CoV-2 severe clinical disease in hamsters. Nat Med 2020;26(11): 1694–700.

79. Zheng J, Wong LYR, Li K, et al. COVID-19 treatments and pathogenesis including anosmia in K18-hACE2 mice. Nature 2020. https://doi.org/10.1038/s41586-020-2943-z.

80. Matute-Bello G, Downey G, Moore BB, et al. An official American Thoracic Society workshop report: features and measurements of experimental acute lung injury in animals. Am J Respir Cell Mol Biol 2011;44(5):725–38.
81. Ashbaugh DG, Bigelow DB, Petty TL, et al. Acute respiratory distress in adults. Lancet 1967;2(7511):319–23.
82. Hue S, Beldi-Ferchiou A, Bendib I, et al. Uncontrolled innate and impaired adaptive immune responses in patients with COVID-19 acute respiratory distress syndrome. Am J Respir Crit Care Med 2020;202(11):1509–19.
83. Matthay MA, Leligdowicz A, Liu KD. Biological Mechanisms of COVID-19 acute respiratory distress syndrome. Am J Respir Crit Care Med 2020;202(11): 1489–91.
84. Grant RA, Morales-Nebreda L, Markov NS, et al. Circuits between infected macrophages and T cells in SARS-CoV-2 pneumonia. Nature 2021. https://doi.org/10.1038/s41586-020-03148-w.

Pathophysiology of the Acute Respiratory Distress Syndrome: Insights from Clinical Studies

Pratik Sinha, MB ChB, PhD[a],*, Lieuwe D. Bos, MD, PhD[b]

KEYWORDS

• ARDS • Pathophysiology • COVID-19 • Human studies • Phenotypes

KEY POINTS

- ARDS the clinical entity encompasses a broad spectrum of pathophysiological abnormalities.
- Recent advances in biological measurements and data science have allowed novel insights into subgroups of patients with uniform biological or clinical characteristics that may be targeted for specific therapies.

Acute respiratory distress syndrome (ARDS) is a frequently encountered clinical syndrome associated with unacceptably high morbidity and mortality.[1] Since its first description in 1967 by Ashbaugh and colleagues,[2] numerous strides have been made in our understanding of the pathophysiology of ARDS,[3] which can be simply summarized as an acute inflammatory injury of the lungs. Broadly, the milieu of severe inflammation, locally in the lungs, systemically, or both, triggers an injurious cascade of molecular and cellular responses that lead to epithelial, endothelial, and interstitial/extracellular matrix (ECM) injury.[4] These responses manifest macroscopically as alveolar flooding, interstitial edema leading to increased extravascular lung water, and thromboembolic phenomena in the microvasculature of the lungs. At the bedside, these abnormalities lead to hypoxemia, loss of lung compliance, increased dead space, and the pathognomonic radiological changes of ARDS.

Despite decades of experimental insights into the biology of ARDS, few, if any, have translated into successful therapies.[5] In part, these failures can be attributed to the vast heterogeneity introduced due to the nonspecific clinical definition of ARDS, which subsumes numerous etiologic insults (**Table 1**). Another important, and often

[a] Division of Clinical and Translational Research, Department of Anesthesia, Washington University School of Medicine, 660 S. Euclid Avenue, Campus Box 8054, St Louis, MO 63110, USA;
[b] Department of Respiratory Medicine, Infection and Immunity, Amsterdam University Medical Center, AMC, Meibergdreef 9, Amsterdam 1105AZ, The Netherlands
* Corresponding author.
E-mail address: p.sinha@wustl.edu

Crit Care Clin 37 (2021) 795–815
https://doi.org/10.1016/j.ccc.2021.05.005
0749-0704/21/© 2021 Elsevier Inc. All rights reserved.

Table 1
Common risk factors (causes) leading to acute respiratory distress syndrome

Direct (Pulmonary) Risk Factors	Indirect (Extrapulmonary) Risk Factor
Pneumonia (bacterial, viral, fungal)	Sepsis
COVID-19 (SARS-CoV-2 infection)	Nonthoracic major trauma
Aspiration	Pancreatitis
Inhalation injury	Cardiopulmonary bypass
Pulmonary contusion	Transfusion of blood products
Vasculitis	Major burns injury
Drowning	

Abbreviations: COVID-19, coronavirus disease 2019; SARS-CoV-2, severe acute respiratory syndrome coronavirus 2.

overlooked, factor for the failure of these biological interventions may be that many of the insights about ARDS pathophysiology were made in experimental and preclinical studies and the translation of these models from animals to humans has been challenging,[6,7] not least because many of the animal models focus on studying dysfunctional pathways following a single etiologic insult.[8] Assumptions that there is uniformity of injury and severity across all the components of the alveolar unit regardless of the precipitating insult is clearly not valid; however, most ARDS clinical trials do not discriminate according to aetiology.

Consequently, there has been a growing trend toward studying ARDS in human subjects in real world conditions based on pragmatic sample acquisition.[9,10] Advances in novel biological measurements and data science methods have seen a rapid upsurge in translational and clinical studies in human subjects that has brought new insights into the pathophysiology of ARDS. Given the pace of innovation in both these disciplines, we may be entering a new era of learning in ARDS biology based on in vivo human subject studies. Moreover, such translational studies proffer paradigm-changing approaches to experimental studies in ARDS, where the traditional linear bench to bedside approach is replaced by a cyclic exchange of ideas from these research domains (**Fig. 1**). In this review, some of the recent advances made in our understanding of the pathophysiology of ARDS based on human studies are summarized. Furthermore, the pathophysiology of lung injury in coronavirus disease 2019

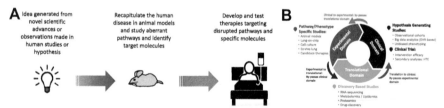

Fig. 1. Basic conceptual model of a circular and iterative research cycle form bedside to bench through translational domains of research. (**A**) Traditional linear flow of ideas and research from bench through to bedside. (**B**) A new approach to conducting research, which is perpetual and iterative. The primary flow is clockwise; however, flow of research can be counterclockwise such that all 3 research domains are platforms for both hypothesis generation and causal inferences. EHR, electronic health record; HTE, heterogeneous treatment effect.

(COVID-19), the disease manifest by severe acute respiratory syndrome coronavirus 2 (SARS-CoV-2), is reviewed.

CLINICAL DIAGNOSIS OF ACUTE RESPIRATORY DISTRESS SYNDROME

The formalization of a clinical diagnosis for ARDS constitutes a pivotal moment in our understanding of its pathophysiology. In 1994, ARDS was given its first consensus diagnosis at the American-European Consensus Conference (AECC).[11] In the absence of a tissue or biological diagnosis, investigators in the consensus panel set clinical criteria to diagnose patients with ARDS as acute onset of symptoms, Pao/fraction of inspired oxygen (Fio_2) 300 mm Hg or less classified as acute lung injury and 200 mm Hg or less as ARDS, bilateral opacification on chest radiograph, and a pulmonary occlusion pressure of 18 mm Hg or less or no evidence of raised left atrial pressure. Since 2012, ARDS is clinically diagnosed using the Berlin definition (**Table 2**), which iterated on the AECC definition by introducing 3 distinct categories of ARDS based on Pao_2/Fio_2: mild 300 mm Hg or less, moderate 200 mm Hg or less, and severe 100 mm Hg or less.[12] Acuteness of the symptoms was time-bound to 7 days and a patient must be receiving 5 cm H_2O of positive end-expiratory pressure (PEEP) at the time of diagnosis. Finally, the absence of cardiac failure need not be established formally and a clinical assessment would suffice. The introduction of these broad clinical diagnoses that are agnostic to the initiating insult makes the pursuit of uniform biological responses in ARDS seem counterintuitive, if not entirely unrealistic. Therefore, there has been a growing trend toward seeking more uniform subgroups within which to study ARDS biology.[13]

HISTOPATHOLOGY IN ACUTE RESPIRATORY DISTRESS SYNDROME

First described by Katzenstein and colleagues,[14] the term diffuse alveolar damage (DAD) refers to the histopathological findings of alveolar epithelial and endothelial cell injury with fluid and cellular exudate and presence of hyaline membranes and/or fibrosis. DAD has long been considered the hallmark histologic finding in ARDS. Bachofen and Weibel[15] differentiated these histopathological changes in ARDS temporally into the following 3 phases: (1) exudative (early) phase characterized by interstitial

Table 2
The Berlin definition for clinical diagnosis of acute respiratory distress syndrome

Variable	Criteria
Timing	Within 1 wk of clinical insult or worsening respiratory symptoms
Chest imaging[a]	Bilateral opacities not fully explained by effusion, collapse, or nodules
Origin of pulmonary edema	Respiratory failure not fully explained by a cardiac cause or fluid overload
Oxygenation	
Mild	200 mm Hg < $Pao_2/Fio_2 \leq$ 300 mm Hg with PEEP or CPAP $\geq$ 5 cm H_2O
Moderate	100 mm Hg < $Pao_2/Fio_2 \leq$ 200 mm Hg with PEEP $\geq$ 5 cm H_2O
Severe	$Pao_2/Fio_2 \leq$ 100 mm Hg with PEEP $\geq$ 5 cm H_2O

Abbreviations: PEEP, positive end-expiratory pressure; CPAP, continuous positive airway pressure.
  [a] Either chest radiograph or computed tomographic scans could be used for the imaging criteria.

edema and capillary and neutrophilic infiltrates, (2) proliferative (subacute) phase characterize by proliferation of alveolar type II cells and fibroblast infiltration, and (3) fibrotic (late) phase associated with collagen deposition, macrophage infiltrates, and resolution of the exudative phase. More recently, Thille and colleagues[16] studied 159 patients who corroborated these histologic phases of ARDS in the presence of DAD; albeit, there is considerably greater overlap between the phases than previously described.

During the development of the Berlin definitions, the investigators considered DAD a key morphologic finding in ARDS and part of the conceptual framework the definition intended to capture. Yet, given the nonspecificity of the Berlin definition and its predecessor, the AECC definition, it is likely that while DAD is being captured, so are many other pathologic morphologies, including those unrelated to ARDS. To that end, only approximately half the patients who meet the clinical criteria for ARDS have DAD on autopsy.[17–21] Even in open biopsy studies, DAD was observed in the same proportion of patients.[22–24] Consistent among these studies was that DAD was more prevalent in severe ARDS and associated with worse outcomes. In a meta-analysis of patients who met ARDS criteria and underwent open lung biopsies, Cardinal-Fernandez and colleagues[25] found an array of heterogeneous morphologies in those meeting patients without DAD, with no single entity featuring in greater than 10% of the samples. Among specimens without DAD, most were consistent with histologic patterns of infective pneumonia.

From these studies, it is difficult to ascertain whether DAD, a consistent finding in experimental animal models of ARDS[26] and in human autopsies pre-AECC/Berlin definition, was inaccurately described historically or whether the clinical definitions of ARDS are poorly specific of acute inflammatory lung injury. Furthermore, the clinical utility of histopathology studies is naturally limited due to either being performed at autopsy or necessitating invasive biopsies. Nonetheless, further autopsy studies are needed to better map cellular abnormalities at different phases of ARDS. Incorporating innovative methods to studying lung tissue, such as next-generation sequencing[27] and cryomicro-computed tomographic (CT) imaging,[28] offers opportunities to gain novel insights in ARDS pathophysiology and should be considered in future investigations.

CLINICAL RADIOLOGY IN ACUTE RESPIRATORY DISTRESS SYNDROME
Quantitative Chest Radiograph

The chest radiograph is included in the definition of ARDS to assess the presence of alveolar edema, and bilateral opacification is used as a qualitative surrogate. A quantitative assessment of the amount of edema would reflect severity of ARDS. The Lung Injury Score (LIS) was an early attempt at quantification that integrated the number of affected quadrants with physiologic parameters into a risk score.[29] LIS was used to enrich the study population in the CESAR (conventional ventilatory support versus extracorporeal membrane oxygenation for severe adult respiratory failure) trial, which tested veno-venous extracorporeal membrane oxygenation to conventional ventilatory support in severe ARDS.[30]

More recently, the Radiographic Assessment of Lung Edema (RALE) score has been developed to further quantify chest radiographic abnormalities in ARDS.[31] The RALE score is calculated by summing the products of the consolidation and density for each radiograph quadrant. The RALE gives a maximal score of 12 for each quadrant resulting in a maximum total score of 48. The consolidation score quantifies the extent of alveolar opacities in each quadrant: (none: 0 points; < 25%: 1 point; 25%–50%: 2 points; 50%–75%: 3 points; > 75%: 4 points), whereas alveolar opacification in each quadrant is scored up to 3 points (hazy: 1 point; moderate: 2 points; dense: 3 points).[31] The RALE score correlated significantly with extravascular lung water in donor lungs and was found to predict survival at the time of ARDS diagnosis. Changing scores over time added to these predictions, where an increasing RALE score had a higher mortality than those with an improving score.[32] Use of the RALE score provides empirical evidence for a common observation in clinical practice, namely, that patients with progressive infiltrative abnormalities have worse outcomes. In future trials, the RALE score may be used as a surrogate end point for therapeutic response or provide objective prognostic enrichment of patients with ARDS.

Chest Computer Tomography

Chest CT provides considerable information additional to chest radiographs. CT is considered the gold standard tool for quantification gas volumes and weight of consolidated lung tissue.[33] With this purpose, it has been used to monitor the effect of recruitment maneuvers on lung volume and reaeration of consolidations.[34] Since the early days of chest CT, considerable heterogeneity in morphology has been observed in ARDS, and for more than 20 years investigators have sought methods to identify meaningful subgroups.[35]

The following three morphologic patterns are differentiated: (1) a focal morphology with a basal-dorsal dominance of consolidations, (2) a patchy morphology with islands of consolidation or ground glass separated by spared areas throughout all lobes, and (3) a diffuse morphology with similar involvement of all lobes without any clear gradient.[36] Patients with patchy and diffuse morphology are nowadays grouped together into a nonfocal phenotype. Lungs with nonfocal morphology are easier to recruit and less prone to overdistention compared with focal morphology.[37]

In the LIVE (Personalised mechanical ventilation tailored to lung morphology versus low positive end-expiratory pressure for patients with ARDS) study, patients were randomized to receive uniform lung protective mechanical ventilation or a lung morphology-driven ventilation. In the personalized ventilation group patients with a nonfocal lung morphology received small tidal volume of 6 mL/kg predicted body weight (PBW) and routine recruitment maneuvers and prone positioning was used as a rescue therapy. Patients with focal lung morphology received higher tidal volumes of 8 mL/kg PBW and lower PEEP strategy and prone positioning was mandatory.[38] The study showed no benefit of the personalized ventilation strategy in the intention-to-treat analysis. However, the morphologic pattern misclassification by the treating physician was 21% and personalized intervention was associated with harm in this group, whereas the control group was not. Taken together, the results of this study provide a strong warning against premature classification of patients into subphenotypes because of the possibility of harm and the real-world challenges of CT interpretation.

Lung Ultrasonography

Lung ultrasonography (LUS) is an attractive alternative to radiation-dependent imaging techniques because images can be obtained at the bedside and provide a comprehensive and rapid overview of subpleural lung aeration. The global LUS score correlates well with extravascular lung water measured using invasive techniques[39] and can be used to estimate reaeration of the lung after a recruitment maneuver.[40] Given the nonspecificity of chest radiographs and complexity of CT imaging, an algorithmic approach based on LUS might be an attractive alternative, although this has yet to be systematically investigated.

Perfusion Scanning

With the increased availability of chest CT scanning, our knowledge about lung aeration and its response to PEEP has increased considerably. Yet, impaired oxygenation secondary to functional shunt encountered in ARDS is insufficiently understood.[41] Perfusion remains the dark side of ventilation-perfusion matching owing to a lack of tools for anatomic assessment of perfusion in critically ill patients. CT chest images acquired during intravenous contrast infusion have been used to estimate regional perfusion with a subsequent mathematical estimation of the match between ventilation (aeration) and perfusion. Dakin and colleagues used this approach and found that the amount of perfusion to consolidated lung areas (a surrogate for functional shunt) negatively correlated with Pa_{O_2}/Fi_{O_2}.[42] Few other such studies, however, have been applied in critical care. Assessing and understanding functional perfusion abnormalities in relation to heterogeneity of lung aeration, and in response to ventilatory changes, represents a key unmet challenge toward better understanding ARDS pathogenesis.

BIOMARKERS IN ACUTE RESPIRATORY DISTRESS SYNDROME

Although bronchoalveolar lavage fluid (BALF) is most proximal to the site of injury and likely the most relevant sample to study, the requirement of a bronchoscopy and inconsistencies in sample dilution have meant that BALF analysis is not routinely performed clinically and remains poorly studied in human subjects. Recent reviews have covered the role of biomarkers in BALF in understanding the pathogenesis of ARDS including animal studies[13,43] and a meta-analysis in human subjects.[44] In this section of the review, we focus primarily on plasma biomarkers.

The Injured Alveoli

A biological marker for ARDS is sorely lacking; however, finding such a biomarker is extremely challenging. We know that endothelial and epithelial cell injury is integral in ARDS pathogenesis and several biomarkers exist that are informative of injury to these cells. However, the extent to which each of these cells is injured is variable and dependent on the severity and mechanism of injury.

Calfee and colleagues[45] observed that levels of circulating biomarkers of epithelial injury, such as surfactant protein-D (SP-D) and soluble receptor for advanced glycation endproducts (sRAGE), were higher in direct injury (eg, pneumonia or aspiration), whereas the level of angiopoietin-2 (ang-2), a marker of endothelial injury, was higher in indirect injury (eg, sepsis). sRAGE levels in the plasma have been studied extensively in ARDS, and elevated levels are associated with disease severity, adverse clinical outcomes, and diffuse changes on CT scans of the lungs.[46–49] Although sRAGE is promising, its specificity to ARDS remains uncertain and has been implicated as a marker of severity in community-acquired pneumonia[50] and in sepsis.[51,52]

Markers of endothelial injury are also elevated in ARDS and specifically sepsis-associated ARDS.[53] Elevated level of Ang-2 is known to be associated with increased risk of developing ARDS[54] and associated with worse clinical outcomes.[55] Similarly, elevated levels of plasma von Willebrand factor (vWF), another marker of endothelial activation, were associated with worse outcomes in ARDS.[56]

Biomarkers of coagulopathy/fibrinolysis and the extracelllular matrix (ECM) are other components of the alveolar unit that have been studied in ARDS. Taking coagulopathy first, plasminogen activator inhibitor-1 and protein C have both been associated with adverse clinical outcomes.[57] In the pediatric population, plasma matrix metalloproteinases 8 and 9, markers of ECM injury, have been associated with prolonged ventilation in ARDS[58] and used to identify clusters with divergent clinical outcomes.[59] Inflammasome activity, as measured by interleukin (IL)-18 levels, is also known to be associated with adverse outcomes in ARDS.[60,61]

Despite several biomarkers of endothelial and epithelial injury known to be elevated in ARDS, these findings have yet to translate to meaningful therapies. In part, this is because the linkage of elevated biomarkers to function remains unestablished. The described pragmatic human translational studies are not the suitable experimental domain to address mechanistic roles for these molecules and highlight a major limitation of such approaches.

Inflammatory Biomarkers: A Special Case for Phenotyping

Given ARDS is an acute inflammatory condition, it is unsurprising that proinflammatory and anti-inflammatory cytokines have been extensively studied in ARDS.[62] IL-1β, IL-1, IL-6, IL-8, IL-10, and soluble tumor necrosis factor (sTNFR)-1 have all been associated with clinical outcomes in ARDS. However, none of these biomarkers are specific to ARDS and are known to be elevated in other inflammatory conditions. Furthermore, it is unclear whether elevated levels of these biomarkers are contributing to pathogenesis of ARDS or merely reflecting an increased burden of systemic inflammation.

To maximize the informative potential of protein biomarkers, increasingly, investigators are using a combination of biomarkers to identify subgroups or clusters within ARDS populations using unbiased approaches. This genre of research, known as phenotyping, has become prominent in ARDS[63] and critical care research.[64] Work from our group has used a combination of protein biomarkers, vital signs, ventilatory variables, laboratory variables, and demographics to identify unmeasured clusters using latent class analysis (LCA). LCA is an unbiased probabilistic modeling algorithm that seeks to identify uniform subgroups in multivariate distributions.[65] Consistently, in independent secondary analyses of 5 randomized controlled trials (RCTs), we have identified 2 phenotypes of ARDS called the hypoinflammatory and hyperinflammatory phenotypes.[66–69] The hyperinflammatory phenotype is associated with higher levels of proinflammatory cytokines including IL-6, IL-8, sTNFR-1, and intracellular adhesion molecule-1. In addition, the hyperinflammatory phenotype is also associated with increased incidence of shock, lower protein C levels, and elevated markers of end-organ dysfunction including creatinine and bilirubin (**Fig. 2**). From a pathophysiological standpoint, proportions of patients with nonpulmonary sepsis were significantly higher in hyperinflammatory phenotype, whereas pulmonary infections were significantly higher in the hypoinflammatory phenotype. Markers of endothelial activation (ang-2, vWF) were higher in the hyperinflammatory phenotype,[67] whereas the epithelial marker SP-D was lower.[66] sRAGE another epithelial marker was higher in the hyperinflammatory phenotype.

Expectedly, mortality and ventilator days were significantly higher in the hyperinflammatory phenotype in all analyses (**Table 3**). Furthermore, divergent outcomes were observed in the phenotypes to randomized interventions in 3 of these trials to PEEP strategy,[66] fluid management strategy,[67] and statin therapy.[68] The complexity of the LCA models, however, is a barrier to the identification of these phenotypes prospectively. To circumnavigate this, we developed models that either use a parsimonious set of biomarkers[70] or readily available clinical data only.[71] Both approaches were able to classify phenotypes accurately, and the divergent treatment responses were also observable using these clinically practical models. The models require prospective validation before they can be used in the clinical setting.

Bos and colleagues[72] used a similar panel of biomarkers (IL-1β, IL-6, IL-8, TNF-α, IL-10, IL-13, interferon gamma, etc) to identify clusters in ARDS. Their approach

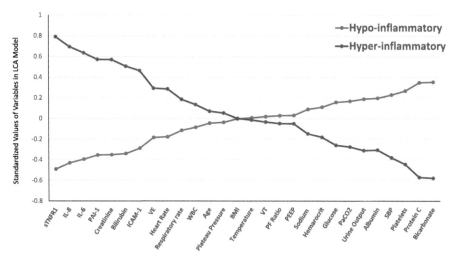

Fig. 2. Standardized values for continuous class-predicting variables. The variables are sorted from left to right in descending order for the difference in values between the hyper-inflammatory and hypoinflammatory subphenotype. Standardized values were calculated by assigning the mean of the variables as 0 and standard deviation as 1. The variables at the extreme left and right of the horizontal axis are the most important phenotype-defining variables. BMI, body mass index; SBP, systolic blood pressure; ICAM-1, intercellular adhesion molecule-1; IL, interleukin; PAI-1, plasminogen activator inhibitor-1; PEEP, positive end-expiratory pressure; sTNFR1, soluble tumor necrosis factor receptor-1; VE, minute ventilation; VT, tidal volume; WBC, white blood cell count.

differed from the above-mentioned phenotyping scheme in that they restricted their predictor variables to protein biomarker and used hierarchical clustering. The investigators also observed 2 clusters of ARDS, which they termed inflamed and uninflamed.[72] As with the hyperinflammatory phenotype, the inflamed phenotype was associate with elevated proinflammatory cytokines and worse clinical outcomes. It remains unclear how much overlap there is between these different approaches of identifying clusters in ARDS. However, from a multitude of these studies, it seems

Table 3
Mortality at day 90 in the 2 latent class analysis-derived acute respiratory distress syndrome phenotypes

Trials	Hypo-inflammatory	Hyper-inflammatory	P Value
ARMA (low vs high V$_T$)	23%	44%	.006
ALVEOLI (low vs high PEEP)	19%	51%	< .0001
FACTT (conservative vs liberal fluid management)	22%	45%	< .0001
HARP2 (simvastatin vs placebo)	22%	47%	< .0001
SAILS (rosuvastatin vs placebo)	21%	38%	< .0001

Abbreviations: ARMA, low tidal volume versus high tidal volume trial; ALVEOLI, Assessment of Low Tidal Volume and Elevated End-Expiratory Pressure to Obviate Lung Injury; FACTT, Fluids and Catheters Treatment Trial; HARP-2, Hydroxymethylglutaryl-CoA Reductase Inhibition in Acute Lung Injury to Reduce Pulmonary Dysfunction; SAILS, Statins for Acutely Injured Lungs from Sepsis.

apparent that concealed within ARDS are 2 biologically distinct subgroups that are primarily differentiated by their circulating inflammatory responses.

Among the remaining questions, 4 require urgent consideration. (1) Are these phenotypes temporally stable and over what period of time? (2) Are these phenotypes specific to ARDS or generalizable to other inflammatory conditions? (3) Among the various approaches, which scheme should be used to uniformly identify the hyperinflammatory state in the clinical setting or clinical trial? (4) What are the optimal candidate interventions that could be evaluated in phenotype-specific trial? From a biological standpoint, it is unclear if the observed responses that define the phenotypes are always deleterious or whether they are part of a well-conserved inflammatory response. Addressing these issues will mostly likely lead to successful therapies in ARDS.

GENOMICS AND TRANSCRIPTOMICS IN ACUTE RESPIRATORY DISTRESS SYNDROME
Genomic Predisposition for Lung Injury

Several genomic approaches have been used to assess predisposition to ARDS. Genome-wide association studies may facilitate our understanding of ARDS pathogenesis by identifying genes that increase the likelihood of ARDS development. However, because ARDS is a complication from an underlying condition, these analyses require correction for the likelihood of common risk factors such as sepsis or pneumonia. An additional concern with these studies is the lack of reproducibility in independent datasets.[73] An important next step toward understanding the genuine implication of a genetic variant in the pathogenesis of ARDS is Mendelian randomization studies, an approach that allows evaluation of causal of a modifiable exposure on disease based on genetic variance.[74]

ANGPT2, the gene that encodes for ANG2 expression, was found to be related to the development of ARDS in a sepsis population.[75] Importantly, this risk was mediated via an increase in plasma ANG2 concentration, suggesting a possible causal pathway. A similar approach was taken for sRAGE. Plasma sRAGE was strongly related to genetic variation and to the occurrence of ARDS in a sepsis cohort, suggesting that it acts as a causal intermediate in ARDS development.[76] Now that this approach has been taken for a marker of endothelial and epithelial injury, likely additional markers implicated as central in the pathogenesis of ARDS need evaluating through such studies.

Transcriptomic Alterations Related to Lung Injury

Transcriptomics analysis is the comprehensive assessment of messenger RNA from blood or tissue and provides insight in the complex interaction between genomics (providing the genetic potential) and exposures (resulting in the protein transcription of those genes). Therefore, it could potentially provide more information on the state a patient is in than genomic analysis alone. Gene expression of blood leukocytes has frequently been used to quantify the host response in critical illness in general and ARDS more specifically. In an analysis of multiple observational ARDS cohorts, Sweeney and colleagues[77] found that 30 genes were associated with ARDS; however, after adjusting for severity of systemic inflammation, none of these genes were significant, leading the investigators to conclude that plasma transcriptomics is unlikely to be a meaningful tool in ARDS. It is worth noting that this was a retrospective analysis of data extracted from public repositories where the ARDS diagnosis was uncertain, and the populations included adults and children. Two approaches may provide further insight into the gene expression in ARDS: (1) focus more on gene expression in the organ of interest, the lung, and (2) account for the biological heterogeneity observed in ARDS when analyzing blood gene expression profiles.

A limited number of studies have focused on gene expression in pulmonary samples from ARDS. In a hallmark study, Morrell and colleagues[78] simultaneously evaluated expression profiles of alveolar macrophages to those of peripheral blood monocytes (PBMs) in ARDS. The investigators observed that gene expression was profoundly different between these compartments and that enrichment of immune-inflammatory gene sets was associated with a favorable outcome in alveolar macrophages but an unfavorable outcome in PBMs, demonstrating distinct implication of inflammatory responses that may be compartment and cell specific.

The second approach was taken by Bos and colleagues[79] in a posthoc analysis of blood leukocyte expression obtained from patients with suspected sepsis and ARDS. Patients were classified into 2 subphenotypes based on plasma biomarkers of inflammation, coagulation, and endothelial injury as discussed in the section on Biomarkers in acute respiratory distress syndrome. Subsequently, expression profiles were compared between subphenotypes rather than with and without ARDS. The investigators reported that around 30% of genes were differentially expressed between the subphenotypes, with an enrichment of neutrophil-related genes in the reactive (inflamed) subphenotype. Furthermore, the genes that were most upregulated in the reactive subphenotype also discriminated between ARDS and a control group with sepsis but without ARDS. These data suggest that patients with the reactive subphenotype have a distinct gene expression profile related to neutrophil activation, oxidative phosphorylation, and cholesterol metabolism.

INSIGHTS FROM NOVEL BIOLOGICAL MEASUREMENT SYSTEMS
Metabolomics

The advent of mass spectrometry (MS) and nuclear magnetic resonance (NMR) to study high-throughput metabolites has seen the emergence of the field metabolomics over the past 2 decades. Despite its growing use to study human biology, its application in ARDS remains in its infancy.[80] In a small pilot study, Stringer and colleagues[81] studied plasma metabolites using NMR in sepsis-induced ARDS versus healthy volunteers, and metabolites pertaining to oxidant stress, energy homeostasis, apoptosis, and endothelial barrier function distinguished ARDS from healthy volunteers. Other investigators have subsequently studied differences between plasma metabolites in ARDS versus ventilated controls,[82] or healthy controls,[83] with similar findings. MS has been used to study metabolites in edema fluid or BALF in patients with ARDS. When compared with controls, metabolites of oxidative stress (glutamate and proline) were elevated in ARDS.[84,85] Differences in ARDS from controls were consistently observed; however, most of these described studies are limited by samples size (<30).

In the largest study of its kind, Viswan and colleagues[86] took a different approach to see whether they can differentiate severity and etiologic sites (pulmonary vs extrapulmonary) of ARDS using metabolic profile. Both serum (n = 176) and BALF (n = 146) metabolic profiles showed good performance metric at differentiating ARDS severity; however, the ability to discriminate site of injury was poor. These findings were correspondent with an earlier work of Bos and colleagues[87] who studied the discriminatory properties of exhaled breath metabolites in ARDS.

Lipidomics is another growing field in human biology and uses MS/NMR to study high-throughput quantification of lipids in biological compartments. Fatty acid-derived lipid mediators are critical in the regulation of the inflammatory response. Specifically, the role of lipid proresolving mediators in the resolution and homeostatic normalization of inflammation is being increasingly recognized.[88,89] Lipidomics in critical illness is largely unexplored and perhaps represents a new frontier in our understanding of systems biology, particularly, given the ubiquity of these molecules both intracellularly and extracellularly. Future studies in human subjects profiling the lipidome in ARDS and their functional role are eagerly anticipated.

MICROBIOME IN ACUTE RESPIRATORY DISTRESS SYNDROME
Lung Microbiome is Altered by Invasive Mechanical Ventilation

Until about a decade ago, the lung was considered sterile under normal conditions. Since then, culture-independent techniques for the detection and identification of microbiota have provided expansive insights into the lung microbiome in health and disease. The lung microbiome is shaped by 3 factors: (1) immigration of microorganism into the lung, (2) elimination of microorganisms through microbial killing and immigration via cough and mucocilliairy clearance, and (3) locoregional growth circumstances that act as selective pressures on certain types of microorganisms.[90] During intubation and invasive mechanical ventilation, these forces are disturbed significantly.[91] Therefore, it is unsurprising that duration of mechanical ventilation is one of the most important factors driving the change in lung microbiome in critically ill patients.[92]

The Complex Relation Between Lung Injury and Microbial Composition

As lung injury occurs, additional nutrients become heterogeneously available in the lung and may further perpetuate regional growth differences and impose selective pressures toward specific microorganisms.[93,94] Simultaneously, specific bacteria seem to be enriched in the lung microbiome at the moment ARDS is diagnosed and invasive mechanical ventilation is initiated.[95,96] Furthermore, in these 2 independent studies, performed on 2 different continents, the same enrichment of gut bacteria was found to be related to ARDS and predicted unfavorable outcome.[95,96] Taken together these findings suggest that (1) changes in microbial composition in the lung may precede lung injury and play a role in ARDS pathogenesis and (2) findings of microbiome disruption are agnostic to interindividual and regional heterogeneity in microbial composition and antimicrobial practices. Future studies need to further clarify the causal relation between microbial dysbiosis and lung injury.

CORONAVIRUS DISEASE 2019

COVID-19, the disease caused by SARS-CoV-2 virus, has transformed the clinical landscape of ARDS. At the time of writing, 74 million people have been infected with more than 1.6 million deaths. Many, if not most, patients who were admitted to the intensive care unit (ICU) with COVID-19 have met the criteria for ARDS. Currently, there are more than 21,000 patients admitted to the ICU in the United States, and the annual incidence of ARDS will have increased by several folds, if not by an order of magnitude, in 2020. Despite these staggering numbers, the precise pathophysiology of COVID-19 ARDS remains largely unmapped.

As with all causes of acutely injured lungs, the central schema of pathophysiological abnormalities in the COVID-19 remains the same, that is, injury of the epithelia, endothelia, and ECM. To what extent each of these architectural domains is injured and what the principal drivers of this injury may be require further elucidating.

Insights from Histopathology

Given the biosafety constraints of studying SARS-COV-2 in experimental models, findings at autopsy have been singularly informative in appreciating the pathophysiology of lung injury in COVID-19. Consistent among almost all studies that report autopsy finding of the lungs is DAD.[97] Borczuk and colleagues[98] in a multicenter study reported autopsy findings in 68 deceased patients and observed DAD in most patients with virus detectable in alveolar type II cells and airway epithelia. It has been postulated that as SARS-CoV-2 spike protein binds to angiotensin-converting enzyme (ACE)-2 receptor to gain cellular entry and given the abundance of these receptors on endothelial cells, COVID-19 is associated with increased endothelial activation and thromboembolic phenomena. To that end, these investigators also observed thrombi present in large vessel of the lungs in the 42% of the cases at autopsy.

Elsewhere, in a case series of 80 patients, Edler and colleagues observed large vessel thrombi in the lungs in only 21% of the patients; however, if they included deep vein thrombosis, the cumulative large vessel thrombi were 40%.[99] In a small study comparing COVID-19 to influenza at autopsy, the findings of thromboembolic phenomena were almost double in the former,[100] and these findings were corroborated when rates were compared between COVID-19 and historical influenza data.[101] It is unclear whether the thromboembolic phenomena are due to direct invasion of the endothelial cells or a hypercoagulable state or both. The presence of virus in endothelial cells[102] and in organs outside of the respiratory tract[103] would suggest that direct viral pathogenicity is a plausible theory.

Insights from Imaging

Early reports on CT images from patients with COVID-19 ARDS speculated that it was characterized by normal lung volumes with severe hypoxemia.[104] Subsequent studies were unable to show that lung volumes are preserved and showed no relation between compliance of the respiratory system and the extent of parenchymal involvement.[105,106] In line with histopathological findings, perfusion defects have been consistently detected on lung imaging of COVID-19 ARDS (**Fig. 3**) irrespective of the presence of pulmonary embolism and are likely reflective of the microthrombi.[107–109]

Insights from Biomarkers

A frequently described theory in COVID-19 is that a cytokine storm is the key driver of disease severity.[110,111] Closer scrutiny of the described levels of proinflammatory cytokines such as IL-6 in COVID-19 would suggest that, although elevated above normal, they were much lower than those described in historical cohorts of ARDS.[112] In a systematic review, when proinflammatory cytokine levels in COVID-19 were compared with the hyperinflammatory phenotype of ARDS, sepsis, or cytokine release syndrome (post chiemeric antigen receptor T cell therapy), the levels were significantly lower.[113] D-dimer levels in severe COVID-19 were higher compared with historical critical care cohorts, suggesting a common theme of a hypercoagulable state. Other investigators have similarly observed attenuated IL-6 and IL-8 levels in COVID-19 compared with non-COVID-19 ARDS.[114,115]

A prospective exploratory analysis of COVID-19 ARDS suggested that the prevalence of the hyperinflammatory phenotype was between 11% and 21% compared with 30% observed in non-COVID-19 ARDS.[116] Together, these findings suggest that circulating inflammatory biomarkers may not be critical or unique in the pathophysiology of COVID-19 ARDS. Yet, mortality in COVID-19 ARDS is considerably higher. Rather than ruminating on the cytokine storm, a more intriguing question to ask is what biological phenomenon is driving injury in the lung and the observed excess mortality? As a unifying biological hypothesis, we speculate that COVID-19 ARDS is associated with a more immunosuppressive state, either systemically or locally in the lungs, which in turn leads to impaired

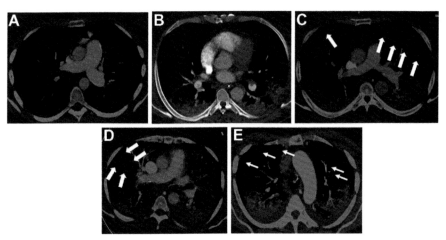

Fig. 3. CT pulmonary angiography and dual-energy CT (DECT) perfusion in coronavirus disease 2019 (COVID-19)-related ARDS. (*A*) DECT perfused volume map of a patient without COVID-19 and no pulmonary embolism (control). The image is notable for homogeneous coloring throughout both lungs (indicating normal iodine distribution and normal perfusion). (*B*) Soft tissue reconstruction showing filling defects in lower lobe pulmonary arteries (*arrows*) in a 42-year patient with COVID-19. (*C*) Corresponding DECT color map showing widespread perfusion defects (*arrows*) in the same patient 42-year-old patient. (*D*) Example of wedge-shaped perfusion defect on DECT color map. (*E*) Example of mottled generalized perfusion defect on DECT color map. (*Courtesy of* Dr Brijesh V. Patel and Professor Sujal R. Desai, London, UK).

viral clearance and the ensuing epithelial injury and hypercoagulable state that are consistently observed. The absence/attenuation of interferon responses have been observed in COVID-19 and are shown to be associated with adverse outcomes.[117] This hypothesis needs testing in both the lung and circulating compartments.

FUTURE DIRECTIONS

In the context of the current understanding of ARDS with its clinical diagnosis, conceptually, it is perhaps easiest to comprehend its pathophysiology as a graded permutation of injuries to the 4 components of the alveolar unit: the epithelium, endothelium, extracellular matrix, and coagulopathy of the microvasculature. The prototype injury of each anatomic domain is represented in **Fig. 4**. Clearly, these are not mutually exclusive injury types; however, the extent to which a domain principally drives the global lung injury is likely to be dependent on the original insult. Among these staggering numbers of patients with COVID-19, it is worth acknowledging that all cases are due to a single pathogen; this is noteworthy because critical care is accustomed to managing nebulous clinical syndromes with multiple causes. Yet, from a biological standpoint, understanding a unifying pathophysiology in COVID-19 has been exceedingly challenging. It is then worth asking, what are the probabilities of making such a biological discovery in ARDS if we persist with its clinical diagnosis?

Regardless, the steps needed to better understand the biology of the disease and the clinical syndrome are the same. Studies are needed where biological measurements are simultaneously made in the lungs and the circulation and over multiple timepoints using multidimensional data types. The heterogeneity subsumed within these diagnoses needs to be broken down into biologically intuitive subgroups that are empirically derived. Finally, a central challenge facing the specialty is to harness these

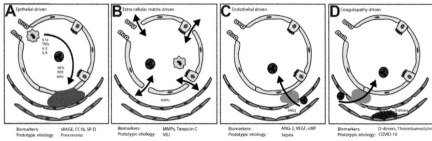

Fig. 4. Prototype injury schema in the anatomic components of the alveolar unit in ARDS. (*A*) Epithelial-dominant injury: associated with cellular infiltrates and alveolar flooding, prototypically seen in pneumonia-associated ARDS and may be neutrophil driven. (*B*) Extracellular matrix-dominant injury: associated with persistent inflammatory signaling due to stress to the extracellular matrix, prototypically seen with in ventilator-induced lung injury (VILI). (*C*) Endothelial-dominant injury: associated with endothelial dysfunction and interstitial edema and proteinaceous exudates leading to increased extravascular lung water; prototypically seen in sepsis-induced ARDS. (*D*) Coagulopathy-dominant injury: this is associated with intravascular thromboembolic phenomena with extensive microthrombi in the pulmonary microvasculature; prototypically seen in COVID-19-associated ARDS. It is worth emphasizing that these figures represent extreme prototypes of the anatomic injuries and most ARDS cases are combination of the injuries to these sites. IL, interleukin; TNF, tumor necrosis factor receptor; NET, neutrophil extracellular traps; ROS, reactive oxygen species; MPO, myeloperoxidase; sRAGE, soluble receptor for advanced glycation endproduct; CC16, Clara cell 16; SP-D, surfactant protein-D; MMP, matrix metalloproteinases; Ang-2, angiopoeitin-2; VEGF, vascular endothelial growth factor; vWF, von Willebrand factor.

high-throughput data and translate it into a therapy that benefits patients with lung injury testing hypotheses in more experimental models.

CLINICS CARE POINTS

- Radiological assessment of patients with CT scans, perfusion scans, and LUS may offer novel insights into the pathologic and physiologic abnormalities in ARDS
- Bedside quantification of protein biomarkers can lead to diagnosis of phenotypes or disease states that may be amenable to phenotype-specific trials in the near future
- In COVID-19 and non-COVID-19, the mainstay of the management of patients with ARDS remains delivery of high-quality critical care with the least injurious support of mechanical ventilation

ACKNOWLEDGMENTS

Fig. 3 was courtesy of Dr Brijesh V Patel and Professor Sujal R Desai, Departments of Adult Critical Care Units and Radiology, Royal Brompton & Harefield NHS Foundation Trust, London, UK.

DISCLOSURE

Dr P. Sinha has no conflict of interest to declare. Dr L.D. Bos reports grants from the Dutch Lung Foundation (Young Investigator grant), grants from the Dutch Lung Foundation and Health-Holland (Public-Private Partnership grant), grants from the Dutch Lung Foundation (Dirkje Postma Award), grants from IMI COVID19 initiative, and grants from Amsterdam UMC fellowship, outside the submitted work.

REFERENCES

1. Bellani G, Laffey JG, Pham T, et al. Epidemiology, patterns of care, and mortality for patients with acute respiratory distress syndrome in intensive care units in 50 countries. JAMA 2016;315(8):788–800.
2. Ashbaugh DG, Bigelow DB, Petty TL, et al. Acute respiratory distress in adults. Lancet 1967;2(7511):319–23.
3. Matthay MA, Zemans RL, Zimmerman GA, et al. Acute respiratory distress syndrome. Nat Rev Dis Primers 2019;5(1):18.
4. Thompson BT, Chambers RC, Liu KD. Acute respiratory distress syndrome. N Engl J Med 2017;377(6):562–72.
5. Matthay MA, McAuley DF, Ware LB. Clinical trials in acute respiratory distress syndrome: challenges and opportunities. Lancet Respir Med 2017;5(6):524–34.
6. Bonniaud P, Fabre A, Frossard N, et al. Optimising experimental research in respiratory diseases: an ERS statement. Eur Respir J 2018;51(5).
7. Bain W, Matute-Bello G. Should we shift the paradigm of preclinical models for ARDS therapies? Thorax 2019;74(12):1109–10.
8. Matute-Bello G, Frevert CW, Martin TR. Animal models of acute lung injury. Am J Physiol Lung Cell Mol Physiol 2008;295(3):L379–99.
9. Juffermans NP, Schultz M, Bos LD, et al. Why translational research matters: proceedings of the third international symposium on acute lung injury translational research (INSPIRES III). Intensive Care Med Exp 2019;7(Suppl 1):40.
10. Meyer NJ, Calfee CS. Novel translational approaches to the search for precision therapies for acute respiratory distress syndrome. Lancet Respir Med 2017;5(6):512–23.
11. Acute Respiratory Distress Syndrome N, Brower RG, Matthay MA, et al. Ventilation with lower tidal volumes as compared with traditional tidal volumes for acute lung injury and the acute respiratory distress syndrome. N Engl J Med 2000;342(18):1301–8.
12. Force ADT, Ranieri VM, Rubenfeld GD, et al. Acute respiratory distress syndrome: the Berlin Definition. JAMA 2012;307(23):2526–33.
13. Matthay MA, Arabi YM, Siegel ER, et al. Phenotypes and personalized medicine in the acute respiratory distress syndrome. Intensive Care Med 2020;46(12):2136–52.
14. Katzenstein AL, Bloor CM, Leibow AA. Diffuse alveolar damage–the role of oxygen, shock, and related factors. A review. Am J Pathol 1976;85(1):209–28.
15. Bachofen M, Weibel ER. Alterations of the gas exchange apparatus in adult respiratory insufficiency associated with septicemia. Am Rev Respir Dis 1977;116(4):589–615.
16. Thille AW, Esteban A, Fernandez-Segoviano P, et al. Chronology of histological lesions in acute respiratory distress syndrome with diffuse alveolar damage: a prospective cohort study of clinical autopsies. Lancet Respir Med 2013;1(5):395–401.
17. Esteban A, Fernandez-Segoviano P, Frutos-Vivar F, et al. Comparison of clinical criteria for the acute respiratory distress syndrome with autopsy findings. Ann Intern Med 2004;141(6):440–5.
18. Pinheiro BV, Muraoka FS, Assis RV, et al. Accuracy of clinical diagnosis of acute respiratory distress syndrome in comparison with autopsy findings. J Bras Pneumol 2007;33(4):423–8.
19. de Hemptinne Q, Remmelink M, Brimioulle S, et al. ARDS: a clinicopathological confrontation. Chest 2009;135(4):944–9.

20. Sarmiento X, Guardiola JJ, Almirall J, et al. Discrepancy between clinical criteria for diagnosing acute respiratory distress syndrome secondary to community acquired pneumonia with autopsy findings of diffuse alveolar damage. Respir Med 2011;105(8):1170–5.

21. Thille AW, Esteban A, Fernandez-Segoviano P, et al. Comparison of the Berlin definition for acute respiratory distress syndrome with autopsy. Am J Respir Crit Care Med 2013;187(7):761–7.

22. Patel SR, Karmpaliotis D, Ayas NT, et al. The role of open-lung biopsy in ARDS. Chest 2004;125(1):197–202.

23. Guerin C, Bayle F, Leray V, et al. Open lung biopsy in nonresolving ARDS frequently identifies diffuse alveolar damage regardless of the severity stage and may have implications for patient management. Intensive Care Med 2015;41(2):222–30.

24. Park J, Lee YJ, Lee J, et al. Histopathologic heterogeneity of acute respiratory distress syndrome revealed by surgical lung biopsy and its clinical implications. Korean J Intern Med 2018;33(3):532–40.

25. Cardinal-Fernandez P, Bajwa EK, Dominguez-Calvo A, et al. The presence of diffuse alveolar damage on open lung biopsy is associated with mortality in patients with acute respiratory distress syndrome: a systematic review and meta-analysis. Chest 2016;149(5):1155–64.

26. Matute-Bello G, Downey G, Moore BB, et al. An official American Thoracic Society workshop report: features and measurements of experimental acute lung injury in animals. Am J Respir Cell Mol Biol 2011;44(5):725–38.

27. Nienhold R, Ciani Y, Koelzer VH, et al. Two distinct immunopathological profiles in autopsy lungs of COVID-19. Nat Commun 2020;11(1):5086.

28. Vasilescu DM, Phillion AB, Tanabe N, et al. Nondestructive cryomicro-CT imaging enables structural and molecular analysis of human lung tissue. J Appl Physiol (1985) 2017;122(1):161–9.

29. Murray JF, Matthay MA, Luce JM, et al. An expanded definition of the adult respiratory distress syndrome. Am Rev Respir Dis 1988;138(3):720–3.

30. Peek GJ, Mugford M, Tiruvoipati R, et al. Efficacy and economic assessment of conventional ventilatory support versus extracorporeal membrane oxygenation for severe adult respiratory failure (CESAR): a multicentre randomised controlled trial. Lancet 2009;374(9698):1351–63.

31. Warren MA, Zhao Z, Koyama T, et al. Severity scoring of lung oedema on the chest radiograph is associated with clinical outcomes in ARDS. Thorax 2018; 73(9):840–6.

32. Jabaudon M, Audard J, Pereira B, et al. Early changes over time in the radiographic assessment of lung edema score are associated with survival in ARDS. Chest 2020;158(6):2394–403.

33. Gattinoni L, Caironi P, Pelosi P, et al. What has computed tomography taught us about the acute respiratory distress syndrome? Am J Respir Crit Care Med 2001;164(9):1701–11.

34. Gattinoni L, Caironi P, Cressoni M, et al. Lung recruitment in patients with the acute respiratory distress syndrome. N Engl J Med 2006;354(17):1775–86.

35. Spragg RG, Levin D. ARDS and the search for meaningful subgroups. Intensive Care Med 2000;26(7):835–7.

36. Puybasset L, Cluzel P, Gusman P, et al. Regional distribution of gas and tissue in acute respiratory distress syndrome. I. Consequences for lung morphology. CT Scan ARDS Study Group. Intensive Care Med 2000;26(7):857–69.

37. Constantin JM, Grasso S, Chanques G, et al. Lung morphology predicts response to recruitment maneuver in patients with acute respiratory distress syndrome. Crit Care Med 2010;38(4):1108–17.
38. Constantin JM, Jabaudon M, Lefrant JY, et al. Personalised mechanical ventilation tailored to lung morphology versus low positive end-expiratory pressure for patients with acute respiratory distress syndrome in France (the LIVE study): a multicentre, single-blind, randomised controlled trial. Lancet Respir Med 2019; 7(10):870–80.
39. Shyamsundar M, Attwood B, Keating L, et al. Clinical review: the role of ultrasound in estimating extra-vascular lung water. Crit Care 2013;17(5):237.
40. Bouhemad B, Brisson H, Le-Guen M, et al. Bedside ultrasound assessment of positive end-expiratory pressure-induced lung recruitment. Am J Respir Crit Care Med 2011;183(3):341–7.
41. Cressoni M, Caironi P, Polli F, et al. Anatomical and functional intrapulmonary shunt in acute respiratory distress syndrome. Crit Care Med 2008;36(3):669–75.
42. Dakin J, Jones AT, Hansell DM, et al. Changes in lung composition and regional perfusion and tissue distribution in patients with ARDS. Respirology 2011;16(8): 1265–72.
43. Blondonnet R, Constantin JM, Sapin V, et al. A pathophysiologic approach to biomarkers in acute respiratory distress syndrome. Dis Markers 2016;2016: 3501373.
44. Wang Y, Wang H, Zhang C, et al. Lung fluid biomarkers for acute respiratory distress syndrome: a systematic review and meta-analysis. Crit Care 2019; 23(1):43.
45. Calfee CS, Janz DR, Bernard GR, et al. Distinct molecular phenotypes of direct vs indirect ARDS in single-center and multicenter studies. Chest 2015;147(6): 1539–48.
46. Calfee CS, Ware LB, Eisner MD, et al. Plasma receptor for advanced glycation end products and clinical outcomes in acute lung injury. Thorax 2008;63(12): 1083–9.
47. Jabaudon M, Blondonnet R, Roszyk L, et al. Soluble forms and ligands of the receptor for advanced glycation end-products in patients with acute respiratory distress syndrome: an observational prospective study. PLoS One 2015;10(8): e0135857.
48. Jabaudon M, Futier E, Roszyk L, et al. Soluble form of the receptor for advanced glycation end products is a marker of acute lung injury but not of severe sepsis in critically ill patients. Crit Care Med 2011;39(3):480–8.
49. Mrozek S, Jabaudon M, Jaber S, et al. Elevated plasma levels of sRAGE are associated with nonfocal CT-based lung imaging in patients with ARDS: a prospective multicenter study. Chest 2016;150(5):998–1007.
50. Narvaez-Rivera RM, Rendon A, Salinas-Carmona MC, et al. Soluble RAGE as a severity marker in community acquired pneumonia associated sepsis. BMC Infect Dis 2012;12:15.
51. Brodska H, Malickova K, Valenta J, et al. Soluble receptor for advanced glycation end products predicts 28-day mortality in critically ill patients with sepsis. Scand J Clin Lab Invest 2013;73(8):650–60.
52. Bopp C, Hofer S, Weitz J, et al. sRAGE is elevated in septic patients and associated with patients outcome. J Surg Res 2008;147(1):79–83.
53. Hendrickson CM, Matthay MA. Endothelial biomarkers in human sepsis: pathogenesis and prognosis for ARDS. Pulm Circ 2018;8(2). 2045894018769876.

54. Agrawal A, Matthay MA, Kangelaris KN, et al. Plasma angiopoietin-2 predicts the onset of acute lung injury in critically ill patients. Am J Respir Crit Care Med 2013;187(7):736–42.

55. Li F, Yin R, Guo Q. Circulating angiopoietin-2 and the risk of mortality in patients with acute respiratory distress syndrome: a systematic review and meta-analysis of 10 prospective cohort studies. Ther Adv Respir Dis 2020;14. 1753466620905274.

56. Ware LB, Eisner MD, Thompson BT, et al. Significance of von Willebrand factor in septic and nonseptic patients with acute lung injury. Am J Respir Crit Care Med 2004;170(7):766–72.

57. Ware LB, Koyama T, Billheimer DD, et al. Prognostic and pathogenetic value of combining clinical and biochemical indices in patients with acute lung injury. Chest 2010;137(2):288–96.

58. Kong MY, Li Y, Oster R, et al. Early elevation of matrix metalloproteinase-8 and -9 in pediatric ARDS is associated with an increased risk of prolonged mechanical ventilation. PLoS One 2011;6(8):e22596.

59. Zinter MS, Delucchi KL, Kong MY, et al. Early plasma matrix metalloproteinase profiles. A novel pathway in pediatric acute respiratory distress syndrome. Am J Respir Crit Care Med 2019;199(2):181–9.

60. Dolinay T, Kim YS, Howrylak J, et al. Inflammasome-regulated cytokines are critical mediators of acute lung injury. Am J Respir Crit Care Med 2012;185(11): 1225–34.

61. Rogers AJ, Guan J, Trtchounian A, et al. Association of elevated plasma interleukin-18 level with increased mortality in a clinical trial of statin treatment for acute respiratory distress syndrome. Crit Care Med 2019;47(8):1089–96.

62. Cross LJ, Matthay MA. Biomarkers in acute lung injury: insights into the pathogenesis of acute lung injury. Crit Care Clin 2011;27(2):355–77.

63. Sinha P, Calfee CS. Phenotypes in acute respiratory distress syndrome: moving towards precision medicine. Curr Opin Crit Care 2019;25(1):12–20.

64. Reddy K, Sinha P, O'Kane CM, et al. Subphenotypes in critical care: translation into clinical practice. Lancet Respir Med 2020;8(6):631–43.

65. Sinha P, Calfee CS, Delucchi KL. Practitioner's guide to latent class analysis: methodological considerations and common pitfalls. Crit Care Med 2021; 49(1):e63–79.

66. Calfee CS, Delucchi K, Parsons PE, et al. Subphenotypes in acute respiratory distress syndrome: latent class analysis of data from two randomised controlled trials. Lancet Respir Med 2014;2(8):611–20.

67. Famous KR, Delucchi K, Ware LB, et al. Acute respiratory distress syndrome subphenotypes respond differently to randomized fluid management strategy. Am J Respir Crit Care Med 2017;195(3):331–8.

68. Calfee CS, Delucchi KL, Sinha P, et al. Acute respiratory distress syndrome subphenotypes and differential response to simvastatin: secondary analysis of a randomised controlled trial. Lancet Respir Med 2018;6(9):691–8.

69. Sinha P, Delucchi KL, Thompson BT, et al. Latent class analysis of ARDS subphenotypes: a secondary analysis of the statins for acutely injured lungs from sepsis (SAILS) study. Intensive Care Med 2018;44(11):1859–69.

70. Sinha P, Delucchi KL, McAuley DF, et al. Development and validation of parsimonious algorithms to classify acute respiratory distress syndrome phenotypes: a secondary analysis of randomized controlled trials. Lancet Respir Med 2020; 8(3):247–57.

71. Sinha P, Churpek MM, Calfee CS. Machine learning classifier models can identify acute respiratory distress syndrome phenotypes using readily available clinical data. Am J Respir Crit Care Med 2020;202(7):996–1004.

72. Bos LD, Schouten LR, van Vught LA, et al. Identification and validation of distinct biological phenotypes in patients with acute respiratory distress syndrome by cluster analysis. Thorax 2017;72(10):876–83.

73. N-NWGoRiA Studies, Chanock SJ, Manolio T, et al. Replicating genotype-phenotype associations. Nature 2007;447(7145):655–60.

74. Davies NM, Holmes MV, Davey Smith G. Reading Mendelian randomisation studies: a guide, glossary, and checklist for clinicians. BMJ 2018;362:k601.

75. Reilly JP, Wang F, Jones TK, et al. Plasma angiopoietin-2 as a potential causal marker in sepsis-associated ARDS development: evidence from Mendelian randomization and mediation analysis. Intensive Care Med 2018;44(11):1849–58.

76. Jones TK, Feng R, Kerchberger VE, et al. Plasma sRAGE acts as a genetically regulated causal intermediate in sepsis-associated acute respiratory distress syndrome. Am J Respir Crit Care Med 2020;201(1):47–56.

77. Sweeney TE, Thomas NJ, Howrylak JA, et al. Multicohort analysis of whole-blood gene expression data does not form a robust diagnostic for acute respiratory distress syndrome. Crit Care Med 2018;46(2):244–51.

78. Morrell ED, Radella F 2nd, Manicone AM, et al. Peripheral and alveolar cell transcriptional programs are distinct in acute respiratory distress syndrome. Am J Respir Crit Care Med 2018;197(4):528–32.

79. Bos LDJ, Scicluna BP, Ong DSY, et al. Understanding heterogeneity in biologic phenotypes of acute respiratory distress syndrome by leukocyte expression profiles. Am J Respir Crit Care Med 2019;200(1):42–50.

80. Rogers AJ, Matthay MA. Applying metabolomics to uncover novel biology in ARDS. Am J Physiol Lung Cell Mol Physiol 2014;306(11):L957–61.

81. Stringer KA, Serkova NJ, Karnovsky A, et al. Metabolic consequences of sepsis-induced acute lung injury revealed by plasma (1)H-nuclear magnetic resonance quantitative metabolomics and computational analysis. Am J Physiol Lung Cell Mol Physiol 2011;300(1):L4–11.

82. Singh C, Rai RK, Azim A, et al. Metabolic profiling of human lung injury by H-1 high-resolution nuclear magnetic resonance spectroscopy of blood serum. Metabolomics 2015;11(1):166–74.

83. Lin SH, Yue X, Wu H, et al. Explore potential plasma biomarkers of acute respiratory distress syndrome (ARDS) using GC-MS metabolomics analysis. Clin Biochem 2019;66:49–56.

84. Evans CR, Karnovsky A, Kovach MA, et al. Untargeted LC-MS metabolomics of bronchoalveolar lavage fluid differentiates acute respiratory distress syndrome from health. J Proteome Res 2014;13(2):640–9.

85. Rogers AJ, Contrepois K, Wu M, et al. Profiling of ARDS pulmonary edema fluid identifies a metabolically distinct subset. Am J Physiol Lung Cell Mol Physiol 2017;312(5):L703–9.

86. Viswan A, Ghosh P, Gupta D, et al. Distinct metabolic endotype mirroring acute respiratory distress syndrome (ARDS) subphenotype and its heterogeneous biology. Sci Rep 2019;9(1):2108.

87. Bos LD, Weda H, Wang Y, et al. Exhaled breath metabolomics as a noninvasive diagnostic tool for acute respiratory distress syndrome. Eur Respir J 2014;44(1):188–97.

88. Serhan CN. Pro-resolving lipid mediators are leads for resolution physiology. Nature 2014;510(7503):92–101.

89. Colas RA, Shinohara M, Dalli J, et al. Identification and signature profiles for proresolving and inflammatory lipid mediators in human tissue. Am J Physiol Cell Physiol 2014;307(1):C39–54.

90. Dickson RP, Erb-Downward JR, Martinez FJ, et al. The microbiome and the respiratory tract. Annu Rev Physiol 2016;78:481–504.

91. Martin-Loeches I, Dickson R, Torres A, et al. The importance of airway and lung microbiome in the critically ill. Crit Care 2020;24(1):537.

92. Zakharkina T, Martin-Loeches I, Matamoros S, et al. The dynamics of the pulmonary microbiome during mechanical ventilation in the intensive care unit and the association with occurrence of pneumonia. Thorax 2017;72(9):803–10.

93. Scales BS, Dickson RP, Huffnagle GB. A tale of two sites: how inflammation can reshape the microbiomes of the gut and lungs. J Leukoc Biol 2016;100(5):943–50.

94. Dickson RP. The lung microbiome and ARDS. It is time to broaden the model. Am J Respir Crit Care Med 2018;197(5):549–51.

95. Panzer AR, Lynch SV, Langelier C, et al. Lung microbiota is related to smoking status and to development of acute respiratory distress syndrome in critically ill trauma patients. Am J Respir Crit Care Med 2018;197(5):621–31.

96. Dickson RP, Schultz MJ, van der Poll T, et al. Lung microbiota predict clinical outcomes in critically ill patients. Am J Respir Crit Care Med 2020;201(5):555–63.

97. Maiese A, Manetti AC, La Russa R, et al. Autopsy findings in COVID-19-related deaths: a literature review. Forensic Sci Med Pathol 2020.

98. Borczuk AC, Salvatore SP, Seshan SV, et al. COVID-19 pulmonary pathology: a multi-institutional autopsy cohort from Italy and New York City. Mod Pathol 2020;33(11):2156–68.

99. Edler C, Schroder AS, Aepfelbacher M, et al. Dying with SARS-CoV-2 infection-an autopsy study of the first consecutive 80 cases in Hamburg, Germany. Int J Leg Med 2020;134(4):1275–84.

100. Ackermann M, Verleden SE, Kuehnel M, et al. Pulmonary vascular endothelialitis, thrombosis, and angiogenesis in covid-19. N Engl J Med 2020;383(2):120–8.

101. Hariri LP, North CM, Shih AR, et al. Lung histopathology in coronavirus disease 2019 as compared with severe acute respiratory sydrome and H1N1 influenza: a systematic review. Chest 2020.

102. Varga Z, Flammer AJ, Steiger P, et al. Endothelial cell infection and endotheliitis in COVID-19. Lancet 2020;395(10234):1417–8.

103. Hanley B, Naresh KN, Roufosse C, et al. Histopathological findings and viral tropism in UK patients with severe fatal COVID-19: a post-mortem study. Lancet Microbe 2020;1(6):e245–53.

104. Gattinoni L, Coppola S, Cressoni M, et al. COVID-19 does not lead to a "typical" acute respiratory distress syndrome. Am J Respir Crit Care Med 2020;201(10):1299–300.

105. Bos LDJ, Paulus F, Vlaar APJ, et al. Subphenotyping acute respiratory distress syndrome in patients with COVID-19: consequences for ventilator management. Ann Am Thorac Soc 2020;17(9):1161–3.

106. Grasselli G, Tonetti T, Protti A, et al. Pathophysiology of COVID-19-associated acute respiratory distress syndrome: a multicentre prospective observational study. Lancet Respir Med 2020;8(12):1201–8.

107. Beenen LFM, Bos LD, Scheerder MJ, et al. Extensive pulmonary perfusion defects compatible with microthrombosis and thromboembolic disease in severe Covid-19 pneumonia. Thromb Res 2020;196:135–7.
108. Grillet F, Busse-Cote A, Calame P, et al. COVID-19 pneumonia: microvascular disease revealed on pulmonary dual-energy computed tomography angiography. Quant Imaging Med Surg 2020;10(9):1852–62.
109. Patel BV, Arachchillage DJ, Ridge CA, et al. Pulmonary angiopathy in severe COVID-19: physiologic, imaging, and hematologic observations. Am J Respir Crit Care Med 2020;202(5):690–9.
110. Tay MZ, Poh CM, Renia L, et al. The trinity of COVID-19: immunity, inflammation and intervention. Nat Rev Immunol 2020;20(6):363–74.
111. Fajgenbaum DC, June CH. Cytokine storm. N Engl J Med 2020;383(23):2255–73.
112. Sinha P, Matthay MA, Calfee CS. Is a "cytokine storm" relevant to COVID-19? JAMA Intern Med 2020;180(9):1152–4.
113. Leisman DE, Ronner L, Pinotti R, et al. Cytokine elevation in severe and critical COVID-19: a rapid systematic review, meta-analysis, and comparison with other inflammatory syndromes. Lancet Respir Med 2020;8(12):1233–44.
114. Kox M, Waalders NJB, Kooistra EJ, et al. Cytokine levels in critically ill patients with COVID-19 and other conditions. JAMA 2020.
115. Mudd PA, Crawford JC, Turner JS, et al. Distinct inflammatory profiles distinguish COVID-19 from influenza with limited contributions from cytokine storm. Sci Adv 2020;6(50):eabe3024.
116. Sinha P, Calfee CS, Cherian S, et al. Prevalence of phenotypes of acute respiratory distress syndrome in critically ill patients with COVID-19: a prospective observational study. Lancet Respir Med 2020;8(12):1209–18.
117. Hadjadj J, Yatim N, Barnabei L, et al. Impaired type I interferon activity and inflammatory responses in severe COVID-19 patients. Science 2020;369(6504):718–24.

Genetics of Acute Respiratory Distress Syndrome: Pathways to Precision

Heather M. Giannini, MD, MS, Nuala J. Meyer, MD, MS*

KEYWORDS

- Acute respiratory distress syndrome (ARDS) • Genetic association
- Genome-wide association study • RNA sequencing

KEY POINTS

- Acute respiratory distress syndrome (ARDS) is a complex genetic trait requiring both a severe environmental insult and a host susceptibility.
- Both DNA-focused and RNA-focused studies have implicated numerous genes and genetic pathways that may contribute to ARDS risk and mortality.
- The coronavirus disease 2019 (COVID-19) pandemic is accelerating the application of genomic tools to the study of ARDS.

INTRODUCTION

Despite 5 decades of research dedicated to understanding the complexities of the acute respiratory distress syndrome (ARDS), much work remains to fully explain ARDS risk or the risk of dying of ARDS.[1] There is now a deeper understanding of risk factors, precipitants, and pathogenic contributors to development and progression of ARDS.[2] Although there are no pedigrees of ARDS to suggest a classic monogenic inheritance of risk, clinical factors alone fail to explain why certain patients develop ARDS and others exposed to the same pathogen or injury do not, suggesting that individual factors exist that contribute to ARDS risk or mortality. To better understand this individualized risk, genetic association studies, whole-blood and lung lavage transcriptomic studies, and profiling of plasma proteins and metabolites have been completed, implicating specific pathways that may enable precision treatment approaches. Although therapy tailored to patients' individualized risks is ultimately the goal, the heterogeneity of the ARDS population in most cohorts creates a unique challenge and requires additional considerations.[3] Furthermore, translating

University of Pennsylvania Perelman School of Medicine, 3400 Spruce Street, 5038 Gates Building, Philadelphia, PA 19104, USA
* Corresponding author.
E-mail address: nuala.meyer@pennmedicine.upenn.edu

Crit Care Clin 37 (2021) 817–834
https://doi.org/10.1016/j.ccc.2021.05.006
0749-0704/21/© 2021 Elsevier Inc. All rights reserved.

the information gleaned from genetic studies in ARDS has yet to yield true precision therapy. Randomized controlled trials have proved the superiority of ventilation strategies,[4,5] but have yet to identify an effective therapeutic drug. The mission to identify ARDS therapeutics has never been more critical, because a once-in-a-century global pandemic virus capable of inducing ARDS has affected infected millions of individuals, frequently with deadly consequences.

This article considers genetic and genomic tools to advance the understanding of individualized risk, refine diagnosis and subclassifications, and discover new and novel pathways that may point to therapeutic targets. It examines the current state of genomic research in ARDS and discusses methods that will facilitate making the crucial leaps from association to function and causation. In addition, it posits that there are emerging treatment paradigms to be pursued in ARDS along biologically defined phenotypes that will lead to meaningful changes in outcomes.

UNIQUE HURDLES FOR ACUTE RESPIRATORY DISTRESS SYNDROME GENOMICS

A central tenet of all successful genetic studies, in ARDS and other critical care syndromes, is accurately identifying the population of interest and applying a careful and accurate phenotype. In ARDS specifically, there are unique challenges to accomplishing this goal. The clinical definitions of ARDS, developed initially by the American-European Consensus Conference in 1994[6] and the subsequent refinement by Berlin Criteria,[7] are easily applied in the clinical setting when blood gases are available, but providers frequently do not recognize or code ARDS, and no validated algorithm using administrative codes exists.[8,9] An important component of successful genetic association studies is selecting noncase patients who are at risk for the condition. For ARDS genetic studies, this necessitates decisions about which disease precipitants to include, and whether to broadly enroll patients with any potential inciting cause or to focus only on those with 1 entity, such as pneumonia, sepsis, trauma, or toxic inhalants, to reduce heterogeneity. A broader approach increases overall power, but there may be distinct biological drivers to different precipitants or other subgroups of ARDS, both obvious or unrecognized. The cost of maximizing power while increasing heterogeneity may be that a signal is harder to find because it is only relevant to the subpopulation. In ARDS, distinct genetic variants have been identified in pulmonary and nonpulmonary ARDS risk[10] and between sepsis and trauma.[11] In addition, because genetic architecture has been shaped by ancestral migration patterns, attention to the genetic ancestry of study participants is also vital.[12] Far too few studies have included sufficient subjects from African, South and Southeast Asian, Pacific Island, or admixed genetic ancestries, and this limits the knowledge of whether genetic findings are broadly relevant to all populations.

IDENTIFYING GENES CONFERRING INDIVIDUAL RISK

ARDS behaves as a complex genetic trait requiring both an extreme environmental insult, such as pneumonia, aspiration, sepsis, sterile inflammation, or trauma, and an inherited predisposition. Before the coronavirus disease 2019 (COVID-19) pandemic, there were no reported families in which ARDS had clustered, thus uncovering the inherited element relied on studies between unrelated individuals, looking for an enrichment of variants within the case or noncase population. In broad terms, genetic association testing can proceed by a knowledge-based approach, investigating genes hypothesized to play a role in the syndrome, or by a discovery approach, whereby all genes are assessed.

Candidate Gene Studies

Candidate gene studies are a reasonable approach to investigate the link between genetic inheritance and phenotype or disease risk. Candidate genetic loci are typically proposed after observing dysregulated downstream biomarkers detected in gene expression or proteomic studies, and a working-backwards theory that the expression is dictated largely by the locus and local regulatory elements.[13,14] Some candidate genes are also proposed by in vitro or animal models that recapitulate features of lung injury.[15,16] The candidate approach may be faster for therapeutic translation because the gene product is known and finding a signal may be feasible with smaller sample sizes, potentially conferring lower cost.[17] However, selecting a limited number of candidates a priori is risky in a complex trait such as ARDS. In complex traits, multiple smaller associations contribute to the development of disease, making it difficult to identify significant interactions. In addition, the candidate approach requires that the investigator not only select the correct gene but genotype or sequence the correct variants that regulate the gene's expression. Much has to go right for a candidate gene association study to detect significant enrichment; the investigator must select the correct gene, correct variant, and the appropriate case and control populations, and the effect size must be large enough to be detected in a modest sample. In ARDS, protein and transcript investigation from both plasma and bronchoalveolar lavage (BAL) fluid has suggested numerous candidates, including a varied selection of inflammatory markers and endothelial activators, which were pursued in genomic studies (**Fig. 1**).

One of the first and most replicated candidate genes tested has been interleukin 6 (*IL6*), after numerous cytokine analyses across both animal and human samples studies showed a consistent upregulation of this and other proinflammatory cytokines in ARDS and experimental lung injury, as well as an association with increased risk of mortality.[18–20] Initial work identified an *IL6* locus polymorphism,[14,21] which was subsequently expanded to an *IL6* haplotype associated with ARDS,[22] and this was successfully replicated in a larger targeted study that also replicated other candidate genes in ARDS, including *IL10*, *IRAK3*, and *VEGFA*.[23]

Other notable candidate genes identified in this fashion include variants in the surfactant protein B (*SFTPB*) gene,[24] as well as the angiotensin-converting enzyme (*ACE*) locus, both candidates that were tested given their high expression in the lung and potential for regulating lung epithelial or endothelial function, respectively.[13,14] Using a medium-throughput candidate gene array, which assayed approximately 2000 candidate genes, replicated associations were also identified for the genes *IL1RN*,[25] the gene that encodes interleukin (IL)-1 receptor antagonist, and *ANGPT2*,[26] the gene encoding angiopoietin-2 protein. Highlighting the potential translation of candidate genes, both the *IL1RN* and the *ANGPT2* variants associated with altered plasma protein expression of their gene products and clinical trials to modify both the IL-1 and angiopoietin pathway are currently underway for COVID-19–related ARDS and are listed on clinicaltrials.gov. After a decade or more of candidate studies with inconsitent replication and small effects attributed to single nucleotide polymorphisms (SNPs) within these candidates, as well as the increasingly accessible whole-genome technology, the field has largely pivoted to discovery-based methods, such as genome-wide association studies (GWAS), to further characterize associations between genotype and phenotype in ARDS.

Genome-Wide Association Studies

GWAS have been used as a broader discovery technique to examine susceptibility to and severity of ARDS. Although still knowledge-based in that genome-wide arrays use

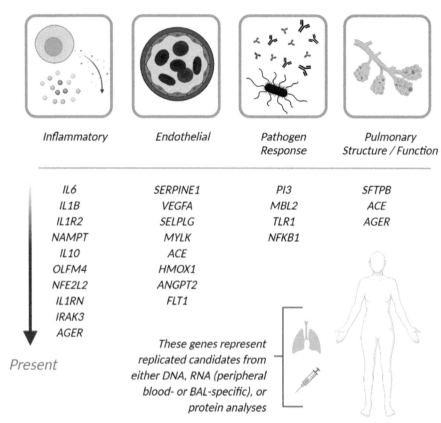

Inflammatory	Endothelial	Pathogen Response	Pulmonary Structure / Function
IL6	SERPINE1	PI3	SFTPB
IL1B	VEGFA	MBL2	ACE
IL1R2	SELPLG	TLR1	AGER
NAMPT	MYLK	NFKB1	
IL10	ACE		
OLFM4	HMOX1		
NFE2L2	ANGPT2		
IL1RN	FLT1		
IRAK3			
AGER			

Present

These genes represent replicated candidates from either DNA, RNA (peripheral blood- or BAL-specific), or protein analyses

Fig. 1. Candidate genes identified via genetic and/or proteomic investigations of plasma and bronchoalveolar lavage fluid that have been replicated and proposed to have implications in the pathogenesis or progression of ARDS. IL, interleukin.

probes assessing known genetic variants from genetic sequencing in global populations,[27] the implications of linkage disequilibrium in multiple global populations allows imputation of SNPs that are not directly assessed, such that an array of 500,000 to 750,000 variants can provide high-quality estimates of the genetic variation at more than 2 million sites in the genome. Genome-wide thus refers to having some confidence in the genetic variation across all known genes. There is ample evidence that, although ARDS is not a Mendelian or classic monogenic trait, there is a clear interaction between the host response to infection/injury and genetic variation between individuals. There are significant challenges to executing large-scale ARDS GWAS, including issues with diagnosis and coding, physiologically diverse precipitants of acute lung injury that may have different genetic regulation, and appropriate selection of control populations. As such, these efforts have been limited in their capabilities to detect the statistically extreme genotype effects required to declare GWAS significance. As previously mentioned, not all variants show a consistent effect size in populations from different precipitants, or across different genetic ancestries. Although 1 interpretation is that a failure to replicate indicates a type I error, it may be that the variant has different effects under different biological conditions and discriminating between these possibilities requires ever-larger populations with deeper and broader genotyping.

In the first ARDS GWAS, performed in 2 trauma-induced ARDS populations, Christie and colleagues[28] identified a variant regulating expression of liprin-alpha (PPFIA1), a cell-adhesion molecule that influences cell-matrix interactions. This SNP did not reach genome-wide significance but did consistently associate with increased trauma-associated ARDS risk and with increased expression of messenger RNA (mRNA) expression of PPFIA, providing a potential mechanistic link between gene variation and altered ARDS risk. A more recent GWAS examined 232 African American patients with ARDS compared with 162 at-risk control subjects. They used a prioritization schema to identify an exonic variant in SELPLG (selectin P ligand gene), which encodes P-selectin (or CD24), and although the specific variant did not replicate, 2 additional coding SELPLG variants manifested ARDS association in a second population.[29] Subsequent functional studies using murine models of lung injury show significantly increased SELPLG gene expression, and neutralization of this pathway attenuates inflammation in the LPS-induced model. Thus SELPLG represents a strong candidate gene. In addition, in the largest GWAS performed to date, the FMS-related tyrosine kinase 1 (FLT1) gene, which encodes vascular endothelial growth factor receptor-1 (VEGFR-1), reached GWAS significance (P<5E-08), implicating endothelial mediators in inherited risk for acute lung injury[30] and further supporting a prior candidate study that had identified a significant FLT1 SNP in a targeted approach.[31]

Few GWAS of ARDS have been published. Although ARDS was not strictly described, 2 reports on the genetic associations of sepsis may shed light on ARDS also, although admittedly not all patients with pneumonia develop ARDS. A large European collaborative effort to investigate the genetics of sepsis (GenOSept) published a GWAS of pneumonia-associated sepsis in which they identified a consistent signal in the FER gene associated with improved survival in 3 cohorts, with a meta-analysis P value of 10E-08.[32] The FER gene (Fps/Fes related tyrosine kinase) encodes a nonreceptor tyrosine kinase and, similar to other ARDS candidate genes, has a role in the regulation of actin cytoskeleton and cell adhesion as well as potentially an immune regulatory role.[32] Interestingly, the results for this genetic locus were not different in sepsis survivors and nonsurvivors when the populations were modified to include abdominal sepsis, suggesting some specificity for pulmonary sepsis. A more recent ARDS cohort study replicated the association between this FER variant and risk for ARDS mortality, although the effect was limited to subjects with severe ARDS caused by pneumonia.[33] A second sepsis GWAS used a small discovery population (740 subjects with sepsis from any cause who were enrolled in clinical trials for antibiotics or fluid and insulin therapy) and replicated in a hospitalized pneumonia population.[34] The proportion of deaths was only 20% in the discovery population and only 10% in the pneumonia population, thus not directly comparable with ARDS mortality. No variants met genome-wide significance, but an exonic, or coding, variant in the gene VSP13A (vacuolar protein sorting 13 homolog A), a gene with potential roles regulating autophagy, showed a consistent signal in the replication population and had an excess of coding variants in an exome sequencing study.[34]

Although the progress to date with ARDS GWAS is disappointing, with only a few variants and inconsistent effects across different populations, there may yet be reason to keep pursuing such studies. Importantly, the lack of consistency across different ARDS precipitants and phenotypes may indicate different biological roles in varied contexts, or it may reflect decisions made about who constitutes a control population. To move forward, the field will need much larger studies with more diverse populations and to phenotype patients consistently for ARDS. In tandem, efforts to simultaneously apply large-scale proteomic or transcriptomic phenotyping may help to crystallize different biological subgroups of ARDS, and testing for genetic differences between subclasses, or between a subclass and non-ARDS, will be critically important. The scale of the current COVID-19 pandemic may accelerate genomic discoveries for ARDS, at least for ARDS precipitated by the severe acute respiratory syndrome coronavirus-2 (SARS-CoV-2) virus. In a remarkable feat of translational research and multinational scientific collaboration, more than 1 GWAS of severe COVID-19 has already been published. In the first study, a GWAS of severe COVID-19 with respiratory failure identified 2 signals with genome-wide significance, in the gene *ABO*, which encodes the histoblood group ABO transferases, and at chromosome 3p21.31, a locus encompassing a 6-gene cluster that encompasses several promising candidates.[35] The *ABO* gene has previously been implicated in ARDS caused by sepsis and trauma, with evidence that the variants that determine blood type A also associate with higher evoked levels of vascular injury markers in plasma.[36,37] A second massive undertaking was recently published that leveraged a large United Kingdom consortium, the Genetics of Mortality in Critical Care (GenOMICC) study, as well as the UK Biobank, and linked results to the Genotype-Tissue Expression (GTEx) project.[38] The result is a GWAS of more than 2000 critically ill patients with COVID-19 compared with ancestry-matched controls that suggested 15 independent association signals with severe COVID-19 and 4 signals replicated in a second population. To investigate potentially causal mRNA transcripts by Mendelian randomization (described later), the investigators then searched for local expression quantitative trait loci (eQTL; DNA variants that are associated with a different mRNA level of the same gene in at least 1 tissue) for a list of 26 genes that might be targeted by proposed treatments for severe COVID-19, such as anti–IL-1, anti–IL-6, anti–tumor necrosis factor, anti–monocyte colony-stimulating factor, interferon modifiers, Janus kinase (JAK) inhibitors, and Bruton tyrosine kinase inhibitors. Two transcripts, the interferon receptor subunit IFNAR2 and TYK2, a target for JAK inhibitors, showed consistent effect-size estimates between severe COVID-19 and genetic regulation of gene expression.[38] In addition, the investigators identified additional potential genetic associations by using GTEx to infer the expression of mRNA in whole blood or lung based on DNA variation, which suggested that the genes *CCR2*, *CCR3*, and *CXCR6* were each dysregulated in lung tissue, and *ICAM5* and *TNFSF15* were dysregulated in whole blood.[38] The COVID-19 pandemic may also dramatically shift ARDS genomic investigation in that, for the first time, some pedigree analysis may be possible, because multiple affected family members may express varying levels of severity. An early study of Chinese patients included 35 pedigrees from among 332 recruited subjects with severe COVID19 and used DNA sequencing to find rare variants that might be missed on a typical GWAS platform.[39] Although the small size limits the statistical power for this study and results need to be replicated, it is another example of how the pandemic urgency has amplified ARDS research (**Table 1**).

Whole-Exome Sequencing (Genome-Wide Exome Sequencing)

Although expanded in discovery capabilities, DNA array–based genotyping, such as the aforementioned studies, is limited by the design of the array and those probes contained therein. To expand discovery to the entire genome and include rare or private variations, which may be present in only 1 family, whole-exome sequencing has been applied to sequence the entire protein-coding region. This approach has been theorized as more efficient than sequencing the entire genome, given that the analysis is limited to probable functional regions where genetic variation may have potentially large effect by affecting protein sequence. Thus, exome sequencing may find new candidates that could quickly translate to mechanistic understanding of the disease, and to therapeutics. In 1 study linked to the National Heart, Lung, and Blood Institute (NHLBI) Exome Sequencing Project, 96 patients with sepsis-induced ARDS were

Table 1
Genomic studies focused on coronavirus disease 2019 are accelerating acute respiratory distress syndrome research

First Author	Date	Genetic Tool	Tissue Analyzed	Proposed Key Mediators
Xiong et al,[91] 2020	March 2020	RNA-seq (bulk)	Peripheral blood and BAL	CCL2/MCP-1, CXCL10/IP-10, CCL3/MIP-1A, and CCL4/MIP1B; activation of apoptosis and P53 signaling pathway in lymphocytes
Wen et al,[92] 2020	May 2020	RNA-seq (single cell)	Peripheral blood	JUN, FOS, JUNB, and KLF6; IL-1B, CCL3, IRF1, DUSP1
Wilk et al,[93] 2020	June 2020	RNA-seq (single cell)	Peripheral blood	Upregulation of IFN-stimulated genes; highly dependent on cell type
Overmyer et al,[94] 2020	October 2020	RNA-seq (single cell)	Peripheral blood	PRTN3, LCN2, CD24, BPI, CTSG, DEFA1, DEFA4, MMP8, and MPO
Xu et al,[95] 2020	October 2020	RNA-seq (single cell)	Paired peripheral blood and BAL	IFN-stimulating genes (ISG15, IFITM1, IFITM3, MX1, IRF7, IFI27), neutrophil activation (S100A8, S100A9, S100A12, CLU, RNASE2)
Ellinghaus et al,[35] 2020	October 2020	GWAS	Peripheral blood	SLC6A20, LZTFL1, CCR9, FYCO1, CXCR6, and XCR1; ABO blood group locus (3p21.31)
Mick et al,[96] 2020	November 2020	RNA-seq (bulk)	Upper airway (nasopharyngeal swab)	Pronounced IFN response; IFI6, IFI44L, IFI27, IFI44, HERC6, OAS2, and IFIT1
Wang et al,[39] 2020	November 2020	GWAS; eQTL	Peripheral blood	(SNP) rs6020298, LINC01273, TMEM189; HLA-A*11:01, B*51:01, and C*14:02 alleles
Pairo-Castineira et al,[38] 2020	December 2020	GWAS, expression eQTL, Mendelian randomization	Peripheral blood	IFNAR2 and TYK2; OAS gene cluster, CCR2, CCR3 and CXCR6, MTA2B; replication of 3p21.31 locus

Abbreviations: HLA, human leukocyte antigen; IFN, interferon; RNA-seq, RNA sequencing. Genes are named in convention with the HUGO human gene nomenclature committee.

compared with whole-exome sequencing to 440 healthy control subjects without ARDS. Two SNPs were found to be highly associated with ARDS, including variants in genes encoding X-linked gene arylsulfatase D (ARSD) and XK Kell blood group complex member 3 (XKR3), the functional significance of which remains unclear.[40] Further, exome sequencing is a type of rare variant analysis whereby the effect may be large but is limited to only a few individuals, or a few families. Although the potential to broaden understanding is great, the impact on patients may not be realized unless the pathway identified replicates in a general population.

In addition, whole-genome sequencing (WGS) is also possible given efficiencies of scale and reduced time and cost. In this strategy, all DNA elements are sequenced, both coding and noncoding. Advantages to this approach are that it is truly discovery based, and it is not constrained by the current understanding of genetic architecture or linkage. Thus, this method may be powerful to discover new DNA species or genetic regions associated with ARDS risk or outcome. However, sequencing also tends to highlight regions of the genome that are not annotated to a specific gene, gene product, or function. Although it is likely that, with time, these gaps in the knowledge of genome science will be addressed, at present, there is little published activity for WGS in ARDS. The COVID-19 pandemic, with the potential for pedigree designs, may change that.[39]

GENE EXPRESSION: IS IT THE MESSAGE THAT COUNTS?
Gene Expression Microarray

The transcriptome represents the expression of inherited genetic risk, revealing how existing genetic elements manifest in the context of host response for both sterile and nonsterile triggers of ARDS. Gene expression is highly variable, in a temporal and tissue-specific sense. The investigation of gene transcripts in a tissue at a particular time in the disease course has highlighted dysregulation and pathway activation in ARDS, but replicative efforts are challenging and inconsistent. Furthermore, genes implicated in DNA variant analysis do not always show differential regulation at the mRNA level, and vice versa, simply because the two techniques assay different aspects of the genome. In many studies, transcript profiles are extracted from whole blood, thus representing a weighted sum of patterns from the myriad of cell types (leukocytes) populating circulating blood. Thus, a DNA variant in an endothelial-restricted gene such as *ANGPT2* will not be detected in the whole-blood transcriptome; *ANGPT2* mRNA may be dysregulated if lung vasculature is sampled, or lung homogenate including vessels, but it would not be detected on a whole-blood platform because leukocytes do not express *ANGPT2*. Although lung tissue might yield valuable gene expression patterns for ARDS pathology, obtaining these specimens is risky and thus rare,[41] making peripheral blood a more accessible option. Whole-blood or leukocyte cell fractions (neutrophils or peripheral blood mononuclear cells) still have potential utility in ARDS, because the host response to infection or injury seems a dominant factor in ARDS development. In addition, multiple studies have used the immune cells obtained from BAL, and particularly alveolar macrophages, which are key ARDS immune responders that regulate proinflammatory and antiinflammatory fate.[42,43] Gene expression microarray, made possible through microchips coated with thousands of oligonucleotide probes specific to a complementary DNA (cDNA) library of between 20,000 and 40,000 known genes, is one technique for this query.

Delineating dysregulated gene expression can be revealing in the pathobiology of ARDS.[44] Initial microarray studies based on whole blood in sepsis-associated ARDS identified CD24, the granulocyte receptor for P-selectin,[45] the candidate gene prioritized in a prior GWAS,[29] further implicating the platelet-neutrophil interaction in ARDS.[46,47] Neutrophil-associated transcripts were consistently upregulated in this study as well, including lipocalin2 (LCN2, also known as neutrophil gelatinase-associated lipocalin, NGAL), bactericidal permeability-increasing protein (BPI), and matrix-metalloprotein 8 (MMP-8), and these transcripts were not correlated with absolute neutrophil count.[45] A group expert in neutrophil biology identified both transcriptional and functional changes in both circulating neutrophils and BAL neutrophils from patients with ARDS, identifying a milieu of neutrophil-specific differentially expressed genes that implicated the phosphoinositide 3-kinase pathway.[48,49] Still other array-based studies have identified inflammasome mediators caspase 1 and IL-1 and IL-18, also providing evidence in the same study of elevated IL-18 protein levels in plasma of patients with ARDS that distinguished ARDS from sepsis without ARDS.[50]

mRNA signatures in specific tissues and diseases have emerged as a powerful molecular tool with not only diagnostic and prognostic information but also the possibility of subclassifying disease, permitting a more elegant and precise splitting of previously lumped diagnoses with the identification of subphenotypes, or, ideally, biologically defined endotypes.[51] This approach has been particularly fruitful in asthma, where demonstration of the unique T-helper (Th) 2 expression profile in respiratory epithelial cells has led to effective endotyping in patients with asthma and now increased specificity of therapy.[52,53] The signature approach has also been moderately successful in sepsis, where there are now industry-led efforts for bedside diagnostics that can predict, using a small amount of peripheral blood, the likelihood of bacterial and viral infection to define sepsis based on a proprietary mRNA algorithm.[54] ARDS transcriptional signatures have been less consistent, despite several efforts. An initial study of whole blood from 13 patients with sepsis and acute lung injury, compared with 20 controls with sepsis, developed an 8-transcript mRNA classifier that also accurately parsed a small validation population, but has since not been replicated.[55] A subsequent small and carefully phenotyped sepsis population reported a microarray study of peripheral leukocyte expression and suggested a distinguishable ARDS signature compared with that of sepsis alone, although the statistical significance of each transcript was not robust, with false discovery rate (FDR) ~20%. Importantly, each gene expression study deposits publicly accessible raw and adjusted data, and thus the Kangelaris[45] study was able to identify potential modest replication of transcripts reported in the prior Howrylak and colleagues[55] study (ARF3, CDKN1A, PNPLA2), although again with FDR ~20%. These early efforts set the stage for a larger multicohort study, which remains the largest to date at more than 400 subjects, but it failed to establish a reliable ARDS classifier despite identification of approximately 30 differentially expressed genes (odds ratio >1.3 and FDR<20%).[56] No transcripts were significantly dysregulated in ARDS after accounting for severity of illness. Performance of the classifier yielded poor diagnostic utility, with an area under the receiver operating curve of only 0.63.[56] The question remains as to whether a robust signature for ARDS will be reproducible as sample sizes increase, or perhaps the differential gene expression patterns are a recapitulation of critical illness phenotypes on a larger scale.[56] The confounding effects of widespread systemic inflammation and the heterogeneous spectrum of ARDS across multiple precipitants and severities may prove too difficult to overcome to identify a universal ARDS transcriptional signature.

Although peripheral blood is more accessible and potentially revealing, other investigations have focused on the lung compartment, obtaining BAL samples and isolating alveolar macrophage for gene expression. In a comparison of transcripts in ARDS from peripheral blood buffy coat compared with alveolar macrophage isolated from BAL, S100A12 and IL-2R were identified as shared upregulated transcripts, both of which are strongly implicated in inflammatory pathways.[57] The expression patterns were divergent, as expected given the highly varied cell types and tissue compartments. Additional BAL studies since then have confirmed and expanded the description of alveolar macrophage profiles in ARDS.[58,59] An elegant longitudinal study, performed by obtaining multiple bronchoscopy samples over time through ARDS disease course, dichotomized ARDS severity and identified an interesting temporal dynamic. The investigators found that ARDS persistence was characterized by continued and progressive inflammatory signatures, whereas inflammatory programming was promptly downregulated in patients with shorter mechanical ventilation needs.[58] This direct evidence from the lung compartment provides important temporal details in the regulated host response to infection, which has, to date, been elusive to characterize. Neutrophils are also plentiful but functionally dysregulated in the BAL fluid of patients with ARDS,[60] suggesting that restoring the resting lung neutrophil phenotype could have therapeutic benefit. Continued investigations of the lung space and resident macrophage may help in understand the pathobiology of ARDS at a deeper level, whereas peripheral blood sampling may encourage development of diagnostics and prognostics in this syndrome. Furthermore, although microarray has been an extremely valuable tool, the increasingly cost-effective next-generation sequencing (NGS) technology has facilitated the expansion of RNA sequencing (RNA-seq) as the de facto methodology in transcriptomic studies. Single-cell transcriptomics, where the transcriptome can be reliably attributed to a known cell constituent and compared between different cells, further allows a more detailed characterization of the multiple contributions to disease than has ever been possible.

RNA Sequencing

RNA-seq has gained traction as the leading method for interrogation of gene expression over the past decade.[61] This technique is a true discovery model akin to WGS of DNA, using next-generation technology to directly sequence RNA, typically via conversion to cDNA. RNA-seq fueled the discovery of numerous RNA species that were previously unrecognized and largely under-researched, such as micro-RNAs, Piwi-interacting RNAs, short interfering RNAs, and longer noncoding RNAs, among others not discussed here.[62] The role these unique transcripts play in the larger scope of ARDS remains unclear, although a recent study focused on the long noncoding RNA THRIL identified increased expression in ARDS sepsis compared with sepsis controls, which also correlated with severity and mortality.[63]

Again, as with any gene expression study, RNA-seq depends entirely on tissue specificity. In ARDS, there have so far been a limited number of RNA-seq studies, using a range of tissues, including whole blood, purified neutrophils, BAL samples, and lung biopsy from animal models. In peripheral blood, the transcriptome is most representative of the circulating leukocyte response, and varies over the course of disease, particularly in critical illness syndromes.[64] An important single-cell RNA-seq effort of peripheral blood mononuclear cells in ARDS caused by pneumonia compared with pneumonia sepsis without ARDS detected numerous interesting changes, particularly in the monocyte populations, with downregulation of *SOCS3* and upregulation of the interferon response genes *IFI44L* and *IFITM3*. Furthermore, they validated 17 transcripts in independent populations.[65] This study is notable for the marriage of high-dimensional cytometric data with RNA-seq to understand both cell composition and transcriptional status, an important step toward a systems biology approach in ARDS. The once-in-a-century severe acute respiratory syndrome coronavirus-2 (SARS-COV-2) pandemic has prompted an expansion of genetic investigations, including many interesting RNA-seq efforts for ARDS related to COVID-19 (see **Table 1**). These efforts contain a wealth of revealing information about this pathogen-driven ARDS and potentially ARDS as a syndrome, although the field's rapid evolution places a comprehensive discussion beyond the scope of this article.

INFERRING CAUSALITY OF QUANTITATIVE TRAITS USING GENOMICS

The huge amount of data created by these genomic techniques presents unique challenges with respect to data storage, organization, manipulation, and analysis.

Extracting meaningful signals requires a cautious and thoughtful computational approach. DNA sequencing and RNA-seq generate a staggering amount of observational data, largely designed for discovery of new targets and signals that either define biology or provide therapeutic inspiration. Although these studies can suggest association between ARDS and a specific gene or gene product, they do not, and cannot alone, extend to causation. Although a gene product or protein may be much higher (or lower) in patients with ARDS than in those without ARDS, this observation alone is insufficient to declare that changes in that feature contribute to ARDS. Short of randomized controlled trials, it remains challenging to show causal relationships from studies involving humans. Further, randomized trials are not always practical or ethical, such as randomizing patients to receive exogenous cytokine supplementation. However, there may be opportunities to make some causal inference from observational data, and genomic tools have unique advantages to accomplish this.

Several genomic causal inference techniques can be applied to quantitative intermediates, or traits that can be measured and add value toward ARDS diagnosis, prognosis, or molecular subtype.[66] If causal intermediates can be identified, these markers would have very strong rationale to be targeted pharmacologically and may facilitate either target population identification (precision medicine to only treat patients showing pathway dysregulation) and more efficient pharmacology screens.[67,68] For example, drug screens to reduce plasma low-density lipoprotein levels are more efficient than screening for agents that improve coronary disease in an animal model. However, in ARDS, only a few quantitative traits have used causal inference methodology to test whether they may have a causal role.

Some quantitative traits are highly genetically predictable; 1 or several DNA variants explain a high proportion of the variation in the marker. When this is the case, genetics can offer a unique opportunity to test relationships between genetic variant and intermediate, intermediate and outcome, and genetic variant and outcome, using this information to make inferences about whether the intermediate contributes to the outcome. In a mediation analysis, these relationships are used to formally explain the proportion of an association between genetic variants and outcome that are mediated by a change in a third variable.[69] Essentially, the association is mathematically deconvoluted into a direct effect of genetic variant on the outcome, and an indirect effect mediated by the intermediate (third variable). If the proportion of observed risk explained by the intermediate is substantial, it provides statistical support for the intermediate to be causally involved in the disease outcome. One group has applied the mediation framework to test whether changes in platelet count explain differential ARDS risk or ARDS mortality. Thrombocytopenia is associated with ARDS,[46,70,71] and platelet count in ambulatory subjects is genetically predictable.[72,73] Wei and colleagues[70,74] interrogated relationships between platelet count–determining genes and ARDS, and identified SNPs in the gene LRRC16A and both ARDS risk and ARDS mortality. Further, his team confirmed that a significant portion of the SNP-ARDS and SNP-mortality associations was mediated by each SNP's effect on either platelet count or platelet trajectory, respectively.[70,74] Although work remains to explain the precise mechanism by which these effects occur, these studies focus attention on platelet count and stability as a novel avenue for ARDS prevention or treatment.

An alternative approach is to consider genetics akin to a natural experiment that has randomized individuals to being high-expressing or low-expressing biomarker phenotypes by virtue of genetic recombination. In this framework, termed Mendelian randomization, genetic variation is used as an instrument to estimate a proportion of the variation in the intermediate variable. This instrumental variable method controls for threats to the internal validity of the association between ARDS and the intermediate, such as confounding variables, measurement error, spuriousness, simultaneity, and reverse causality.[75,76] The genetic assignment always precedes ARDS, and the genetically predicted portion of an intermediate is less confounded by being randomly assigned by parental allele assortment. If the genetically predicted portion of the intermediate marker shows association with outcome, then it is assumed that the measured marker has a causal true effect on the outcome. The methodology relies on specific assumptions, including a genetically predictable intermediate, which can be challenging to confirm for evoked traits during acute illness[77]; an association between the intermediate and outcome; and that there are no confounders acting on both the SNP (instrument) and the intermediate.[78,79] To date, Mendelian randomization studies have implicated potential causal roles for several plasma proteins on the risk for ARDS: angiopoietin-2 (ANG2), soluble receptor for advanced glycation end-products (sRAGE), and insulinlike growth factor–binding protein-7 (IGFBP-7).[80–82] Thus, each of these proteins is a candidate for modification of ARDS risk. As mentioned earlier, the recent GenOMICC COVID-19 publication also applied Mendelian randomization to infer true causal effects of mRNA abundance of *IFNAR2* and *TYK2*, both transcripts that are potentially targetable, on severe COVID-19.[38]

METAGENOMICS: COMMENSALS AND PATHOGENS

Although a full consideration of the role of genomic methods to interrogate the microbiome, or microbial communities within individuals, is beyond the scope of this review, a few important studies warrant discussion. The same advances that have allowed cost-effective NGS such as RNA-seq, WES, and WGS facilitate rapid pathogen detection without a reliance on culture positivity,[83] and it seems likely that genomic diagnostics will be in wide use in the near future. Freedom from culture-based microbiologic studies could increase sensitivity for infection, shorten time to diagnosis, detect pathogens that are notoriously challenging to grow in culture, and potentially aid in the fight against antimicrobial resistance by providing high confidence that patients are not infected. However, several potential barriers impede immediate deployment of metagenomic NGS (mNGS) in the clinic. Most of these will be overcome, such as standardization of the methodology, quality control, and workflow validation, but the data interpretation piece may take more time to achieve consensus and utility.[83] Sequencing metagenomic nucleic acids may be overly sensitive, and distinguishing pathogenic from commensal microbes may be challenging. Further, as shown by the COVID-19 pandemic, polymerase chain reaction–based methods cannot easily distinguish actively replicating virus from residual, inactive, or even dead virus.[84,85]

Beyond the potential diagnostic utility of mNGS, metagenomic shotgun sequencing has also yielded important pathophysiologic insights into ARDS. Using first a murine cecal ligation and puncture model of sepsis, then an endotoxin model, investigators showed a shift in the BAL microbiome to being dominated by gut bacteria within days of sepsis.[86] In addition, the microbiome of patients with ARDS undergoing BAL also showed that a surprisingly high proportion (33%) of patients with ARDS had BAL recovery of the gut microbial genus *Bacteroides*, a pathogen that is almost never cultured from patients with ARDS.[86] Neither time since ARDS onset nor source of ARDS, whether pneumonia or bacterial sepsis, explained the detection of *Bacteroides*. Further, alveolar proinflammatory cytokines associated with the detection of *Bacteroides*, suggesting a host response to the microbe. Thus, sepsis may predispose to typically gut-restricted pathogens dominating the lung microbiota in a culture-negative fashion, which may explain ongoing inflammation or failure of recovery in ARDS.

SUMMARY

This article highlights recent works in ARDS genomics that point to improved recognition of novel candidates in ARDS pathogenesis; better molecular subclassification of subtypes in ARDS that may display a unique, and potentially targetable, biology; and a better appreciation for the varied contributions of different cells and tissues to ARDS risk and mortality. Studies are increasingly not only replicating associations but emphasizing functional consequences of genetic or transcriptomic variation, which brings investigators a step closer to naming the dysregulated pathway and testing whether a strategy to manipulate expression improves outcomes in animal or in vitro models.

Subphenotypes exist in ARDS that are not always easily identifiable based on clinical features alone,[87,88] and more biological subtypes may be identified in the future. As new subphenotypes are discovered, retroactively applying genetic tools may help uncover regulatory elements that contribute to the underlying biology.

In future studies, to optimize the benefit gained from the enormous effort of implementing clinical and translational trials for patients with ARDS, an investment to collect and preserve DNA and RNA could facilitate retroactive identification of subpopulations that react differently to the same treatment.[89,90] If such subpopulations can be replicated and prospectively identified, then precision medicine for ARDS may be a testable strategy. These types of studies may accrue slowly, and have smaller target populations, but are likely to move clinicians closer to treatment based on a predicted individual response to treatment, the ultimate goal in personalized medicine.

DISCLOSURE

Dr. Meyer is funded by NIH HL137915, HL137006, HL155804, and GM115553. Dr. Giannini is funded by NIH HL007586.

REFERENCES

1. Luyt CE, Combes A, Becquemin MH, et al. Long-term outcomes of pandemic 2009 influenza A(H1N1)-associated severe ARDS. Chest 2012;142(3):583–92.
2. Matthay MA, Zemans RL, Zimmerman GA, et al. Acute respiratory distress syndrome. Nat Rev Dis Primers 2019;5(1):18.
3. Prescott HC, Calfee CS, Thompson BT, et al. Toward smarter lumping and smarter splitting: rethinking strategies for sepsis and acute respiratory distress syndrome clinical trial design. Am J Respir Crit Care Med 2016;194(2):147–55.
4. Amato MBP, Barbas CSV, Medeiros DM, et al. Effect of a protective-ventilation strategy on mortality in the acute respiratory distress syndrome. N Engl J Med 1998;338(6):347–54.
5. Beitler JR, Shaefi S, Montesi SB, et al. Prone positioning reduces mortality from acute respiratory distress syndrome in the low tidal volume era: a meta-analysis. Intensive Care Med 2014;40(3):332–41.
6. Bernard GR, Artigas A, Brigham KL, et al. The American-European Consensus Conference on ARDS. Definitions, mechanisms, relevant outcomes, and clinical trial coordination. Am J Respir Crit Care Med 1994;149(3 Pt 1):818–24.
7. Ranieri VM, Rubenfeld GD, Thompson BT, et al. Acute respiratory distress syndrome: the Berlin Definition. JAMA 2012;307(23):2526–33.
8. Bellani G, Laffey JG, Pham T, et al. Epidemiology, patterns of care, and mortality for patients with acute respiratory distress syndrome in intensive care units in 50 countries. JAMA 2016;315(8):788–800.

9. Weissman GE, Harhay MO, Lugo RM, et al. Natural language processing to assess documentation of features of critical illness in discharge documents of acute respiratory distress syndrome survivors. Ann Am Thorac Soc 2016;13(9): 1538–45.

10. Tejera P, Meyer NJ, Chen F, et al. Distinct and replicable genetic risk factors for acute respiratory distress syndrome of pulmonary or extrapulmonary origin. J Med Genet 2012;49(11):671–80.

11. Meyer NJ, Christie JD. Genetic heterogeneity and risk for ARDS. Semin Respir Crit Care Med 2013;34(4):459–74.

12. Akey JM. Constructing genomic maps of positive selection in humans: where do we go from here? Genome Res 2009;19(5):711–22.

13. Marshall RP, Webb S, Bellingan GJ, et al. Angiotensin converting enzyme insertion/deletion polymorphism is associated with susceptibility and outcome in acute respiratory distress syndrome. Am J Respir Crit Care Med 2002;166(5):646–50.

14. Marshall RP, Webb S, Hill MR, et al. Genetic polymorphisms associated with susceptibility and outcome in ARDS. Chest 2002;121(3 Suppl):68S–9S.

15. Ma SF, Grigoryev DN, Taylor AD, et al. Bioinformatic identification of novel early stress response genes in rodent models of lung injury. Am J Physiol Lung Cell Mol Physiol 2005;289(3):L468–77.

16. Grigoryev DN, Ma SF, Irizarry RA, et al. Orthologous gene-expression profiling in multi-species models: search for candidate genes. Genome Biol 2004;5(5):R34.

17. Daly AK, Day CP. Candidate gene case-control association studies: advantages and potential pitfalls. Br J Clin Pharmacol 2001;52(5):489–99.

18. Meduri GU, Headley S, Kohler G, et al. Persistent elevation of inflammatory cytokines predicts a poor outcome in ARDS. Plasma IL-1 beta and IL-6 levels are consistent and efficient predictors of outcome over time. Chest 1995;107(4): 1062–73.

19. Park WY, Goodman RB, Steinberg KP, et al. Cytokine balance in the lungs of patients with acute respiratory distress syndrome. Am J Respir Crit Care Med 2001; 164(10 Pt 1):1896–903.

20. Takala A, Jousela I, Takkunen O, et al. A prospective study of inflammation markers in patients at risk of indirect acute lung injury. Shock 2002;17(4):252–7.

21. Nonas SA, Finigan JH, Gao L, et al. Functional genomic insights into acute lung injury. Proc Am Thorac Soc 2005;2(3):188–94.

22. Flores C, Ma SF, Maresso K, et al. IL6 gene-wide haplotype is associated with susceptibility to acute lung injury. Transl Res 2008;152(1):11–7.

23. Meyer NJ, Daye ZJ, Rushefski M, et al. SNP-set analysis replicates acute lung injury genetic risk factors. BMC Med Genet 2012;13(1):52.

24. Lin Z, Pearson C, Chinchilli V, et al. Polymorphisms of human SP-A, SP-B, and SP-D genes: association of SP-B Thr131Ile with ARDS. Clin Genet 2000;58(3): 181–91.

25. Meyer NJ, Feng R, Li M, et al. IL1RN coding variant is associated with lower risk of acute respiratory distress syndrome and increased plasma IL-1 receptor antagonist. Am J Respir Crit Care Med 2013;187(9):950–9.

26. Meyer NJ, Li M, Feng R, et al. ANGPT2 genetic variant is associated with trauma-associated acute lung injury and altered plasma angiopoietin-2 isoform ratio. Am J Respir Crit Care Med 2011;183(10):1344–53.

27. Visscher Peter M, Brown Matthew A, McCarthy Mark I, et al. Five years of GWAS discovery. Am J Hum Genet 2012;90(1):7–24.

28. Christie JD, Wurfel MM, Feng R, et al. Genome wide association identifies PPFIA1 as a candidate gene for acute lung injury risk following major trauma. PLoS One 2012;7(1):e28268.

29. Bime C, Pouladi N, Sammani S, et al. Genome-wide association study in African Americans with acute respiratory distress syndrome identifies the selectin P ligand gene as a risk factor. Am J Respir Crit Care Med 2018;197(11):1421–32.

30. Guillen-Guio B, Lorenzo-Salazar JM, Ma SF, et al. Sepsis-associated acute respiratory distress syndrome in individuals of European ancestry: a genome-wide association study. Lancet Respir Med 2020;8(3):258–66.

31. Hernandez-Pacheco N, Guillen-Guio B, Acosta-Herrera M, et al. A vascular endothelial growth factor receptor gene variant is associated with susceptibility to acute respiratory distress syndrome. Intensive Care Med Exp 2018;6(1):16.

32. Rautanen A, Mills TC, Gordon AC, et al. Genome-wide association study of survival from sepsis due to pneumonia: an observational cohort study. Lancet Respir Med 2015;3(1):53–60.

33. Hinz J, Büttner B, Kriesel F, et al. The FER rs4957796 TT genotype is associated with unfavorable 90-day survival in Caucasian patients with severe ARDS due to pneumonia. Sci Rep 2017;7(1):9887.

34. Scherag A, Schöneweck F, Kesselmeier M, et al. Genetic factors of the disease course after sepsis: a genome-wide study for 28Day mortality. EBioMedicine 2016;12:239–46.

35. Ellinghaus D, Degenhardt F, Bujanda L, et al. Genomewide association study of severe Covid-19 with respiratory failure. N Engl J Med 2020;383(16):1522–34.

36. Reilly JP, Meyer NJ, Shashaty MG, et al. The ABO Histo-Blood Group, endothelial activation, and acute respiratory distress syndrome risk in critical illness. J Clin Invest 2020;131(1):e139700.

37. Reilly JP, Meyer NJ, Shashaty MGS, et al. ABO blood type A is associated with increased risk of ARDS in whites following both major trauma and severe sepsis. Chest 2014;145(4):753–61.

38. Pairo-Castineira E, Clohisey S, Klaric L, et al. Genetic mechanisms of critical illness in Covid-19. Nature 2020;591(7848):92–8.

39. Wang F, Huang S, Gao R, et al. Initial whole-genome sequencing and analysis of the host genetic contribution to COVID-19 severity and susceptibility. Cell Discov 2020;6(1):83.

40. Shortt K, Chaudhary S, Grigoryev D, et al. Identification of novel single nucleotide polymorphisms associated with acute respiratory distress syndrome by exome-seq. PLoS One 2014;9(11):e111953.

41. Palakshappa JA, Meyer NJ. Which patients with ARDS benefit from lung biopsy? Chest 2015;148(4):1073–82.

42. Frank JA, Wray CM, McAuley DF, et al. Alveolar macrophages contribute to alveolar barrier dysfunction in ventilator-induced lung injury. Am J Physiol Lung Cell Mol Physiol 2006;291(6):L1191–8.

43. Guo L, Xie J, Huang Y, et al. Higher PEEP improves outcomes in ARDS patients with clinically objective positive oxygenation response to PEEP: a systematic review and meta-analysis. BMC Anesthesiol 2018;18(1):172.

44. Thompson BT, Chambers RC, Liu KD. Acute respiratory distress syndrome. N Engl J Med 2017;377(6):562–72.

45. Kangelaris KN, Prakash A, Liu KD, et al. Increased expression of neutrophil-related genes in patients with early sepsis-induced ARDS. Am J Physiol Lung Cell Mol Physiol 2015;308(11):L1102–13.

46. Bozza FA, Shah AM, Weyrich AS, et al. Amicus or adversary. Am J Respir Cell Mol Biol 2009;40(2):123–34.
47. Lefrançais E, Ortiz-Muñoz G, Caudrillier A, et al. The lung is a site of platelet biogenesis and a reservoir for haematopoietic progenitors. Nature 2017;544:105.
48. Juss JK, House D, Amour A, et al. Acute respiratory distress syndrome neutrophils have a distinct phenotype and are resistant to phosphoinositide 3-kinase inhibition. Am J Respir Crit Care Med 2016;194(8):961–73.
49. Juss J, Herre J, Begg M, et al. Genome-wide transcription profiling in neutrophils in acute respiratory distress syndrome. The Lancet 2015;385(Supplement 1):S55.
50. Dolinay T, Kim YS, Howrylak J, et al. Inflammasome-regulated cytokines are critical mediators of acute lung injury. Am J Respir Crit Care Med 2012;185(11):1225–34.
51. Prescott HC, Calfee CS, Thompson BT, et al. Toward smarter lumping and smarter splitting: rethinking strategies for sepsis and acute respiratory distress syndrome clinical trial design. Am J Respir Crit Care Med 2016;194(2):147–55.
52. Kuo CS, Pavlidis S, Loza M, et al. A transcriptome-driven analysis of epithelial brushings and bronchial biopsies to define asthma phenotypes in U-BIOPRED. Am J Respir Crit Care Med 2017;195(4):443–55.
53. Fajt ML, Wenzel SE. Asthma phenotypes and the use of biologic medications in asthma and allergic disease: the next steps toward personalized care. J Allergy Clin Immunol 2015;135(2):299–310.
54. Sweeney TE, Shidham A, Wong HR, et al. A comprehensive time-course-based multicohort analysis of sepsis and sterile inflammation reveals a robust diagnostic gene set. Sci Transl Med 2015;7(287):287ra271.
55. Howrylak JA, Dolinay T, Lucht L, et al. Discovery of the gene signature for acute lung injury in patients with sepsis. Physiol Genomics 2009;37(2):133–9.
56. Sweeney TE, Thomas NJ, Howrylak JA, et al. Multicohort analysis of whole-blood gene expression data does not Form a robust diagnostic for acute respiratory distress syndrome. Crit Care Med 2018;46(2):244–51.
57. Kovach MA, Stringer KA, Bunting R, et al. Microarray analysis identifies IL-1 receptor type 2 as a novel candidate biomarker in patients with acute respiratory distress syndrome. Respir Res 2015;16(1):29.
58. Morrell ED, Bhatraju PK, Mikacenic CR, et al. Alveolar macrophage transcriptional programs are associated with outcomes in acute respiratory distress syndrome. Am J Respir Crit Care Med 2019;200(6):732–41.
59. Morrell ED, Radella F 2nd, Manicone AM, et al. Peripheral and alveolar cell transcriptional programs are distinct in acute respiratory distress syndrome. Am J Respir Crit Care Med 2018;197(4):528–32.
60. Juss JK, House D, Amour A, et al. Acute respiratory distress syndrome neutrophils have a distinct phenotype and are resistant to phosphoinositide 3-kinase inhibition. Am J Respir Crit Care Med 2016;194(8):961–73.
61. Lowe R, Shirley N, Bleackley M, et al. Transcriptomics technologies. PLoS Comput Biol 2017;13(5):e1005457.
62. Wang Z, Gerstein M, Snyder M. RNA-Seq: a revolutionary tool for transcriptomics. Nat Rev Genet 2009;10(1):57–63.
63. Wang Ye, Fu X, Yu B, et al. Long non-coding RNA THRIL predicts increased acute respiratory distress syndrome risk and positively correlates with disease severity, inflammation, and mortality in sepsis patients. J Clin Lab Anal 2019;33(6):e22882.
64. Maslove DM, Wong HR. Gene expression profiling in sepsis: timing, tissue, and translational considerations. Trends Mol Med 2014;20(4):204–13.

65. Jiang Y, Rosborough BR, Chen J, et al. Single cell RNA sequencing identifies an early monocyte gene signature in acute respiratory distress syndrome. JCI Insight 2020;5(13):e135678.
66. Mackay TFC, Stone EA, Ayroles JF. The genetics of quantitative traits: challenges and prospects. Nat Rev Genet 2009;10(8):565–77.
67. Meyer NJ, Calfee CS. Novel translational approaches to the search for precision therapies for acute respiratory distress syndrome. Lancet Respir Med 2017;5(6): 512–23.
68. Tejera P, Christiani DC. Deconstructing ARDS Variability: platelet count, an ARDS intermediate phenotype and novel mediator of genetic effects in ARDS. Semin Respir Crit Care Med 2019;40(1):12–8.
69. Imai K, Keele L, Tingley D. A general approach to causal mediation analysis. Psychol Methods 2010;15(4):309–34.
70. Wei Y, Wang Z, Su L, et al. Platelet count mediates the contribution of a genetic variant in LRRC 16A to ARDS risk. Chest 2015;147(3):607–17.
71. Yadav H, Kor DJ. Platelets in the pathogenesis of acute respiratory distress syndrome. Am J Physiol 2015;309(9):L915–23.
72. Qayyum R, Snively BM, Ziv E, et al. A meta-analysis and genome-wide association study of platelet count and mean platelet volume in african americans. PLoS Genet 2012;8(3):e1002491.
73. Shameer K, Denny JC, Ding K, et al. A genome- and phenome-wide association study to identify genetic variants influencing platelet count and volume and their pleiotropic effects. Hum Genet 2014;133(1):95–109.
74. Wei Y, Tejera P, Wang Z, et al. A missense genetic variant in LRRC16A/CARMIL1 improves acute respiratory distress syndrome survival by attenuating platelet count decline. Am J Respir Crit Care Med 2017;195(10):1353–61.
75. Bochud M, Rousson V. Usefulness of Mendelian randomization in observational epidemiology. Int J Environ Res Public Health 2010;7(3):711–28.
76. Lawlor DA, Harbord RM, Sterne JA, et al. Mendelian randomization: using genes as instruments for making causal inferences in epidemiology. Stat Med 2008; 27(8):1133–63.
77. Ferguson JF, Meyer NJ, Qu L, et al. Integrative genomics identifies 7p11.2 as a novel locus for fever and clinical stress response in humans. Hum Mol Genet 2015;24(6):1801–12.
78. Didelez V, Meng S, Sheehan NA. Assumptions of IV methods for observational epidemiology. Stat Sci 2010;25(1):22–40.
79. Sheehan NA, Didelez V. Epidemiology, genetic epidemiology and Mendelian randomisation: more need than ever to attend to detail. Hum Genet 2020;139(1): 121–36.
80. Reilly JP, Wang F, Jones TK, et al. Plasma angiopoietin-2 as a potential causal marker in sepsis-associated ARDS development: evidence from Mendelian randomization and mediation analysis. Intensive Care Med 2018;44(11):1849–58.
81. Jones TK, Feng R, Kerchberger VE, et al. Plasma sRAGE acts as a genetically regulated causal intermediate in sepsis-associated acute respiratory distress syndrome. Am J Respir Crit Care Med 2020;201(1):47–56.
82. Dong X, Zhu Z, Wei Y, et al. Plasma insulin-like growth factor binding protein-7 (IGFBP-7) contributes causally to ARDS 28-day mortality: evidence from multistage Mendelian randomization. Chest 2020;159(3):1007–18.
83. Han D, Li Z, Li R, et al. mNGS in clinical microbiology laboratories: on the road to maturity. Crit Rev Microbiol 2019;45(5–6):668–85.

84. Bullard J, Dust K, Funk D, et al. Predicting infectious SARS-CoV-2 from diagnostic samples. Clin Infect Dis 2020;71(10):2663–6.
85. Abu Raya B, Goldfarb DM, Sadarangani M. What is the role of severe acute respiratory syndrome Coronavirus 2 polymerase chain reaction testing in discontinuation of Transmission-based precautions for Coronavirus disease 2019 patients? Clin Infect Dis 2020;71(16):2304–5.
86. Dickson RP, Singer BH, Newstead MW, et al. Enrichment of the lung microbiome with gut bacteria in sepsis and the acute respiratory distress syndrome. Nat Microbiol 2016;1(10):16113.
87. Calfee CS, Delucchi K, Parsons PE, et al. Subphenotypes in acute respiratory distress syndrome: latent class analysis of data from two randomised controlled trials. Lancet Respir Med 2014;2(8):611–20.
88. Bos LD, Schouten LR, van Vught LA, et al. Identification and validation of distinct biological phenotypes in patients with acute respiratory distress syndrome by cluster analysis. Thorax 2017;72(10):876–83.
89. Antcliffe DB, Burnham KL, Al-Beidh F, et al. Transcriptomic signatures in sepsis and a differential response to steroids: from the VANISH randomized trial. Am J Respir Crit Care Med 2019;199(8):980–6.
90. Meyer NJ, Reilly JP, Anderson BJ, et al. Mortality benefit of recombinant human interleukin-1 receptor antagonist for sepsis varies by initial interleukin-1 receptor antagonist plasma concentration. Crit Care Med 2018;46(1):21–8.
91. Xiong Y, Liu Y, Cao L, et al. Transcriptomic characteristics of bronchoalveolar lavage fluid and peripheral blood mononuclear cells in COVID-19 patients. Emerg Microbes Infect 2020;9(1):761–70.
92. Wen W, Su W, Tang H, et al. Immune cell profiling of COVID-19 patients in the recovery stage by single-cell sequencing. Cell Discov 2020;6:31.
93. Wilk AJ, Rustagi A, Zhao NQ, et al. A single-cell atlas of the peripheral immune response in patients with severe COVID-19. Nat Med 2020;26(7):1070–6.
94. Overmyer KA, Shishkova E, Miller IJ, et al. Large-scale multi-omic analysis of COVID-19 severity. Cell Syst 2020;12(1):23–40.e7.
95. Xu G, Qi F, Li H, et al. The differential immune responses to COVID-19 in peripheral and lung revealed by single-cell RNA sequencing. Cell Discov 2020;6:73.
96. Mick E, Kamm J, Pisco AO, et al. Upper airway gene expression reveals suppressed immune responses to SARS-CoV-2 compared with other respiratory viruses. Nat Commun 2020;11(1):5854.

Acute Kidney Injury and Acute Respiratory Distress Syndrome

Bryan D. Park, MD[a], Sarah Faubel, MD[b],*

KEYWORDS

- Acute kidney injury • Acute respiratory distress syndrome • COVID-19
- Intensive care unit

KEY POINTS

- AKI is a common complication of ARDS and portends a poor prognosis.
- AKI is associated with numerous traditional and nontraditional complications that conspire to adversely affect the lungs.
- Key considerations in the management of AKI complicating ARDS include close attention to fluid balance, maintenance of euvolemia, avoidance of hypophosphatemia while on RRT, and continuous dialogue between nephrologists and critical care specialists.
- Clinicians should recognize that patients with AKI can be expected to require mechanical ventilation longer and wean longer than other patient populations.
- AKI is common in COVID-19 disease and is predominantly caused by sepsis pathophysiology.

INTRODUCTION

Acute kidney injury (AKI) is a common complication in patients with acute respiratory distress syndrome (ARDS) with studies reporting up to 35% incidence rate. The combination of AKI and ARDS portends worse outcomes including higher mortality and increased hospital length-of-stay.[1–3] Recently, the novel SARS-CoV-2 (or COVID-19) has emerged as the most significant viral pandemic in the modern era, and has further highlighted the important relationship of organ-organ crosstalk in the critically ill. In this article, we explore the interrelationship between the kidneys and the lungs in the setting of ARDS. We emphasize key clinical information including definition,

ª Division of Pulmonary Sciences and Critical Care Medicine, Department of Internal Medicine, University of Colorado, Anschutz Medical Campus, 12700 East 19th Avenue, Box C272, Aurora, CO 80045, USA; ᵇ Division of Renal Diseases and Hypertension, Department of Internal Medicine, University of Colorado, Anschutz Medical Campus, 12700 East 19th Avenue, Box C281, Aurora, CO 80045, USA
* Corresponding author.
E-mail address: sarah.faubel@cuanschutz.edu

Crit Care Clin 37 (2021) 835–849
https://doi.org/10.1016/j.ccc.2021.05.007
0749-0704/21/© 2021 Elsevier Inc. All rights reserved.

criticalcare.theclinics.com

epidemiology, pathophysiology, and treatment strategies important for any critical care clinician. Finally, we also describe the current understanding of AKI in SARS-CoV-2 infection given the high incidence of AKI in this population.

DEFINITIONS OF ACUTE KIDNEY INJURY

Early studies of hospital and intensive care unit (ICU)-acquired AKI were limited by the lack of a uniform, standard definition.[4,5] Before 2004, more than 30 different definitions of AKI had been described, which created difficulties in validating diagnostic and therapeutic interventions.[5] The first collaborative efforts to define and stage AKI was performed by an international, multidisciplinary group in 2004 by the Acute Dialysis Quality Initiative (ADQI)[5] and then in 2005 by the Acute Kidney Injury Network.[4] More recently, the Kidney Disease: Improving Global Outcomes (KDIGO) society developed rigorous evidence-based clinical practice guidelines in 2012 for the evaluation and management of AKI.[6] Their proposal included a modified definition of AKI by combining the ADQI and Acute Kidney Injury Network definitions, and is now the most used definition and classification system (**Table 1**).

Although the 2012 KDIGO criteria for AKI have now been successfully implemented, some limitations exist.[7] First, these criteria do not include identification of an underlying cause. AKI is a heterogeneous disease with a variety of causes requiring different diagnostic and therapeutic interventions. As such, the clinical context is always key, and outcomes may differ depending on the underlying cause. Second, the heavy reliance on serum creatinine in the AKI definition has several drawbacks.[7] Although serum creatinine is routinely available and its measurement is standardized across institutions, creatinine may be affected by many nonrenal disease states,[8–10] is a late marker of kidney function decline, and does not rise until a substantial amount of kidney function has been lost.[11] As a result, the contributions of AKI to systemic diseases may be underappreciated because AKI is typically diagnosed late in the hospital course and may be incorrectly regarded as a consequence of systemic disease even though it may occur simultaneously or even before other complications.[12] Third, oliguria is an excellent early marker of AKI,[13] but it is less readily studied.

Table 1 KDIGO diagnosis and staging criteria for AKI		
Stage	**Serum Creatinine**	**Urine Output**
1	1.5–1.9 times baseline or ≥0.3 mg/dL (≥26.5 μmol/L) increase	<0.5 mL/kg/h for 6–12 h
2	2.0–2.9 times baseline	<0.5 mL/kg/h for ≥12 h
3	3 times baseline or ≥4.0 mg/dL (≥353.6 μmol/L) increase or Initiation of renal-replacement therapy or Patients <18 y, decrease in estimated glomerular filtration rate <35 mL/min/1.73 m²	< 0.3 mL/kg/h for ≥24 h or Anuria ≥12 h

Data from Kellum JA, Lameire N, Group KAGW. Diagnosis, evaluation, and management of acute kidney injury: a KDIGO summary (Part 1). Crit Care. 2013;17(1):204.

CLINICAL OUTCOMES OF ACUTE KIDNEY INJURY AND ACUTE RESPIRATORY DISTRESS SYNDROME

AKI is a common complication and associated with a high mortality in the hospital and ICU settings. AKI may complicate up to 20% of all hospital admissions.[14] In the ICU, up to 57% of patients develop AKI, and approximately 13% require renal-replacement therapy (RRT).[15,16] More importantly, AKI is associated with a high mortality,[14] and an international study evaluating more than 23 countries and 54 ICUs found that the hospital mortality ranged between 40% and 60%.[17] Another multinational cross-sectional study investigating AKI using the KDIGO criteria demonstrated that AKI is an independent predictor of in-hospital mortality across all stages of AKI with exponential increase in hazard ratios from mild/stage 1 disease (hazard ratio, 1.7) to severe/stage 3 disease (hazard ratio, 6.7) even after adjustment for covariates.[15] Strong associations with mortality in AKI is also true across many different settings and populations, including aortic surgery,[18] cardiac surgery,[19] decompensated cirrhosis,[20] and bone marrow transplant.[21] Furthermore, AKI can increase the risk of long-term adverse outcomes with one large systematic review demonstrating an increased risk of mortality, myocardial infarction, and development of end-stage renal disease.[22]

Clinical Outcomes of Acute Kidney Injury Complicating Acute Respiratory Distress Syndrome

AKI is a common complication in patients with ARDS. A secondary analysis from the landmark ARDSnet trial demonstrated that approximately 24% of participants with ARDS developed AKI.[23] One prospective, multicenter ICU study showed that 44.3% of ARDS patients also had AKI with a median time to diagnosis of 2 days after ARDS.[24] After adjustment for cofounders, mechanical ventilation (MV) with ARDS had a high likelihood of developing AKI.

AKI complicating ARDS portends a poor prognosis. In the ARDSnet trial, the 180-day mortality rate was much higher in those with AKI versus those without (58% vs 28%)[25] and this association was confirmed in other prospective studies.[24] Similarly, another study evaluating oliguric renal failure and lung injury found that the survival rate was much lower compared with the entire cohort of patients studied (**Fig. 1**).[26]

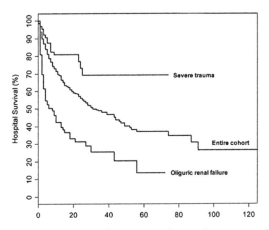

Fig. 1. ARDS complicated by severe AKI has increased mortality compared with ARDS alone. (*Adapted from* Cooke CR, Kahn JM, Caldwell E, et al. Predictors of hospital mortality in a population-based cohort of patients with acute lung injury. Crit Care Med. 2008;36(5):1412-1420; with permission.)

Severe AKI requiring RRT was associated with up to 50% mortality,[27] and one retrospective study demonstrated increased ventilator days (10 vs 7 days) and duration of weaning (41 vs 21 hours) in those with ARDS complicated by AKI versus ARDS alone.[28]

THE EFFECT OF ACUTE KIDNEY INJURY ON THE LUNGS

Traditional complications of AKI, such as electrolyte derangements, uremia, and fluid overload, have long been considered to contribute to the poor pulmonary outcomes associated with AKI; however, research over the last two decades highlights the importance of nontraditional consequences of AKI (**Table 2**).[29] The importance of nontraditional complications to outcomes after AKI is evidenced by the fact that RRT is well known to correct the traditional complications of AKI, yet the mortality of AKI requiring RRT in the ICU is 50% to 60%.[30–33] Thus, improving mortality rates in patients with AKI requires therapies targeted beyond modifications and improvements to RRT.

AKI and its effects on the lungs has been well studied in animal models.[34,35] AKI-mediated lung injury is associated with lung inflammation characterized by increased levels of pulmonary cytokines, chemokines, and neutrophil accumulation.[36–39] The proinflammatory cytokine interleukin (IL)-6 increases in the plasma by 2 hours of AKI[36,37] and is a major mediator of lung inflammation post-AKI.[36,40] These findings are clinically relevant because patients with AKI develop increased plasma IL-6 within 2 hours[41] and increased IL-6 is associated with prolonged MV[41] and increased mortality.[42] Additional characteristics of AKI-mediated lung injury in animal models include dysregulation of salt and water channels,[43] pulmonary vascular congestion,[39] T-cell accumulation,[44] and apoptotic and necrotic cell death.[45,46] Unlike direct lung injury, AKI lung injury is not characterized by significant epithelial injury and the alveolar space is devoid of inflammatory cytokines and neutrophils.[47]

THE EFFECT OF ACUTE RESPIRATORY DISTRESS SYNDROME ON THE KIDNEYS

Around the time of the ARDSnet trial, several papers demonstrated that protective lung strategies were associated with reduced serum cytokine/chemokine levels and

Table 2
Traditional and nontraditional complications of AKI

Traditional Complications of AKI	Nontraditional Complications of AKI
Recognized for >50 y	Newly appreciated and studied in the past 20 y
May contribute to increased mortality of AKI	May contribute greatly to AKI mortality
Typically corrected by renal-replacement therapy	Requires therapy beyond renal-replacement therapy

Include
  Hyperkalemia
  Acidosis
  Hyperphosphatemia
  Hypocalcemia
  Fluid overload
  Pericarditis
  Uremic bleeding
	Include
	  Respiratory complications/inflammatory lung injury
	  Sepsis
	  Cardiac dysfunction/injury
	  Intestinal injury
	  Liver injury
	  Immunoparalysis

Adapted from Faubel S, Edelstein CL. Mechanisms and mediators of lung injury after acute kidney injury. Nat Rev Nephrol. 2016;12(1):48-60; with permission.

decreased organ dysfunction, including a reduced rate of AKI.[23,48,49] The reduced rate of AKI with low tidal volume ventilation may be caused by the known effects of MV on renal function.[50] Positive pressure ventilation was first shown to decrease renal perfusion in 1947.[51] Since then, several studies in experimental models and clinical cohorts have shown that the use of positive end-expiratory pressure can decrease urine output likely caused by a reduction in cardiac output.[52–55] Positive end-expiratory pressure has also been shown to alter the normal neurohormonal homeostasis (ie, renin-angiotensin-aldosterone axis) important for regulation of normal kidney function,[55] resulting in decreased renal perfusion, glomerular filtration rate, and urine output.[52,55–57]

TREATMENT STRATEGIES FOR PATIENTS WITH ACUTE RESPIRATORY DISTRESS SYNDROME AND ACUTE KIDNEY INJURY

Overall, treatment strategies for patients with ARDS and AKI are similar to the treatment of either condition alone. Next we discuss the general approach to ARDS and AKI, and how care of one may influence overall treatment and physiology when the two are together.

Acute Respiratory Distress Syndrome Management at a Glance

In general, the identification and treatment of underlying causes for ARDS (eg, sepsis, trauma, and burns) will ensure optimal outcomes. The supportive treatment options for ARDS have been well-studied.[58,59] First, the landmark ARDSnet trial[23] showed a clinically significant reduction in mortality and more ventilator-free days with the use of low-tidal volume ventilation to prevent significant barotrauma. Second, among patients with severe ARDS, prone positioning significantly reduced 28-day mortality.[60] Third, a conservative fluid management strategy with use of diuretics decreased ventilator-free days, reduced ICU days, and improved lung function, although a statistically significant mortality improvement was not appreciated.[61,62]

Fluid Management in Acute Respiratory Distress Syndrome and Acute Kidney Injury

Fluid overload has consistently been shown to be associated with adverse outcomes and worse mortality in the critically ill in general, and in patients with AKI in particular.[63–65] Maintaining a net negative fluid balance (and therefore, less pulmonary edema) can positively affect lung physiology and outcomes in critically ill ventilated patients[61,66]; however, clinical equipoise is key, and at some point striving for a net negative fluid balance is not beneficial once the patient's dry weight has been achieved. Several studies in septic shock and ARDS patients have demonstrated an association between a positive fluid balance and worse mortality, MV duration, and ICU length of stay.[61,67–70] In the FACTT trial, the conservative fluid cohort (treated with diuretics) was more likely to have a shorter MV duration and shorter ICU stay compared with a liberal fluid strategy.[61] There was also a trend for the conservative fluid group to require dialysis less often compared with the liberal fluid group highlighting that excess fluid administration does not protect against AKI requiring RRT as had been previously thought. Volume overload can also increase the risk of intra-abdominal hypertension and the risk of AKI through an overall reduction in renal blood flow.[71,72] In the absence of intra-abdominal hypertension, excess volume can also increase edema in the renal interstitium thereby leading to worse AKI.[68]

Acute Kidney Injury Management at a Glance

The 2012 KDIGO recommendations for the management of AKI has been widely adopted and serve to help the clinician with prognostication and diagnostic/treatment decisions.[6] Since its publication, several studies have shown that implementation of these guidelines may aid in prompt diagnosis and management of AKI in susceptible populations leading to improved clinical outcomes.[73–75]

The first step is to obtain an accurate diagnosis of AKI and identify the cause of kidney injury whenever possible. Next, the prevention of worsening injury revolves around maintaining adequate organ perfusion, avoiding volume overload, avoiding hyperglycemia, discontinuing nephrotoxic agents, and renally dosing medications. Lastly, when such maneuvers are inadequate and the patient develops worsening complications of AKI (eg, fluid overload, hyperkalemia), RRT is the next appropriate treatment modality to consider.

Approach to Renal-Replacement Therapy in the Critically Ill Patient with Acute Kidney Injury

Initiation of RRT requires astute clinical judgment and the collaboration of nephrologists and intensivists to determine patient suitability. In general, the decision to start RRT depends on (1) the underlying cause, (2) indications for RRT, (3) patient factors guiding modality, and (4) specific treatment variables. We briefly summarize important aspects of RRT for the critical care provider.

First, it is widely accepted that RRT should be initiated in those with severe electrolyte derangements (eg, hyperkalemia), severe acidosis, severe uremia, and pulmonary edema in the setting of oliguria.[6] Even with this recommendation, clinical equipoise must be maintained and current guidelines also recommend considering the broader clinical context when starting dialysis.

Second, the timing of RRT has been well-studied and the current evidence indicates that early initiation has no benefits regarding survival. In general, most randomized controlled trials showed no mortality benefit with an early versus late timing approach to RRT.[30,31,33,76,77] A meta-analysis of seven different randomized clinical trials with 1343 patients showed no benefit with an early RRT approach (95% confidence interval, 0.74 [0.43–1.27]).[78] As such, the ultimate timing decision depends on multiple factors to be addressed and discussed among nephrologists and intensivists.

Third, there is no firm consensus on the optimal RRT modality in AKI. Continuous RRT (CRRT) is generally preferred over intermittent hemodialysis and prolonged intermittent RRT because of perceived hemodynamic instability in the critically ill. One recent meta-analysis comparing CRRT, intermittent hemodialysis, and prolonged intermittent RRT showed no clear advantage of one modality over another on short-term mortality and dialysis dependence.[79]

Hypophosphatemia in Continuous Renal-Replacement Therapy

CRRT is associated with a high incidence of severe hypophosphatemia occurring in up to 70% of patients.[80–82] Phosphate is essential for all cells and is important for cell membrane integrity, bone structure, cell signaling, acid-base buffering, and energy storage in the form of adenosine triphosphate.[83] As such, severe hypophosphatemia has been implicated in respiratory muscle failure and prolonged duration of MV.[84–86] Additionally, reduced levels of phosphate can impair myocardial contractility and lead to arrhythmias, which may be improved once hypophosphatemia is corrected.[83] Hypophosphatemia has been associated with prolonged MV,[87] longer vasopressor duration,[87] longer duration of CRRT use,[82] longer ICU stays,[82] and higher doses of CRRT.[88] Therefore, it is important to monitor and treat the common complication of hypophosphatemia in RRT patients.

ACUTE KIDNEY INJURY AND SARS-CoV-2: CURRENT KNOWLEDGE

SARS-CoV-2 is a novel coronavirus that was first reported in December 2019,[89] and has since become the most significant pandemic in the modern era. Initial reports suggested that the rates of AKI were low[90,91]; however, more recent data suggest AKI to be a common complication with values reported as high as 37%.[91–94] The ICU incidence of AKI is more significantly elevated at more than 50% in multiple studies, and has been associated with significant mortality.[93,95,96] A large registry from the European Renal Association-European Dialysis and Transplant Association has shown a high short-term mortality rate of 20% for dialysis and renal transplant patients.[97] Independent risk factors for AKI included elderly, Black race, diabetes, cardiovascular disease, hypertension, MV, and vasopressor use.[93,98]

The pathophysiologic mechanism underlying AKI in COVID-19 is still incompletely understood. The best evidence to date indicates that the underlying mechanism is similar to severe sepsis with one case series reporting acute tubular necrosis in approximately 66% of cases.[96] Another important consideration is the cytokine storm phenomenon experienced in severe COVID-19 ARDS patients, which may lead to hypotension and sepsis further compromising renal perfusion. Focal kidney fibrin thrombi have been identified in histologic specimens, but are not currently thought to directly contribute to AKI and are instead considered a sequelae of deranged coagulopathy.[99] AKI in COVID-19 patients may also be as a result of prerenal azotemia and tubular injury as a result of toxic insults, such as rhabdomyolysis.[100] Collapsing glomerulopathy is an uncommon, but well-established cause of AKI that is associated with nephrotic syndrome and has been described particularly in the setting of high-risk APOL1 alleles.[101] Other pathologic features described include membranous glomerulopathy, antiglomerular basement membrane nephritis, and exacerbation of preexisting autoimmune glomerulonephritis, but it is unclear whether these features are related to COVID-19 or new/preexisting diagnoses.[102]

Whether SARS-CoV-2 causes direct viral injury to the kidneys is currently controversial. Because SARS-CoV-2 enters cells via the ACE-2 receptors, which are abundant on the renal proximal tubule, it was thought that directly viral entry was probable. Early studies demonstrated viral staining in the proximal tubule, but later studies failed to confirm this. Targeting of ACE-2 receptors by COVID-19 may result in several downstream effects, such as hypercoagulation, innate and adaptive immune pathway activation, and angiotensin dysregulation.[103] However, these studies also report on patient samples that did not demonstrate significant viral particle staining.

At time of submission, there are two therapies approved for use in severe COVID-19 illness (remdesivir and dexamethasone).[104] Of note, remdesivir is currently contraindicated in those with a reduced glomerular filtration rate, but recent evidence suggests that it may be suitable in those receiving RRT.[105] The initial concern for remdesivir use in patients with AKI revolved around the nephrotoxic accumulation of sulfobutylether-β-cyclodextrin, but evidence suggests there is adequate removal of sulfobutylether-β-cyclodextrin with dialysis.[105,106] The risk of venous thromboembolism seems to be higher in this syndrome; however, recent critical care guidelines recommend against full anticoagulation without evidence of venous thromboembolisms, and recommend typical thromboprophylaxis and monitoring as key.[107]

The indications for RRT in the management of severe AKI in the setting of COVID-19 disease are the same as for other critically ill patients.[94,108] One important distinction is the use of anticoagulation because higher incidence of filter clotting during CRRT in COVID-19 disease has been reported.[109–111] Several studies have reported distinct perturbations in the clotting cascade in COVID-19 patients including thrombocytopenia and prolonged prothrombin/partial thromboplastic time, which may contribute to the high incidence of filter clotting.[110,112,113] CRRT filter clotting is an important concern because it can lead to blood loss and lost time on RRT. ADQI guidelines for the management of AKI in COVID-19 patients recommend the use of anticoagulation if not otherwise contraindicated, monitoring for impending signs of circuit failure, and establishing center-specific stepwise escalation options for CRRT anticoagulation.[94] Finally, as the pandemic continues, there is concern about dialysis and CRRT availability, including consumables, machines, and staff.[114] Critical shortages were seen during the initial surge in New York City and similarly experienced abroad; therefore, preparation of resources in the coming months is key.[114,115]

SUMMARY

AKI is a common complication during hospital and ICU stays, and is particularly problematic when coexisting with ARDS. Previous studies have highlighted that AKI is an independent predictor for death in patients who are critically ill with acute lung injury. Clinical and experimental data indicate that there is significant crosstalk between injured kidneys and the lung, and that AKI exerts a multitude of deleterious effects on the lung via fluid overload leading to cardiogenic pulmonary edema, cytokine excess leading to noncardiogenic pulmonary edema, and others. The organ-organ effects of kidney and lung injury have been especially poignant in the era of the novel SARS-CoV-2 virus where the existence of both complications portends a poor prognosis. In summary, AKI complicating ARDS is a common phenomenon that contributes to a significant burden of disease, and clinical recognition of this syndrome aids the clinician in management and prognostication in the critically ill.

CRITICAL CARE POINTS

- AKI in conjunction with ARDS portends a poor prognosis and can help guide the intensivist in goals of care discussion.
- AKI can affect the lungs in multiple ways via traditional (eg, volume overload) and nontraditional (eg, systemic inflammatory mediators) complications.
- Maintaining appropriate fluid balance and ensuring adequate treatment of the underlying cause of ARDS are crucial.
- If a patient becomes anuric, renal-replacement therapy should be considered. Initiation and management of such treatment should involve a continuous dialogue between the intensivist and nephrologist.
- AKI is also a common complication of COVID-19. In general, management of AKI in COVID-19 patients is similar to other disease states. However, special consideration should be made to potential drug toxicities of new SARS-CoV2 agents; and the increased prevalence of hypercoagulability in this population.

DISCLOSURE

None.

REFERENCES

1. Liu KD, Matthay MA. Advances in critical care for the nephrologist: acute lung injury/ARDS. Clin J Am Soc Nephrol 2008;3(2):578–86.
2. Liu KD, Thompson BT, Ancukiewicz M, et al. Acute kidney injury in patients with acute lung injury: impact of fluid accumulation on classification of acute kidney injury and associated outcomes. Crit Care Med 2011;39(12):2665–71.
3. Mehta RL, Pascual MT, Gruta CG, et al. Refining predictive models in critically ill patients with acute renal failure. J Am Soc Nephrol 2002;13(5):1350–7.
4. Mehta RL, Kellum JA, Shah SV, et al. Acute Kidney Injury Network: report of an initiative to improve outcomes in acute kidney injury. Crit Care 2007;11(2):R31.
5. Bellomo R, Ronco C, Kellum JA, et al. Acute Dialysis Quality Initiative w. Acute renal failure - definition, outcome measures, animal models, fluid therapy and information technology needs: the Second International Consensus Conference of the Acute Dialysis Quality Initiative (ADQI) Group. Crit Care 2004;8(4):R204–12.
6. Kellum JA, Lameire N, Group KAGW. Diagnosis, evaluation, and management of acute kidney injury: a KDIGO summary (Part 1). Crit Care 2013;17(1):204.
7. Selby NM, Fluck RJ, Kolhe NV, et al. International criteria for acute kidney injury: advantages and remaining challenges. PloS Med 2016;13(9):e1002122.
8. Caregaro L, Menon F, Angeli P, et al. Limitations of serum creatinine level and creatinine clearance as filtration markers in cirrhosis. Arch Intern Med 1994;154(2):201–5.
9. Racz O, Lepej J, Fodor B, et al. Pitfalls in the measurements and assessment of glomerular filtration rate and how to escape them. EJIFCC 2012;23(2):33–40.
10. Lin J, Fernandez H, Shashaty MG, et al. False-positive rate of AKI using consensus creatinine-based criteria. Clin J Am Soc Nephrol 2015;10(10):1723–31.
11. Vaidya VS, Ferguson MA, Bonventre JV. Biomarkers of acute kidney injury. Annu Rev Pharmacol Toxicol 2008;48:463–93.
12. Palevsky PM, Liu KD, Brophy PD, et al. KDOQI US commentary on the 2012 KDIGO clinical practice guideline for acute kidney injury. Am J Kidney Dis 2013;61(5):649–72.
13. Macedo E, Malhotra R, Bouchard J, et al. Oliguria is an early predictor of higher mortality in critically ill patients. Kidney Int 2011;80(7):760–7.
14. Uchino S, Bellomo R, Goldsmith D, et al. An assessment of the RIFLE criteria for acute renal failure in hospitalized patients. Crit Care Med 2006;34(7):1913–7.
15. Hoste EA, Bagshaw SM, Bellomo R, et al. Epidemiology of acute kidney injury in critically ill patients: the multinational AKI-EPI study. Intensive Care Med 2015;41(8):1411–23.
16. Nisula S, Kaukonen KM, Vaara ST, et al. Incidence, risk factors and 90-day mortality of patients with acute kidney injury in Finnish intensive care units: the FIN-NAKI study. Intensive Care Med 2013;39(3):420–8.
17. Uchino S, Kellum JA, Bellomo R, et al. Acute renal failure in critically ill patients: a multinational, multicenter study. J Am Med Assoc 2005;294(7):813–8.
18. Kashyap VS, Cambria RP, Davison JK, et al. Renal failure after thoracoabdominal aortic surgery. J Vasc Surg 1997;26(6):949–55, discussion 955-947.
19. Chertow GM, Levy EM, Hammermeister KE, et al. Independent association between acute renal failure and mortality following cardiac surgery. Am J Med 1998;104(4):343–8.

20. Aggarwal A, Ong JP, Younossi ZM, et al. Predictors of mortality and resource utilization in cirrhotic patients admitted to the medical ICU. Chest 2001;119(5): 1489–97.

21. Parikh CR, McSweeney P, Schrier RW. Acute renal failure independently predicts mortality after myeloablative allogeneic hematopoietic cell transplant. Kidney Int 2005;67(5):1999–2005.

22. Coca SG, Yusuf B, Shlipak MG, et al. Long-term risk of mortality and other adverse outcomes after acute kidney injury: a systematic review and meta-analysis. Am J Kidney Dis 2009;53(6):961–73.

23. Acute Respiratory Distress Syndrome N, Brower RG, Matthay MA, et al. Ventilation with lower tidal volumes as compared with traditional tidal volumes for acute lung injury and the acute respiratory distress syndrome. N Engl J Med 2000; 342(18):1301–8.

24. Darmon M, Clec'h C, Adrie C, et al. Acute respiratory distress syndrome and risk of AKI among critically ill patients. Clin J Am Soc Nephrol 2014;9(8):1347–53.

25. Liu KD, Glidden DV, Eisner MD, et al. Predictive and pathogenetic value of plasma biomarkers for acute kidney injury in patients with acute lung injury. Crit Care Med 2007;35(12):2755–61.

26. Cooke CR, Kahn JM, Caldwell E, et al. Predictors of hospital mortality in a population-based cohort of patients with acute lung injury. Crit Care Med 2008;36(5):1412–20.

27. Dill J, Bixby B, Ateeli H, et al. Renal replacement therapy in patients with acute respiratory distress syndrome: a single-center retrospective study. Int J Nephrol Renovasc Dis 2018;11:249–57.

28. Vieira JM Jr, Castro I, Curvello-Neto A, et al. Effect of acute kidney injury on weaning from mechanical ventilation in critically ill patients. Crit Care Med 2007;35(1):184–91.

29. Faubel S, Edelstein CL. Mechanisms and mediators of lung injury after acute kidney injury. Nat Rev Nephrol 2016;12(1):48–60.

30. Barbar SD, Clere-Jehl R, Bourredjem A, et al. Timing of renal-replacement therapy in patients with acute kidney injury and sepsis. N Engl J Med 2018;379(15): 1431–42.

31. Gaudry S, Hajage D, Schortgen F, et al. Initiation strategies for renal-replacement therapy in the intensive care Unit. N Engl J Med 2016;375(2): 122–33.

32. Metnitz PG, Krenn CG, Steltzer H, et al. Effect of acute renal failure requiring renal replacement therapy on outcome in critically ill patients. Crit Care Med 2002;30(9):2051–8.

33. Zarbock A, Kellum JA, Schmidt C, et al. Effect of early vs delayed initiation of renal replacement therapy on mortality in critically ill patients with acute kidney injury: the ELAIN randomized clinical trial. J Am Med Assoc 2016;315(20): 2190–9.

34. Grams ME, Rabb H. The distant organ effects of acute kidney injury. Kidney Int 2012;81(10):942–8.

35. Lee SA, Cozzi M, Bush EL, et al. Distant organ dysfunction in acute kidney injury: a review. Am J Kidney Dis 2018;72(6):846–56.

36. Klein CL, Hoke TS, Fang WF, et al. Interleukin-6 mediates lung injury following ischemic acute kidney injury or bilateral nephrectomy. Kidney Int 2008;74(7): 901–9.

37. Hoke TS, Douglas IS, Klein CL, et al. Acute renal failure after bilateral nephrectomy is associated with cytokine-mediated pulmonary injury. J Am Soc Nephrol 2007;18(1):155–64.
38. Awad AS, Rouse M, Huang L, et al. Compartmentalization of neutrophils in the kidney and lung following acute ischemic kidney injury. Kidney Int 2009;75(7): 689–98.
39. Kramer AA, Postler G, Salhab KF, et al. Renal ischemia/reperfusion leads to macrophage-mediated increase in pulmonary vascular permeability. Kidney Int 1999;55(6):2362–7.
40. Altmann C, Ahuja N, Kiekhaefer CM, et al. Early peritoneal dialysis reduces lung inflammation in mice with ischemic acute kidney injury. Kidney Int 2017;92(2): 365–76.
41. Liu KD, Altmann C, Smits G, et al. Serum interleukin-6 and interleukin-8 are early biomarkers of acute kidney injury and predict prolonged mechanical ventilation in children undergoing cardiac surgery: a case-control study. Crit Care 2009; 13(4):R104.
42. Simmons EM, Himmelfarb J, Sezer MT, et al. Plasma cytokine levels predict mortality in patients with acute renal failure. Kidney Int 2004;65(4):1357–65.
43. Rabb H, Wang Z, Nemoto T, et al. Acute renal failure leads to dysregulation of lung salt and water channels. Kidney Int 2003;63(2):600–6.
44. Lie ML, White LE, Santora RJ, et al. Lung T lymphocyte trafficking and activation during ischemic acute kidney injury. J Immunol 2012;189(6):2843–51.
45. Nakazawa D, Kumar SV, Marschner J, et al. Histones and neutrophil extracellular traps enhance tubular necrosis and remote organ injury in ischemic AKI. J Am Soc Nephrol 2017;28(6):1753–68.
46. Hassoun HT, Lie ML, Grigoryev DN, et al. Kidney ischemia-reperfusion injury induces caspase-dependent pulmonary apoptosis. Am J Physiol Renal Physiol 2009;297(1):F125–37.
47. Bhargava R, Janssen W, Altmann C, et al. Intratracheal IL-6 protects against lung inflammation in direct, but not indirect, causes of acute lung injury in mice. PLoS ONE 2013;8(5):e61405.
48. Ranieri VM, Giunta F, Suter PM, et al. Mechanical ventilation as a mediator of multisystem organ failure in acute respiratory distress syndrome. J Am Med Assoc 2000;284(1):43–4.
49. Ranieri VM, Suter PM, Tortorella C, et al. Effect of mechanical ventilation on inflammatory mediators in patients with acute respiratory distress syndrome: a randomized controlled trial. J Am Med Assoc 1999;282(1):54–61.
50. Kuiper JW, Groeneveld AB, Slutsky AS, et al. Mechanical ventilation and acute renal failure. Crit Care Med 2005;33(6):1408–15.
51. Drury DR, Henry JP, Goodman J. The effects of continuous pressure breathing on kidney function. J Clin Invest 1947;26(5):945–51.
52. Annat G, Viale JP, Bui Xuan B, et al. Effect of PEEP ventilation on renal function, plasma renin, aldosterone, neurophysins and urinary ADH, and prostaglandins. Anesthesiology 1983;58(2):136–41.
53. Pannu N, Mehta RL. Effect of mechanical ventilation on the kidney. Best Pract Res Clin Anaesthesiol 2004;18(1):189–203.
54. Priebe HJ, Heimann JC, Hedley-Whyte J. Mechanisms of renal dysfunction during positive end-expiratory pressure ventilation. J Appl Physiol Respir Environ Exerc Physiol 1981;50(3):643–9.
55. Koyner JL, Murray PT. Mechanical ventilation and the kidney. Blood Purif 2010; 29(1):52–68.

56. Andrivet P, Adnot S, Sanker S, et al. Hormonal interactions and renal function during mechanical ventilation and ANF infusion in humans. J Appl Physiol (1985) 1991;70(1):287–92.

57. Bark H, Le Roith D, Nyska M, et al. Elevations in plasma ADH levels during PEEP ventilation in the dog: mechanisms involved. Am J Physiol 1980;239(6): E474–81.

58. Fan E, Del Sorbo L, Goligher EC, et al. An official American Thoracic Society/European Society of Intensive Care Medicine/Society of Critical Care Medicine clinical practice guideline: mechanical ventilation in adult patients with acute respiratory distress syndrome. Am J Respir Crit Care Med 2017;195(9): 1253–63.

59. Thompson BT, Chambers RC, Liu KD. Acute respiratory distress syndrome. N Engl J Med 2017;377(6):562–72.

60. Guerin C, Reignier J, Richard JC, et al. Prone positioning in severe acute respiratory distress syndrome. N Engl J Med 2013;368(23):2159–68.

61. National Heart L, Blood Institute Acute Respiratory Distress Syndrome Clinical Trials N, Wiedemann HP, et al. Comparison of two fluid-management strategies in acute lung injury. N Engl J Med 2006;354(24):2564–75.

62. Silversides JA, Major E, Ferguson AJ, et al. Conservative fluid management or deresuscitation for patients with sepsis or acute respiratory distress syndrome following the resuscitation phase of critical illness: a systematic review and meta-analysis. Intensive Care Med 2017;43(2):155–70.

63. Bagshaw SM, Brophy PD, Cruz D, et al. Fluid balance as a biomarker: impact of fluid overload on outcome in critically ill patients with acute kidney injury. Crit Care 2008;12(4):169.

64. Claure-Del Granado R, Mehta RL. Fluid overload in the ICU: evaluation and management. BMC Nephrol 2016;17(1):109.

65. Selewski DT, Goldstein SL. The role of fluid overload in the prediction of outcome in acute kidney injury. Pediatr Nephrol 2018;33(1):13–24.

66. Seeley EJ. A dry lung is a happy lung: more supporting evidence. J Thorac Cardiovasc Surg 2015;149(1):321–2.

67. Pittard MG, Huang SJ, McLean AS, et al. Association of positive fluid balance and mortality in sepsis and septic shock in an Australian cohort. Anaesth Intensive Care 2017;45(6):737–43.

68. Prowle JR, Echeverri JE, Ligabo EV, et al. Fluid balance and acute kidney injury. Nat Rev Nephrol 2010;6(2):107–15.

69. Rosenberg AL, Dechert RE, Park PK, et al. Review of a large clinical series: association of cumulative fluid balance on outcome in acute lung injury: a retrospective review of the ARDSnet tidal volume study cohort. J Intensive Care Med 2009;24(1):35–46.

70. van Mourik N, Metske HA, Hofstra JJ, et al. Cumulative fluid balance predicts mortality and increases time on mechanical ventilation in ARDS patients: an observational cohort study. PLoS One 2019;14(10):e0224563.

71. Dalfino L, Tullo L, Donadio I, et al. Intra-abdominal hypertension and acute renal failure in critically ill patients. Intensive Care Med 2008;34(4):707–13.

72. Vidal MG, Ruiz Weisser J, Gonzalez F, et al. Incidence and clinical effects of intra-abdominal hypertension in critically ill patients. Crit Care Med 2008; 36(6):1823–31.

73. Meersch M, Schmidt C, Hoffmeier A, et al. Prevention of cardiac surgery-associated AKI by implementing the KDIGO guidelines in high risk patients

identified by biomarkers: the PrevAKI randomized controlled trial. Intensive Care Med 2017;43(11):1551–61.

74. Acosta-Ochoa I, Bustamante-Munguira J, Mendiluce-Herrero A, et al. Impact on outcomes across KDIGO-2012 AKI criteria according to baseline renal function. J Clin Med 2019;8(9):1323–36.

75. Gocze I, Jauch D, Gotz M, et al. Biomarker-guided intervention to prevent acute kidney injury after major surgery: the prospective randomized BigpAK study. Ann Surg 2018;267(6):1013–20.

76. Investigators S-A. Canadian Critical Care Trials G, Australian, et al. Timing of initiation of renal-replacement therapy in acute kidney injury. N Engl J Med 2020;383(3):240–51.

77. Wald R, Adhikari NK, Smith OM, et al. Comparison of standard and accelerated initiation of renal replacement therapy in acute kidney injury. Kidney Int 2015; 88(4):897–904.

78. Bagshaw SM, Wald R. Strategies for the optimal timing to start renal replacement therapy in critically ill patients with acute kidney injury. Kidney Int 2017; 91(5):1022–32.

79. Nash DM, Przech S, Wald R, et al. Systematic review and meta-analysis of renal replacement therapy modalities for acute kidney injury in the intensive care unit. J Crit Care 2017;41:138–44.

80. Yang Y, Zhang P, Cui Y, et al. Hypophosphatemia during continuous venovenous hemofiltration is associated with mortality in critically ill patients with acute kidney injury. Crit Care 2013;17(5):R205.

81. Song YH, Seo EH, Yoo YS, et al. Phosphate supplementation for hypophosphatemia during continuous renal replacement therapy in adults. Ren Fail 2019; 41(1):72–9.

82. Hendrix RJ, Hastings MC, Samarin M, et al. Predictors of hypophosphatemia and outcomes during continuous renal replacement therapy. Blood Purif 2020; 49(6):700–7.

83. Geerse DA, Bindels AJ, Kuiper MA, et al. Treatment of hypophosphatemia in the intensive care unit: a review. Crit Care 2010;14(4):R147.

84. Agusti AG, Torres A, Estopa R, et al. Hypophosphatemia as a cause of failed weaning: the importance of metabolic factors. Crit Care Med 1984;12(2):142–3.

85. Aubier M, Murciano D, Lecocguic Y, et al. Effect of hypophosphatemia on diaphragmatic contractility in patients with acute respiratory failure. N Engl J Med 1985;313(7):420–4.

86. Gravelyn TR, Brophy N, Siegert C, et al. Hypophosphatemia-associated respiratory muscle weakness in a general inpatient population. Am J Med 1988; 84(5):870–6.

87. Lim C, Tan HK, Kaushik M. Hypophosphatemia in critically ill patients with acute kidney injury treated with hemodialysis is associated with adverse events. Clin Kidney J 2017;10(3):341–7.

88. Bellomo R, Cass A, Cole L, et al. The relationship between hypophosphataemia and outcomes during low-intensity and high-intensity continuous renal replacement therapy. Crit Care Resusc 2014;16(1):34–41.

89. Zhu N, Zhang D, Wang W, et al. A novel coronavirus from patients with pneumonia in China, 2019. N Engl J Med 2020;382(8):727–33.

90. Wang L, Li X, Chen H, et al. Coronavirus disease 19 infection does not result in acute kidney injury: an analysis of 116 hospitalized patients from Wuhan, China. Am J Nephrol 2020;51(5):343–8.

91. Guan WJ, Ni ZY, Hu Y, et al. Clinical characteristics of coronavirus disease 2019 in China. N Engl J Med 2020;382(18):1708–20.

92. Chen N, Zhou M, Dong X, et al. Epidemiological and clinical characteristics of 99 cases of 2019 novel coronavirus pneumonia in Wuhan, China: a descriptive study. Lancet 2020;395(10223):507–13.

93. Hirsch JS, Ng JH, Ross DW, et al. Acute kidney injury in patients hospitalized with COVID-19. Kidney Int 2020;98(1):209–18.

94. Nadim MK, Forni LG, Mehta RL, et al. COVID-19-associated acute kidney injury: consensus report of the 25th Acute Disease Quality Initiative (ADQI) Workgroup. Nat Rev Nephrol 2020;16(12):747–64.

95. Chan L, Chaudhary K, Saha A, et al. Acute kidney injury in hospitalized patients with COVID-19. medRxiv 2020.

96. Mohamed MMB, Lukitsch I, Torres-Ortiz AE, et al. Acute kidney injury associated with coronavirus disease 2019 in urban New Orleans. Kidney360. 2020;1(7):614–22.

97. Jager KJ, Kramer A, Chesnaye NC, et al. Results from the ERA-EDTA Registry indicate a high mortality due to COVID-19 in dialysis patients and kidney transplant recipients across Europe. Kidney Int 2020;98(6):1540–8.

98. Xia P, Wen Y, Duan Y, et al. Clinicopathological features and outcomes of acute kidney injury in critically ill COVID-19 with prolonged disease course: a retrospective cohort. J Am Soc Nephrol 2020;31(9):2205–21.

99. Santoriello D, Khairallah P, Bomback AS, et al. Postmortem kidney pathology findings in patients with COVID-19. J Am Soc Nephrol 2020;31(9):2158–67.

100. Sharma P, Uppal NN, Wanchoo R, et al. COVID-19-associated kidney injury: a case series of kidney biopsy findings. J Am Soc Nephrol 2020;31(9):1948–58.

101. Wu H, Larsen CP, Hernandez-Arroyo CF, et al. AKI and collapsing glomerulopathy associated with COVID-19 and APOL 1 high-risk genotype. J Am Soc Nephrol 2020;31(8):1688–95.

102. Kudose S, Batal I, Santoriello D, et al. Kidney biopsy findings in patients with COVID-19. J Am Soc Nephrol 2020;31(9):1959–68.

103. Batlle D, Soler MJ, Sparks MA, et al. Acute kidney injury in COVID-19: emerging evidence of a distinct pathophysiology. J Am Soc Nephrol 2020;31(7):1380–3.

104. Panel C-TG. Coronavirus disease 2019 (COVID-19) treatment guidelines. National Institutes of Health. Available at: https://www.covid19treatment guidelines.nih.gov/. Accessed: December 5, 2020.

105. Thakare S, Gandhi C, Modi T, et al. Safety of remdesivir in patients with acute kidney injury or CKD. Kidney Int Rep 2021;6(1):206–10.

106. Kiser TH, Fish DN, Aquilante CL, et al. Evaluation of sulfobutylether-beta-cyclodextrin (SBECD) accumulation and voriconazole pharmacokinetics in critically ill patients undergoing continuous renal replacement therapy. Crit Care 2015;19:32.

107. Moores LK, Tritschler T, Brosnahan S, et al. Prevention, diagnosis, and treatment of VTE in patients with coronavirus disease 2019: CHEST guideline and Expert Panel report. Chest 2020;158(3):1143–63.

108. Panel C-TG. Coronavirus disease 2019 (COVID-19) treatment guidelines. National Institutes of Health. Available at: https://www.covid19treatment guidelines.nih.gov/. Accessed August 23, 2020.

109. Helms J, Tacquard C, Severac F, et al. High risk of thrombosis in patients with severe SARS-CoV-2 infection: a multicenter prospective cohort study. Intensive Care Med 2020;46(6):1089–98.

110. Endres P, Rosovsky R, Zhao S, et al. Filter clotting with continuous renal replacement therapy in COVID-19. J Thromb Thrombolysis 2021;51(4):966–70.
111. Shankaranarayanan D, Muthukumar T, Barbar T, et al. Anticoagulation strategies and filter life in COVID-19 patients receiving continuous renal replacement therapy: a single-center experience. Clin J Am Soc Nephrol 2020;16(1):124–6.
112. Cui S, Chen S, Li X, et al. Prevalence of venous thromboembolism in patients with severe novel coronavirus pneumonia. J Thromb Haemost 2020;18(6): 1421–4.
113. Klok FA, Kruip M, van der Meer NJM, et al. Incidence of thrombotic complications in critically ill ICU patients with COVID-19. Thromb Res 2020;191:145–7.
114. Hsu CM, Weiner DE. COVID-19 in dialysis patients: outlasting and outsmarting a pandemic. Kidney Int 2020;98(6):1402–4.
115. Mogul F. Shortage of dialysis equipment leads to difficult decisions in New York ICUs [press release]. Natl Public Radio 2020;2020.

Acute Respiratory Distress Syndrome

Ventilator Management and Rescue Therapies

Melissa H. Coleman, MD[a], J. Matthew Aldrich, MD[b],*

KEYWORDS

- Acute respiratory distress syndrome • Lung protective ventilation
- Open lung approach • Driving pressure • Prone positioning
- Extracorporeal membrane oxygenation • COVID-19

KEY POINTS

- Low tidal volume ventilation with a moderate to high positive end-expiratory pressure is the foundation of an evidence-based lung protective approach to management of acute respiratory distress syndrome.
- The same lung protective approach should be applied to patients with coronavirus disease 2019 and acute respiratory distress syndrome.
- Prone positioning is the primary rescue strategy for patients with severe acute respiratory distress syndrome.
- Extracorporeal membrane oxygenation can be considered in patients with acute respiratory distress syndrome refractory to standard lung protective ventilation and prone positioning.

INTRODUCTION

Critical care providers are frequently confronted with the challenges of managing patients with acute respiratory distress syndrome (ARDS). Although noninvasive options like high-flow nasal oxygen (HFNO) are appropriate for select patients with mild ARDS, many will ultimately require intubation and mechanical ventilation. The purpose of this review is to describe an evidence-based approach to ventilatory management that avoids exacerbation of lung injury and offers the best hope for good outcomes—intensive care unit (ICU) and hospital survival, as well as decreased length of stay, days on the ventilator, and avoidance and minimization of the cognitive, physical, and psychological impairments that are common to patients with ARDS and severe critical illness.

[a] Division of Cardiothoracic Surgery, Department of Surgery, Critical Care Medicine, University of California, San Francisco, 500 Parnassus Avenue, MUW-405, Box 0118, San Francisco, CA 94143, USA; [b] Department of Anesthesia and Perioperative Care, Critical Care Medicine, University of California, San Francisco, 505 Parnassus Avenue, M917, San Francisco, CA 94143, USA
* Corresponding author.
E-mail address: matt.aldrich@ucsf.edu

Crit Care Clin 37 (2021) 851–866
https://doi.org/10.1016/j.ccc.2021.05.008
0749-0704/21/© 2021 Elsevier Inc. All rights reserved.

We review the major advances in lung protective ventilation with a focus on low tidal ventilation and the optimal use of positive end-expiratory pressure (PEEP). We explore the conflicting and sometimes controversial literature with regard to recruitment maneuvers and driving pressure as a goal and prognostic factor for patients with ARDS. Because many patients will still deteriorate despite lung protective ventilation, we discuss rescue strategies, including prone positioning and extracorporeal membrane oxygenation (ECMO). Lastly, given the extraordinary situation created by the coronavirus disease 2019 (COVID-19) pandemic and the high volume of patients with critical disease and ARDS, we discuss the evidence for ventilatory management of these patients, as well as the burgeoning literature regarding ECMO strategies and outcomes.

LUNG PROTECTIVE VENTILATORY MANAGEMENT

Since Ashbaugh and colleagues[1] landmark paper in 1967 describing acute respiratory distress in 12 adults, intensivists and respiratory therapists have used varied approaches to the mechanical ventilation of patients with ARDS. Much of the initial focus during this era, both in the operating room and in the ICU, was on optimization of gas exchange and higher tidal volumes were common.[2,3] Researchers, however, demonstrated that mechanical ventilation, especially with high tidal volumes, could cause or exacerbate lung injury.[4] In 1990, Hickling and colleagues[5] demonstrated that a mechanical ventilatory strategy that decreased the peak inspiratory pressure and tolerated hypercapnia could improve mortality in a cohort of patients with ARDS. Over the next decade, several randomized controlled trials investigated lung protective approaches, with mixed but mostly negative results.[6–9]

In 2000, the landmark ARMA trial[10] of patients with ARDS compared a traditional ventilatory approach of 12 mL/kg of predicated body weight with a plateau pressure of less than 50 cm H_2O with a lung protective approach of 6 mL/kg with a plateau pressure target of less than 30 cm H_2O. The trial was halted early after 861 patients were randomized owing to an absolute mortality benefit of 9% 31% versus 40% mortality before hospital discharge. Although this trial established that lung protective ventilation with low tidal volumes and an FiO_2/PEEP scale as the standard ventilatory approach to patients with ARDS,[11] implementation and compliance continued to vary over the next 20 years. LUNG SAFE—a large multinational prospective cohort study of severe respiratory failure—demonstrated both an underdiagnosis of ARDS and widespread noncompliance with lung protective ventilation: fewer than two-thirds of patients with ARDS received less than 8 mL/kg of predicated body weight.[12]

POSITIVE END-EXPIRATORY PRESSURE AND OPEN LUNG APPROACHES

The use and adjustment of moderate to high PEEP is a standard approach to the management of ARDS and severe hypoxemia. However, there is considerable variability among clinicians in the use of PEEP strategies.[12] As mentioned elsewhere in this article, the ARMA trial used an FiO_2/PEEP table to set PEEP levels. Subsequent trials over the next decade investigated the potential benefits of higher levels of PEEP in patients receiving low tidal volume ventilation. Brower and colleagues[13] in the ALVEOLI trial found no difference in mortality or unassisted breathing in their comparison of lung protective ventilation using low versus high PEEP/FiO_2 tables; the mean PEEP values were 8 versus 13. The LOVS trial in 2008 examined an "open lung" approach of higher PEEP and recruitment maneuvers and found no improvement in mortality compared with a standard lung protective ventilation approach similar to the ARMA protocol. The study did demonstrate, however, improvements in secondary outcomes, including hypoxemia and need for rescue therapies.[14] The third major study of PEEP in the management of ARDS—the EXPRESS trial[15]—compared a "minimal distention" approach with an "increased recruitment" approach that maximized PEEP while maintaining plateau pressures of less than 28 to 30 cm H_2O. This trial did not demonstrate any mortality benefits, but patients in the intervention arm did have more ventilator- and organ failure-free days. A subsequent systematic review and meta-analysis of these 3 trials confirmed the absence of a benefit of higher PEEP with regard to hospital mortality among all patients.[16] This meta-analysis highlighted the critique that PEEP trials have failed to detect potential benefits to subgroups with severe ARDS.

Therefore, despite these large, well-designed trials, considerable uncertainty remains about the best approach to PEEP management. Some clinicians favor an individualized approach to PEEP titration based on data showing that the amount of recruitable lung is highly variable[17] and low tidal volume ventilation without appropriate PEEP adjustment can result in significant alveolar decruitment.[18]

One common approach is the use of esophageal pressure monitoring as a surrogate for pleural pressure and calculating transpulmonary pressure ($P_L = P_{alveolar} - P_{pleural}$) (**Fig. 1**). PEEP is usually set to achieve a P_L above zero at end expiration.[19] In the single-center EPVent study, Talmor and colleagues[20] randomized patients with acute lung injury or ARDS to an esophageal pressure–guided approach or a conventional approach of PEEP adjustment using the standard ARDSNet PEEP/FiO_2 scale. This resulted in significant PEEP differences between the groups—17 ± 6 versus 10 ± 4 ($P < .001$)—and higher P/F ratios and respiratory system compliance in the esophageal pressure group. There was no statistically significant difference in mortality although adjustment for severity of illness did result in a significant decrease in 28-day mortality. The follow up multicenter study—EPVent2[21]—also investigated a esophageal pressure–guided approach but compared it to a higher PEEP–FiO_2 table with a maximum PEEP of 24. This trial found no significant difference in the primary end point of death and days free from mechanical ventilation through day 28. Even

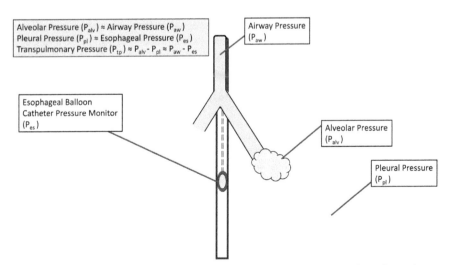

Fig. 1. Transpulmonary pressure (P_{tp}) is the difference between airway and esophageal pressures measured at 2 points in the respiratory cycle: end-inspiration and end-expiration. It is recommended to set PEEP such that the end-inspiratory P_{tp} is less than 25 cm H_2O and the end-expiratory P_{tp} is greater than 0 cm H_2O.

though this was a negative trial, there still may be some rationale for intensivists using esophageal pressure measurements to guide PEEP therapy, especially in patients with a high body mass index or abdominal compression from ascites or other intra-abdominal processes.

RECRUITMENT MANEUVERS

In addition to PEEP, and often used as a combined approach, recruitment maneuvers are a commonly used strategy of applying sustained pressure for a set period of time to open collapsed lung segments and improve oxygenation.[22,23] One challenge in evaluating outcomes is the significant variability in the approaches described in different trials, both in terms of the actual recruitment maneuvers and how the strategy is used with PEEP adjustment.[24] At the University of California–San Francisco, for instance, our standard recruitment maneuvers protocol is to set continuous positive airway pressure to 30 cm H_2O for 35 seconds, but other institutions use pressures of 40 cm H_2O or higher for longer periods of time. Several trials and meta-analyses that investigated recruitment maneuvers, most often as a component of a combined approach with PEEP adjustment, have reported mortality or oxygenation benefit.[14,24–27] A recent American Thoracic Society/European Society of Intensive Care Medicine/Society of Critical Care Medicine guideline provided a conditional recommendation for recruitment maneuvers in patients with ARDS.[11]

More recently, however, the multicenter, multinational ART study of more than 1000 patients investigated a combined recruitment maneuvers and decremental PEEP trial approach compared with a standard ARDSNet low PEEP strategy. The intervention was complex: neuromuscular blockade was initiated and then patients were placed on pressure control ventilation with a driving pressure of 15 cm H_2O followed by a recruitment maneuver via an incremental PEEP technique of 25 cm H_2O for 1 minute, 35 cm H_2O for 1 minute, and 45 cm H_2O for 2 minutes. A decremental PEEP trial was subsequently performed and PEEP set at the level of PEEP with best static compliance plus 2 cm H_2O. A second recruitment maneuver was then performed at 45 cm H_2O for 2 minutes. Despite improvements in oxygenation and driving pressure, the primary outcome—28-day mortality—was higher in the intervention group, and this group also experienced a small decrease in the number of ventilator-free days. An accompanying editorial suggested strong reconsideration of the open lung approach explored in this and previous trials.[28]

DRIVING PRESSURE AND OTHER CONSIDERATIONS WITH VENTILATOR MANAGEMENT

Driving pressure is commonly defined as airway plateau pressure (P_{plat} – PEEP), or the ratio of tidal volume to respiratory system compliance (V_t/C_{rs}). Among the earliest considerations of driving pressure as a concept was as a component of a lung protective intervention in a small 1998 trial.[6] In 2015, Amato and colleagues analyzed 9 previous randomized controlled trials of various mechanical ventilation interventions in patients with ARDS and concluded that driving pressure was the independent variable most strongly associated with survival. Other variables like a decrease in tidal volume and increases in PEEP only demonstrated benefit if associated with decreases in the driving pressure. Another secondary analysis of driving pressure also found it to be a risk factor for mortality with higher survival when the driving pressure was less than 13 cm H_2O at day 1 of mechanical ventilation.[29] This study, however, did not find as strong a correlation with mortality as the study by Amato and colleagues, and determined that driving pressure added little additional value when compared with airway plateau pressure and respiratory system compliance. More recently, a systematic review and meta-analysis of 7 studies and more than 6000 patients receiving mechanical ventilation for ARDS demonstrated that a higher driving pressure is associated with a higher mortality.[30] The authors concluded that a driving pressure of less than 13 to 15 cm H_2O could be a target for clinicians. Although some investigators argue that the driving pressure should be monitored routinely in clinical practice,[19] we agree with the conclusion of other investigators that more research is needed to both confirm its role as a predictor of mortality and to determine how to best incorporate it into a clinical protocol.[31]

Other areas of recent investigation with regard to management of mechanical ventilation include patient self-inflicted lung injury and conservative oxygen strategies. Patient self-inflicted lung injury, a term coined by Brochard and colleagues in 2017,[32] describes the clinical condition in which spontaneous breathing during mechanical ventilation may result in lung injury through a variety of mechanisms: unintended high tidal volumes, high transpulmonary pressure swings owing to vigorous efforts with creation of a "pendelluft" phenomenon, and negative alveolar pressures with concomitant development of lung edema. Although investigators recognize that spontaneous breathing during mechanical ventilation can confer benefits, including the maintenance of respiratory muscle function, improved gas exchange, and lighter sedation requirements, there is increasing concern that spontaneous breathing can contribute to lung injury, especially in severe ARDS.[33,34] However, data from the observational LUNG SAFE study indicate that spontaneous breathing is common early in the course of ARDS, is not associated with increased mortality, and may result in decreased ICU length of stay and earlier weaning from mechanical ventilation.[35] The authors nonetheless urge caution in interpretating the study's results given the greater use of controlled ventilation in severe disease and the absence of measurements of respiratory effort that may provide a better indication of potential harm. There needs to be further study of a structured approach to spontaneous breathing during mechanical ventilation, such as use of a higher PEEP strategy that could confer benefit and avoid some of the harms described elsewhere in this article.[36]

Hyperoxia is common in the management of early stage ARDS, with a prevalence of 30% on day 1 in the LUNG SAFE study. Two recent randomized controlled studies—LOCO2[37] and ICU ROX[38]—investigated whether a conservative oxygen strategy could improve outcomes. LOCO2, which enrolled only patients with ARDS, did not result in an improved 28-day survival and the study was stopped early owing to safety concerns. ICU ROX included a broader range of patients requiring mechanical ventilation, but also did not show any benefit in the primary outcome of ventilator-free days. We agree with the conclusion of the accompanying editorial that hyperoxia is unnecessary and should be avoided, but the lower threshold of 88% used in LOCO2 may be harmful in patients with ARDS.[39]

OTHER VENTILATOR MODES
Airway Pressure Release Ventilation

Airway pressure release ventilation is a ventilatory strategy first described by Stock and Downs in 1987, which allows a patient to breathe spontaneously while providing continuous positive airway pressure with a short, periodic release phase[40,41] (**Fig. 2**). This mode of ventilation uses continuous positive airway pressure to promote and maintain alveolar recruitment, with a partial release phase for ventilation. The implementation of airway pressure release ventilation can vary considerably, which poses a significant challenge when evaluating studies comparing its use with conventional

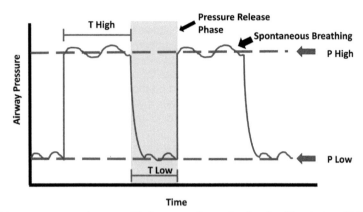

Fig. 2. Airway pressure release ventilation uses alternating levels of inspiratory (P High) and expiratory (P Low) pressures. Inspiratory time is known as T High and expiratory time is known as T low.

mechanical ventilation for patients with ARDS. The duration of the release phase may be fixed or it may be adjusted based on changes in a patient's respiratory mechanics.[41]

To date, there is only 1 randomized control trial that compares airway pressure release ventilation with a low tidal volume mechanical ventilation for patients with ARDS.[42,43] Between May 2015 and October 2016, 138 patients with ARDS were randomized to either airway pressure release ventilation or low tidal volume ventilation with the primary end point of number of ventilator-free days within 28 days of enrollment.[42] Patients randomized to the airway pressure release ventilation group had a median of 19 ventilator-free days compared with 2 ventilator-free days for patients in the low tidal volume group ($P<.001$). The mortality rate in the ICU was 19.7% in the airway pressure release ventilation group and 34.3% in the low tidal volume group; however, this difference was not statistically significant ($P = .053$). This study had several limitations, including the small sample size and investigation only at a single center. Notably, despite randomization, patients in the low tidal volume group had more comorbidities than patients in the airway pressure release ventilation group. Currently, there are no large, multicenter, randomized, controlled trials that demonstrate an improvement in patient outcomes with the use of airway pressure release ventilation versus low tidal volume ventilation for ARDS. Thus, airway pressure release ventilation should not be implemented in standard clinical practice until more evidence is provided for its benefits.

High-Frequency Oscillatory Ventilation

High-frequency oscillatory ventilation (HFOV) is a mode of ventilation that was developed after an incidental finding in 1972, when CO_2 was detected at the mouthpiece of an experimental circuit developed to measure the effects of neuromuscular blockade on lung impedance under anesthesia.[44,45] This observation lead to the development of HFOV, in which ventilation can be modulated by oscillation frequency. HFOV delivers very small tidal volumes that should, in theory, make this method of lung protective ventilation well-suited for patients with ARDS. In 2013, 2 multicenter randomized controlled trials of HFOV versus standard mechanical ventilation were reported. The OSCILLATE trial concluded that HFOV, when compared with low tidal volume ventilation and high PEEP, did not decrease in-hospital mortality.[46] The OSCAR trial showed no significant difference in 30-day mortality between HFOV and standard ventilatory management for patients with ARDS.[47] A subsequent meta-analysis of 6 randomized control trials showed HFOV was not associated with improved survival in patients with ARDS.[48] At this time, HFOV is not recommended for the management of adult patients with ARDS.[49]

RESCUE THERAPIES
Prone Positioning

Prone positioning is associated with improved oxygenation owing to an improved ventilation–perfusion ratio in the setting of the recruitment of dependent portions of the lung with more homogenous ventilation distribution, an increase in lung volume, and improved redistribution of perfusion.[50] In the prone position, the effect of compression from the heart, gravity, and the chest wall are decreased for portions of the lung that are dependent in the supine position.[51] Although prone positioning had previously been used for patients with ARDS, initial trials failed to show an association with improvements in patient outcomes.[52–55]

In 2013, the Prone Positioning in Severe Acute Respiratory Distress Syndrome (PROSEVA) study group published the results of a multicenter, prospective, randomized, controlled trial investigating the effect of early prone positioning on outcomes of patients with severe ARDS.[56] Randomization occurred within 36 hours of intubation. Patients randomized to the prone positioning arm of the trial were proned within 1 hour of randomization and were kept in this position for at least 16 hours per day. Patients in the treatment arm were placed in the prone position an average of 4 ± 4 times. There was a significant difference in 28-day and 90-day mortality rates between the supine and prone positioning groups. At 28 days after inclusion, the mortality rate was 32.8% for the supine group and 16.0% for the prone group. At 90 days, the mortality rate was 41.0% for the supine group versus 23.6% for the prone group. The trial investigators concluded that the use of early prone positioning for at least 16 hours at a time conferred a mortality benefit for patients with severe ARDS. The discrepancy between the findings of the PROSEVA trial and the prior studies has been attributed to the more uniform use of low tidal volumes (6 mL/kg) and neuromuscular blockade.[51,56] The duration of prone position for greater than 12 hours, a focus on patients with severe ARDS, and the fact that the involved hospitals had significant experience with prone positioning may also have contributed to the positive findings of the PROSEVA trial in comparison with prior trials.[51,57]

Extracorporeal Membrane Oxygenation

The results of the initial randomized control trials for ECMO for ARDS did not support the use of ECMO for severe ARDS.[58,59] In 2009, the Conventional ventilation or ECMO for Severe Adult Respiratory failure (CEASAR) trial was conducted in the UK to reevaluate the use of ECMO for ARDS in the setting of modern ventilation strategies and improved patient selection.[60] In this multicenter, randomized, controlled trial, 180 patients were enrolled and assigned randomly to either conventional management or consideration for venovenous (VV)-ECMO. Of the 90 patients randomized to the ECMO arm of the trial, 85 were successfully transferred to a center with ECMO capability and 75% ultimately underwent VV-ECMO cannulation. The primary end point of survival to 6 months after randomization was achieved by 63% of patients within the ECMO consideration group and 47% patients within conventional management group. Because only 75% of the patients within the ECMO consideration arm actually received VV-ECMO, the study investigators did not specifically recommend ECMO for severe ARDS, but instead recommended that these patients be transferred to a center with ECMO capability. These regional centers may have more expertise in applying lung protective ventilation effectively.

Important limitations of the CESAR trial include the use of greater than recommended tidal volumes in the control group and the significant number of patients randomized to the ECMO arm who did not undergo ECMO cannulation.[61] In an effort to address the limitations of prior VV-ECMO for ARDS trials, the international, randomized ECMO to Rescue Lung Injury in Severe ARDS (EOLIA) trial was conducted to study the efficacy of early VV-ECMO versus standard lung protective ventilation for patients with severe ARDS.[62] Early cannulation was defined as endotracheal intubation with fewer than 7 days of mechanical ventilation. The 60-day morality rate was 35% for the VV-ECMO group and 46% for the control group ($P = .09$).[62] The investigators concluded that the mortality at 60 days was not significantly different between patients treated with early VV-ECMO and those treated with conventional management. Of note, the study was stopped early and there was crossover between the VV-ECMO and control groups. Within the control group, 35 patients (28%) underwent VV-ECMO cannulation. For these 35 patients, the time of VV-ECMO cannulation was 6.5 ± 9.7 days after randomization and the 60-day mortality rate was 57%. Although there was no statistically significant difference in mortality, the study did suggest a potential mortality benefit. Further, when considering the secondary outcomes, there was a statistically significant decrease in the number of days of prone positioning and days of renal replacement therapy for patient in the ECMO group. Although this trial did not seem to support the use of VV-ECMO for ARDS definitively, the potential for a mortality benefit that was seen with regard to secondary outcomes has supported the continued use in selected patients. Based on these studies, the Extracorporeal Life Support Organization (ELSO), an international consortium of institutions focusing on providing advanced therapies for organ failure, published guidelines for the use of ECMO for respiratory failure[63] (**Table 1**).

Although many studies focus on the short-term outcomes of ECMO for ARDS, there are fewer studies that focus on long-term outcomes. A retrospective review of patients

Table 1
ELSO guidelines for ECMO for adult respiratory failure

Indications	Risk of mortality $\geq 80\%$
	$Pao_2/Fio_2 <100$ on $Fio_2 >90\%$
	Murray score 3–4
	Hypercarbia with plateau pressure >30 cm H_2O
	Severe air leak
	Patient awaiting lung transplant with need for intubation immediate respiratory collapse unresponsive to optimal emergent management
Relative contraindications	Advanced age
	Immunosuppression
	Central nervous system hemorrhage
	Terminal malignancy
	Severe comorbidity
	Mechanical ventilation for ≥ 7 d

Data from Extracorporeal Life Support Organization. ELSO Guidelines for Cardiopulmonary Extracorporeal Life Support, Version 1.4.; 2017.

in the ELSO registry from 2012 to 2017 who were cannulated for VV-ECMO and successfully weaned was performed to examine long-term outcomes.[64] In this study, 6536 patients were identified and 89.7% survived to discharge. The patients were divided into 2 groups, complete recovery and partial recovery. Complete recovery was defined as discharge to home and partial recovery was defined as ongoing need for hospitalization, transfer to a referral hospital, or discharge to a location other than home. The factors that were noted to have a negative impact on the achievement of complete recovery were age 65 years or greater, cardiac arrest before VV-ECMO cannulation, use of vasopressors, use of neuromuscular blocking agents, renal replacement therapy before VV-ECMO cannulation, ECMO cannulation for 2 or more weeks, and the development of an ECMO-related complication.[64]

CORONAVIRUS DISEASE 2019 AND ACUTE RESPIRATORY DISTRESS SYNDROME
Ventilator Management

Since the beginning of the COVID-19 pandemic, there has been considerable and at times heated debate about the best approach to ventilator management. Several early studies from China, Italy, and the United States described very high mortality in patients requiring mechanical ventilation,[65–69] and mainstream and social media accounts of ICU outcomes were often grim. All of this reporting likely contributed to the belief among some clinicians that mechanical ventilation should be avoided at all costs.[70] Further adding to the debate and confusion, some argued that COVID-19 causes a unique type of lung injury and requires a different approach to ventilator management than standard evidence-based lung protective ventilation.[71]

In contrast, major guidelines from the Society of Critical Care Medicine, the World Health Organization, and the National Institutes of Health recommend an evidence-based approach to lung protective ventilation for COVID-19–induced ARDS, including low tidal volume ventilation, maintaining plateau pressure of less than 30 cm H_2O, and consideration of higher PEEP in those with moderate to severe ARDS.[72–74] Prone positioning for 12 to 16 h/d is recommended by all guidelines for those with severe ARDS and refractory hypoxemia. We strongly agree with the perspective that, in a time of great challenge and uncertainty, we should follow the evidence-based recommendations of these guidelines.[70,75,76]

For those with COVID-19 and acute hypoxemic respiratory failure but not requiring mechanical ventilation, we favor HFNO as the initial approach, largely based on prior institutional experience and strong evidence from non–COVID-19 causes of hypoxemic respiratory failure.[77] There are conflicting studies regarding the role of noninvasive ventilation, either with continuous positive airway pressure or bilevel positive airway pressure.[78–80] Helmet noninvasive ventilation has been of particular interest during the pandemic, and several studies before COVID-19 did demonstrate favorable outcomes compared with face mask noninvasive ventilation,[81] standard supplemental oxygen,[82] and HFNO.[83] The degree of aerosolization with either HFNO or noninvasive ventilation techniques remains unclear.[84] Regardless of the approach, patients should be monitored closely and an experienced airway provider immediately available if urgent intubation is required.

Extracorporeal membrane oxygenation considerations with coronavirus disease 2019
The experience regarding the use of ECMO for COVID-19 in France is captured by a retrospective cohort study of patients within the Paris–Sorbonne ECMO–COVID University Hospital Network.[85] In this study, 492 patients with COVID-19 were treated in the ICU between March 8, 2020, and May 2, 2020. Patients were

Table 2
Paris Sorbonne University hospital network criteria for ECMO cannulation for COVID-19

Indications	ARDS criteria[86,87] plus optimal ventilator management (Fio_2 of $\geq$80%, tidal volume 6 ml/kg of predicated body weight, PEEP of $\geq$10 cm H_2O) and one of the following: 1. Pao_2 to Fio_2 ratio of <50 mm Hg for >3 h 2. Pao_2 to Fio_2 ratio of <80 mm Hg for >6 h 3. Arterial blood pH of <7.25 and $Paco_2$ of $\geq$60 mm Hg for $\geq$6 h
Contraindications	Age >70 y Severe comorbidities Cardiac arrest (unless immediate cardiopulmonary resuscitation is provided and low-flow time < 15 min) Irreversible neurologic injury Mechanical ventilation for >10 d Refractory multiorgan failure Simplified Acute Physiology Score II of >90

Data from Schmidt M, Hajage D, Lebreton G, et al. Extracorporeal membrane oxygenation for severe acute respiratory distress syndrome associated with COVID-19: a retrospective cohort study. Lancet Respir Med. 2020;8(11):1121-1131. https://doi.org/10.1016/S2213-2600(20)30328-3.

considered eligible for ECMO if they had ARDS and despite optimum ventilator management met specific criteria for respiratory failure severity (**Table 2**). Eighty-three of these patients (16.9%) underwent ECMO cannulation, 98% with VV. The median age of the patients with COVID-19 who were cannulated for ECMO was 49 years with a median Simplified Acute Physiology Score II of 45. The median time from intubation to ECMO cannulation was 4 days and the median duration of ECMO support was 20 days. The authors noted that prone positioning after ECMO cannulation was recommended and this strategy was used in 67 patients (81%) in this cohort. The probability of 60-day mortality for COVID patients treated with ECMO was estimated to be 31%.

A recent ELSO registry review investigated ECMO outcomes for COVID patients between January 16, 2020, and May 1, 2020.[86] This cohort study included a total of 1035 patients from 36 countries and 213 hospitals. Of note, 779 of these patients (75%) were reported to have ARDS. Consistent with the Paris experience, the median time from intubation to ECMO cannulation was 4 days with 94% of the patients receiving VV-ECMO. The median duration of ECMO cannulation was 13.9 days and the 90-day in-hospital mortality for patients with ARDS cannulated for VV-ECMO was found to be 38%.

The initial experience with ECMO for ARDS owing to COVID-19 was associated with high mortality and called into question the use of VV-ECMO as a rescue strategy. The Paris and ELSO registry data suggest improved mortality outcomes; however, questions remain as to role of VV-ECMO during the COVID-19 pandemic.[87] With a median duration of cannulation ranging from 14 to 20 days, it is important to consider whether the use of VV-ECMO significantly decreases illness duration and if it is an appropriate use of critical resources for many institutions and health systems. Although patient selection and the timing of ECMO cannulation are important factors, careful consideration of the use of such a resource-intensive treatment during a global pandemic is crucial.

SUMMARY

The use of low tidal volume ventilation has been consistently shown to be the cornerstone of the management of patients with ARDS. Additionally, evidence-based ARDS management supports the use of rescue strategies including neuromuscular blockade and early prone positioning. The use of VV-ECMO for severe ARDS has evolved and increased in the wake of the H1N1 pandemic. As we consider the ongoing use of VV-ECMO for ARDS, now with the growing experience in patients with ARDS owing to COVID-19 infection, it is critical to focus on patient selection, resource allocation and early referral to specialized ECMO centers.

DISCLOSURE

Neither author has financial or commercial conflicts of interest.

REFERENCES

1. Ashbaugh DG, Bigelow DB, Petty TL, et al. Acute respiratory distress in adults. Lancet 1967;2(7511):319–23.
2. Bendixen HH, Hedley-Whyte J, Laver MB. Impaired oxygenation in Surgical patients during General anesthesia with controlled ventilation. A concept of Atelectasis. N Engl J Med 1963;269:991–6.
3. Esteban A, Anzueto A, Alia I, et al. How is mechanical ventilation employed in the intensive care unit? An international utilization review. Am J Respir Crit Care Med 2000;161(5):1450–8.
4. Slutsky AS. History of mechanical ventilation. From Vesalius to ventilator-induced lung injury. Am J Respir Crit Care Med 2015;191(10):1106–15.
5. Hickling KG, Henderson SJ, Jackson R. Low mortality associated with low volume pressure limited ventilation with permissive hypercapnia in severe adult respiratory distress syndrome. Intensive Care Med 1990;16(6):372–7.
6. Amato MB, Barbas CS, Medeiros DM, et al. Effect of a protective-ventilation strategy on mortality in the acute respiratory distress syndrome. N Engl J Med 1998; 338(6):347–54.
7. Brochard L, Roudot-Thoraval F, Roupie E, et al. Tidal volume reduction for prevention of ventilator-induced lung injury in acute respiratory distress syndrome. The Multicenter Trail Group on Tidal Volume reduction in ARDS. Am J Respir Crit Care Med 1998;158(6):1831–8.
8. Stewart TE, Meade MO, Cook DJ, et al. Evaluation of a ventilation strategy to prevent barotrauma in patients at high risk for acute respiratory distress syndrome. Pressure- and Volume-Limited Ventilation Strategy Group. N Engl J Med 1998; 338(6):355–61.
9. Brower RG, Shanholtz CB, Fessler HE, et al. Prospective, randomized, controlled clinical trial comparing traditional versus reduced tidal volume ventilation in acute respiratory distress syndrome patients. Crit Care Med 1999;27(8):1492–8.
10. Acute Respiratory Distress Syndrome N, Brower RG, Matthay MA, et al. Ventilation with lower tidal volumes as compared with traditional tidal volumes for acute lung injury and the acute respiratory distress syndrome. N Engl J Med 2000; 342(18):1301–8.
11. Fan E, Del Sorbo L, Goligher EC, et al. An Official American Thoracic Society/European Society of Intensive Care Medicine/Society of Critical Care Medicine clinical practice guideline: mechanical ventilation in adult patients with acute respiratory distress syndrome. Am J Respir Crit Care Med 2017;195(9):1253–63.

12. Bellani G, Laffey JG, Pham T, et al. Epidemiology, patterns of care, and mortality for patients with acute respiratory distress syndrome in intensive care units in 50 countries. J Am Med Assoc 2016;315(8):788–800.

13. Brower RG, Lanken PN, MacIntyre N, et al. Higher versus lower positive end-expiratory pressures in patients with the acute respiratory distress syndrome. N Engl J Med 2004;351(4):327–36.

14. Meade MO, Cook DJ, Guyatt GH, et al. Ventilation strategy using low tidal volumes, recruitment maneuvers, and high positive end-expiratory pressure for acute lung injury and acute respiratory distress syndrome: a randomized controlled trial. J Am Med Assoc 2008;299(6):637–45.

15. Mercat A, Richard JC, Vielle B, et al. Positive end-expiratory pressure setting in adults with acute lung injury and acute respiratory distress syndrome: a randomized controlled trial. J Am Med Assoc 2008;299(6):646–55.

16. Briel M, Meade M, Mercat A, et al. Higher vs lower positive end-expiratory pressure in patients with acute lung injury and acute respiratory distress syndrome: systematic review and meta-analysis. J Am Med Assoc 2010;303(9):865–73.

17. Gattinoni L, Caironi P, Cressoni M, et al. Lung recruitment in patients with the acute respiratory distress syndrome. N Engl J Med 2006;354(17):1775–86.

18. Richard JC, Maggiore SM, Jonson B, et al. Influence of tidal volume on alveolar recruitment. Respective role of PEEP and a recruitment maneuver. Am J Respir Crit Care Med 2001;163(7):1609–13.

19. Williams EC, Motta-Ribeiro GC, Vidal Melo MF. Driving pressure and transpulmonary pressure: how do we guide safe mechanical ventilation? Anesthesiology 2019;131(1):155–63.

20. Talmor D, Sarge T, Malhotra A, et al. Mechanical ventilation guided by esophageal pressure in acute lung injury. N Engl J Med 2008;359(20):2095–104.

21. Beitler JR, Sarge T, Banner-Goodspeed VM, et al. Effect of titrating positive end-expiratory pressure (PEEP) with an esophageal pressure-guided strategy vs an Empirical high PEEP-Fio2 strategy on death and Days free from mechanical ventilation among patients with acute respiratory distress syndrome: a randomized clinical trial. J Am Med Assoc 2019;321(9):846–57.

22. Liu LL, Aldrich JM, Shimabukuro DW, et al. Special article: rescue therapies for acute hypoxemic respiratory failure. Anesth Analg 2010;111(3):693–702.

23. Pipeling MR, Fan E. Therapies for refractory hypoxemia in acute respiratory distress syndrome. J Am Med Assoc 2010;304(22):2521–7.

24. Goligher EC, Hodgson CL, Adhikari NKJ, et al. Lung recruitment maneuvers for adult patients with acute respiratory distress syndrome. A systematic review and meta-analysis. Ann Am Thorac Soc 2017;14(Supplement_4):S304–11.

25. Fan E, Wilcox ME, Brower RG, et al. Recruitment maneuvers for acute lung injury: a systematic review. Am J Respir Crit Care Med 2008;178(11):1156–63.

26. Kacmarek RM, Villar J, Sulemanji D, et al. Open lung approach for the acute respiratory distress syndrome: a pilot, randomized controlled trial. Crit Care Med 2016;44(1):32–42.

27. Suzumura EA, Figueiró M, Normilio-Silva K, et al. Effects of alveolar recruitment maneuvers on clinical outcomes in patients with acute respiratory distress syndrome: a systematic review and meta-analysis. Intensive Care Med 2014;40(9):1227–40.

28. Sahetya SK, Brower RG. Lung recruitment and titrated PEEP in moderate to severe ARDS: is the door closing on the open lung? J Am Med Assoc 2017;318(14):1327–9.

29. Guerin C, Papazian L, Reignier J, et al. Effect of driving pressure on mortality in ARDS patients during lung protective mechanical ventilation in two randomized controlled trials. Crit Care 2016;20(1):384.

30. Aoyama H, Pettenuzzo T, Aoyama K, et al. Association of driving pressure with mortality among ventilated patients with acute respiratory distress syndrome: a systematic review and meta-analysis. Crit Care Med 2018;46(2):300–6.

31. Aoyama H, Yamada Y, Fan E. The future of driving pressure: a primary goal for mechanical ventilation? J Intensive Care 2018;6(1):64.

32. Brochard L, Slutsky A, Pesenti A. Mechanical ventilation to minimize Progression of lung injury in acute respiratory failure. Am J Respir Crit Care Med 2017;195(4): 438–42.

33. Mauri T, Cambiaghi B, Spinelli E, et al. Spontaneous breathing: a double-edged sword to handle with care. Ann Transl Med 2017;5(14):292.

34. Yoshida T, Fujino Y, Amato MB, et al. Fifty Years of research in ARDS. Spontaneous breathing during mechanical ventilation. Risks, mechanisms, and management. Am J Respir Crit Care Med 2017;195(8):985–92.

35. van Haren F, Pham T, Brochard L, et al. Spontaneous breathing in early acute respiratory distress syndrome: insights from the large observational study to UNderstand the global impact of severe acute respiratory FailurE study. Crit Care Med 2019;47(2):229–38.

36. Yoshida T, Grieco DL, Brochard L, et al. Patient self-inflicted lung injury and positive end-expiratory pressure for safe spontaneous breathing. Curr Opin Crit Care 2020;26(1):59–65.

37. Barrot L, Asfar P, Mauny F, et al. Liberal or conservative oxygen therapy for acute respiratory distress syndrome. N Engl J Med 2020;382(11):999–1008.

38. Investigators I-R, the A. New Zealand Intensive Care Society Clinical Trials G, et al. Conservative Oxygen Therapy during Mechanical Ventilation in the ICU. N Engl J Med 2020;382(11):989–98.

39. Angus DC. Oxygen therapy for the critically ill. N Engl J Med 2020;382(11): 1054–6.

40. Downs JB, Stock MC. Airway pressure release ventilation: a new concept in ventilatory support. Crit Care Med 1987;15(5):459–61.

41. Jain SV, Kollisch-Singule M, Sadowitz B, et al. The 30-year evolution of airway pressure release ventilation (APRV). Intensive Care Med Exp 2016;4(1):11.

42. Zhou Y, Jin X, Lv Y, et al. Early application of airway pressure release ventilation may reduce the duration of mechanical ventilation in acute respiratory distress syndrome. Intensive Care Med 2017;43(11):1648–59.

43. Piraino T, Fan E. Airway pressure release ventilation in patients with acute respiratory distress syndrome: not yet, we still need more data! J Thorac Dis 2018; 10(2):670–3.

44. Bryan AC. The oscillations of HFO. Am J Respir Crit Care Med 2001;163(4): 816–7.

45. Sklar MC, Fan E, Goligher EC. High-frequency oscillatory ventilation in adults with ARDS. Chest 2017;152(6):1306–17.

46. Ferguson ND, Cook DJ, Guyatt GH, et al. High-frequency oscillation in early acute respiratory distress syndrome. N Engl J Med 2013;368(9):795–805.

47. Young D, Lamb SE, Shah S, et al. High-frequency oscillation for acute respiratory distress syndrome. N Engl J Med 2013;368(9):806–13.

48. Gu X, Wu G, Yao Y, et al. Is high-frequency oscillatory ventilation more effective and safer than conventional protective ventilation in adult acute respiratory

distress syndrome patients? A meta-analysis of randomized controlled trials. Crit Care 2014;18(3):R111.

49. Papazian L, Aubron C, Brochard L, et al. Formal guidelines: management of acute respiratory distress syndrome. Ann Intensive Care 2019;9(1):69.

50. Pelosi P, Brazzi L, Gattinoni L. Prone position in acute respiratory distress syndrome. Eur Respir J 2002;20(4):1017–28.

51. Scholten EL, Beitler JR, Prisk GK, et al. Treatment of ARDS with prone positioning. Chest 2017;151(1):215–24.

52. Gattinoni L, Tognoni G, Pesenti A, et al. Effect of prone positioning on the survival of patients with acute respiratory failure. N Engl J Med 2001;345(8):568–73.

53. Taccone P, Pesenti A, Latini R, et al. Prone positioning in patients with moderate and severe acute respiratory distress syndrome: a randomized controlled trial. J Am Med Assoc 2009;302(18):1977.

54. Guerin C, Gaillard S, Lemasson S, et al. Effects of systematic prone positioning in hypoxemic acute respiratory failure: a randomized controlled trial. J Am Med Assoc 2004;292(19):2379.

55. Mancebo J, Fernández R, Blanch L, et al. A multicenter trial of Prolonged prone ventilation in severe acute respiratory distress syndrome. Am J Respir Crit Care Med 2006;173(11):1233–9.

56. Guérin C, Reignier J, Richard J-C, et al. Prone positioning in severe acute respiratory distress syndrome. N Engl J Med 2013;368(23):2159–68.

57. Beitler JR, Shaefi S, Montesi SB, et al. Prone positioning reduces mortality from acute respiratory distress syndrome in the low tidal volume era: a meta-analysis. Intensive Care Med 2014;40(3):332–41.

58. Zapol WM. Extracorporeal membrane oxygenation in severe acute respiratory failure: a randomized prospective study. J Am Med Assoc 1979;242(20):2193.

59. Morris AH, Wallace CJ, Menlove RL, et al. Randomized clinical trial of pressure-controlled inverse ratio ventilation and extracorporeal CO2 removal for adult respiratory distress syndrome. Am J Respir Crit Care Med 1994;149(2):295–305.

60. Peek GJ, Mugford M, Tiruvoipati R, et al. Efficacy and economic assessment of conventional ventilatory support versus extracorporeal membrane oxygenation for severe adult respiratory failure (CESAR): a multicentre randomised controlled trial. The Lancet 2009;374(9698):1351–63.

61. Hardin CC, Hibbert K. ECMO for severe ARDS. N Engl J Med 2018;378(21):2032–4.

62. Combes A, Hajage D, Capellier G, et al. Extracorporeal membrane oxygenation for severe acute respiratory distress syndrome. N Engl J Med 2018;378(21):1965–75.

63. ELSO Guidelines for Cardiopulmonary Extracorporeal Life Support Extracorporeal Life Support Organization, Version 1.4 August 2017 Ann Arbor, MI, USA. Available at: www.elso.org.

64. ELSO Registry Committee, Yeo HJ, Kim YS, Kim D, et al. Risk factors for complete recovery of adults after weaning from veno-venous extracorporeal membrane oxygenation for severe acute respiratory failure: an analysis from adult patients in the Extracorporeal Life Support Organization registry. J Intensive Care 2020;8(1):64.

65. Arentz M, Yim E, Klaff L, et al. Characteristics and outcomes of 21 critically ill patients with COVID-19 in Washington state. J Am Med Assoc 2020;323(16):1612–4.

66. Cummings MJ, Baldwin MR, Abrams D, et al. Epidemiology, clinical course, and outcomes of critically ill adults with COVID-19 in New York City: a prospective cohort study. The Lancet 2020;395(10239):1763–70.
67. Richardson S, Hirsch JS, Narasimhan M, et al. Presenting Characteristics, comorbidities, and outcomes among 5700 patients hospitalized with COVID-19 in the New York city area. J Am Med Assoc 2020;323(20):2052–9.
68. Wu C, Chen X, Cai Y, et al. Risk factors associated with acute respiratory distress syndrome and death in patients with Coronavirus disease 2019 pneumonia in Wuhan, China. JAMA Intern Med 2020;180(7):934–43.
69. Yang X, Yu Y, Xu J, et al. Clinical course and outcomes of critically ill patients with SARS-CoV-2 pneumonia in Wuhan, China: a single-centered, retrospective, observational study. Lancet Respir Med 2020;8(5):475–81.
70. Savel RH, Shiloh AL, Saunders PC, et al. Mechanical ventilation during the Coronavirus disease 2019 pandemic: combating the tsunami of misinformation from mainstream and social media. Crit Care Med 2020;48(9):1398–400.
71. Marini JJ, Gattinoni L. Management of COVID-19 respiratory distress. J Am Med Assoc 2020;323(22):2329–30.
72. Poston JT, Patel BK, Davis AM. Management of critically ill adults with COVID-19. J Am Med Assoc 2020;323(18):1839–41.
73. World Health Organization. COVID-19 Clinical management: living guidance. WHO/2019-nCoV/clinical/2021.1.
74. COVID-19 Treatment Guidelines Panel NI of H. Coronavirus disease 2019 (COVID-19) treatment guidelines 2020. Available at: https://www.covid19treatmentguidelines.nih.gov/. Accessed: January 23, 2021.
75. Mart MF, Ely EW. Coronavirus disease 2019 acute respiratory distress syndrome: guideline-Driven care should Be our Natural Reflex. Crit Care Med 2020. https://doi.org/10.1097/CCM.0000000000004627.
76. Matthay MA, Aldrich JM, Gotts JE. Treatment for severe acute respiratory distress syndrome from COVID-19. Lancet Respir Med 2020;8(5):433–4.
77. Frat JP, Thille AW, Mercat A, et al. High-flow oxygen through nasal cannula in acute hypoxemic respiratory failure. N Engl J Med 2015;372(23):2185–96.
78. Brambilla AM, Prina E, Ferrari G, et al. Non-invasive positive pressure ventilation in pneumonia outside Intensive Care Unit: an Italian multicenter observational study. Eur J Intern Med 2019;59:21–6.
79. Aliberti S, Radovanovic D, Billi F, et al. Helmet CPAP treatment in patients with COVID-19 pneumonia: a multicentre cohort study. Eur Respir J 2020;56(4):2001935.
80. Oranger M, Gonzalez-Bermejo J, Dacosta-Noble P, et al. Continuous positive airway pressure to avoid intubation in SARS-CoV-2 pneumonia: a two-period retrospective case-control study. Eur Respir J 2020;56(2):2001692.
81. Patel BK, Wolfe KS, Pohlman AS, et al. Effect of noninvasive ventilation delivered by Helmet vs face mask on the rate of endotracheal intubation in patients with acute respiratory distress syndrome: a randomized clinical trial. J Am Med Assoc 2016;315(22):2435–41.
82. Ferreyro BL, Angriman F, Munshi L, et al. Association of noninvasive oxygenation strategies with all-cause mortality in adults with acute hypoxemic respiratory failure: a systematic review and meta-analysis. J Am Med Assoc 2020;324(1):57–67.
83. Grieco DL, Menga LS, Raggi V, et al. Physiological comparison of high-flow nasal cannula and helmet noninvasive ventilation in acute hypoxemic respiratory failure. Am J Respir Crit Care Med 2020;201(3):303–12.

84. Haymet A, Bassi GL, Fraser JF. Airborne spread of SARS-CoV-2 while using high-flow nasal cannula oxygen therapy: myth or reality? Intensive Care Med 2020; 46(12):2248–51.

85. Schmidt M, Hajage D, Lebreton G, et al. Extracorporeal membrane oxygenation for severe acute respiratory distress syndrome associated with COVID-19: a retrospective cohort study. Lancet Respir Med 2020;8(11):1121–31.

86. Barbaro RP, MacLaren G, Boonstra PS, et al. Extracorporeal membrane oxygenation support in COVID-19: an international cohort study of the Extracorporeal Life Support Organization registry. Lancet 2020;396(10257):1071–8.

87. Shekar K, Slutsky AS, Brodie D. ECMO for severe ARDS associated with COVID-19: now we know we can, but should we? Lancet Respir Med 2020;8(11):1066–8.

Fluid Therapy and Acute Respiratory Distress Syndrome

Jisoo Lee, MD*, Keith Corl, MD, ScM,
Mitchell M. Levy, MD, MCCM, FCCP*

KEYWORDS

- Acute respiratory distress syndrome • Acute lung injury • Liberal fluid management
- Conservative fluid management • Deresuscitative fluid management
- Phenotypes of acute respiratory distress syndrome
- Hyperinflammatory and hypoinflammatory acute respiratory distress syndrome

KEY POINTS

- The optimal fluid management for acute respiratory distress syndrome (ARDS) is unknown. There are risks and benefits to liberal and conservative fluid management strategies.
- Studies have shown that liberal fluid management may be more harmful in ARDS patients by increasing pulmonary edema and prolonging mechanical ventilation days and intensive care unit and hospital stay. Conservative fluid management has a risk of increasing non-pulmonary end organ damage. Studies suggest preventing fluid overload may lead to improved outcomes, although no prospective randomized controlled trial has shown mortality benefit to date.
- Different phenotypes of ARDS may respond differently to fluid management. Recent research suggests that hypoinflammatory and hyperinflammatory phenotypes may differ in their fluid responsiveness and may be helpful in determining optimum volume status.
- The heterogeneity of treatment effect raises concerns for bedside application of appropriate management. Future studies further refining ARDS phenotypes and their associated differential responses to fluid administration may help guide optimal fluid management strategies in ARDS.

INTRODUCTION

Acute respiratory distress syndrome (ARDS) is a common critical illness encountered in intensive care units (ICUs).[1] ARDS is a heterogenous syndrome characterized by an inflammatory response of the lungs in response to an acute pathophysiologic insult.[2]

Division of Pulmonary, Critical Care & Sleep Medicine, Rhode Island Hospital, 593 Eddy Street, POB Suite 224, Room 222.1, Providence, RI 02903, USA
* Corresponding author.
E-mail addresses: Jisoo_Lee@brown.edu (J.L.); mitchell_levy@brown.edu (M.M.L.)

Crit Care Clin 37 (2021) 867–875
https://doi.org/10.1016/j.ccc.2021.05.012
0749-0704/21/© 2021 Elsevier Inc. All rights reserved.

The acute inflammatory response damages the microvascular endothelium and alveolar epithelium of the alveolar-capillary barrier, leading to increased vascular permeability and subsequent edema. ARDS was first described in 1967 as hypoxemia in the setting of bilateral pulmonary opacities on chest radiograph not attributable to cardiac failure.[3] In 1994, the American-European Consensus Conference (AECC) formally defined ARDS and acute lung injury (ALI).[4] In 2012, the Berlin Definition redefined ARDS using 3 categories (mild, moderate, and severe) to classify patients based on the degree of their hypoxemia.[5] The prevalence of ARDS is 5 to 35 cases per 100,000 individuals annually in the United States, and the incidence continues to rise.[1] The mortality rate ranges from 30% to 50%, although there is a wide variability depending on multiple factors, including patient risk factors, ARDS severity, and the etiology of ARDS.[6,7]

Following an acute insult such as sepsis, pneumonia, aspiration of gastric contents, or severe trauma, a dysregulated inflammatory response leads to increased lung endothelial and epithelial permeability.[8] The pathogenesis occurs in 3 sequential phases with overlapping features: acute exudative/inflammatory phase, proliferative phase, and fibrotic phase.[9] In the acute phase, there is endothelial and epithelial injury to the alveoli and capillaries, alveolar macrophages secrete cytokines such as interleukin-1, 6, 8 and 10 (IL-1, 6, 8, and 10), and tumor necrosis factor α (TNF-α). These immunomodulatory proteins activate neutrophils to release proinflammatory molecules and stimulate the production of the extracellular matrix by fibroblasts.[10] Alveolar-capillary permeability increases, which leads to the accumulation of protein-rich edematous fluid in the alveoli and interstitium.[10] These acute-phase injuries decrease pulmonary compliance and increase ventilation/perfusion (V/Q) mismatch.[9] The protein-rich alveolar fluid also disrupts pulmonary oncotic forces, making the alveoli more vulnerable to increased hydrostatic pressure and the development of noncardiogenic pulmonary edema. During the proliferative phase, type II pneumocytes repopulate alveoli; alveolar edema is resolved by the active sodium and chloride transport and water channels, and protein is cleared from the small airways to restore alveolar architecture and function.[10] A small subset of ARDS patients will progress to the fibrotic phase, which is characterized by the gradual remodeling and resolution of intra-alveolar and interstitial granulation tissue. This phase occurs inconsistently and delays functional recovery, and the presence of fibrosis is associated with increased mortality.[10–12]

This article explores the history of fluid therapy in ARDS, with a focus on liberal versus conservative fluid management strategies. It outlines the challenges and clinical application of the pertinent ARDS literature. Finally, it explores novel study designs such as latent class analysis (LCA) and machine learning to identify ARDS phenotypes.

The History of Fluid Management for Acute Respiratory Distress Syndrome

The optimal fluid management strategy for ARDS is unknown. The American Thoracic Society/European Society of Intensive Care Medicine/Society of Critical Care Medicine (ATS/ESICM/SCCM) Clinical Practice Guidelines make no specific recommendation for fluid management in ARDS patients, and clinical practice varies widely. Experts have debated whether a liberal or conservative fluid management strategy improves clinical outcomes for ARDS patients for over 4 decades.[13–16] Liberal fluid management, historically the conventional practice, does not restrict fluid administration during the resuscitative phase or actively seek to remove fluid during the deresuscitative phase. The theoretic argument for a liberal fluid management strategy is that it can increase stroke volume and thereby improve end organ perfusion and oxygen delivery.[16] This practice pattern prevailed prior to recognition in the 1990s that fluids may worsen refractory hypoxemia in ARDS.[16] Physician-guided early liberal resuscitative practices during that era make it difficult to quantify how much intravenous fluid was routinely given. Data from prior ARDS research provide a window into historic practice patterns. A 1987 randomized controlled trial (RCT) of ARDS patients that allowed for provider practice variation in resuscitative/deresuscitative practices observed 14-day fluid balances ranging from 5 L to 20 L.[17] The 2000 Ventilation with Lower Tidal Volumes as Compared with Traditional Tidal Volumes for Acute Lung Injury and the Acute Respiratory Distress Syndrome (ARMA) and the Higher versus Lower Positive End-Expiratory Pressures in Patients with the 2004 Acute Respiratory Distress Syndrome (ALVEOLI) trials observed more moderate fluid balances of 4 L and 6 L at day 4, respectively.[18,19]

As early as the late 1980s, observational data demonstrated an association between a liberal fluid strategy and worse clinical outcomes for ARDS. In 1 study, a lower cumulative fluid balance and a negative trend in body weight during hospitalization were associated with improved survival.[17] A subsequent observational study found that a 25% reduction in pulmonary capillary wedge pressure (PCWP) among ARDS patients during their ICU course was associated with reduced mortality.[20] However, the observational nature of these studies limits the ability to make any statements of causation. A higher PCWP or more positive fluid balance might be a marker of illness severity and confound the early data. A 1992 RCT of 101 critically ill patients with pulmonary artery catheterization to extravascular lung water (EVLW) group and pulmonary capillary wedge pressure (WP) group and looked at the impact of fluid restriction and diuresis on resolution of EVLW and ventilator and ICU days.[21] Although significantly confounded by including patients with congestive heart failure, fluid restriction and diuresis were associated with lower positive fluid balance and fewer ventilator and ICU days. These studies, although weakened by their observational design and likely confounded by severity, suggest that higher positive fluid balance is associated with worse clinical outcomes in ARDS.

Conservative Fluid Management: a Paradigm Shift

Compared with a liberal fluid management strategy, a conservative strategy restricts fluid administration during the resuscitative phase and employs treatments to reduce the total body fluid balance during the deresuscitative phase. This strategy seeks to reduce the pulmonary ventilation/perfusion mismatch by limiting pulmonary edema but may risk and end-organ damage from decreased cardiac perfusion.[16]

There are few data examining the association of a liberal or conservative intravenous fluid resuscitation strategy and the development of ARDS. A small cohort study of 296 septic patients, in which 25% developed ARDS within 72 hours, showed no association between the amount of resuscitative intravenous fluid administered in the first 24 hours and the development of ARDS.[22] These findings are limited by the small difference in volume of resuscitative fluid between study groups (5.5 vs 4.7 L) and the study's limited sample size. An observational study of 879 patients undergoing elective lung resections found that positive fluid balance was an independent risk factor for developing ARDS.[23] A study of 1366 mechanically ventilated ICU patients, of whom 152 developed ARDS following intubation, found that a positive fluid balance was an independent risk factor for progression to ARDS.[24] Additionally, a case-control study of 414 patients with hospital-acquired ARDS matched with intubated non-ARDS controls found that a greater cumulative fluid balance (7.3 vs 3.6 L) was a modifiable hospital exposure that increased the risk of developing ARDS.[25]

The Crystalloid Liberal or Vasopressors Early Resuscitation in Sepsis (CLOVERS) trial sponsored by the National Heart, Lung and Blood Institute is currently enrolling septic shock patients and randomizing them to a conservative intravenous fluid resuscitation strategy that uses vasopressors to achieve target blood pressure goals versus a liberal intravenous fluid resuscitation strategy for the first 24 hours of care.[26] The primary end point is 28-day mortality. The CLOVERS trial seeks to enroll 2320 participants and will track the development of ARDS over the first 7 days. The primary and anticipated secondary analysis of the CLOVERS participants who develop ARDS and their relationship to intravenous fluids will likely provide the strongest causal data available on the resuscitative phase.

Several RCTs have compared a conservative or deresuscitative fluid to a liberal fluid strategy for septic and/or ARDS patients. These trials, with 1 exception, the Network Fluid and Catheters Treatment Trial (FACTT), were generally smaller proof-of-concept trials. They employed variations of a conservative/deresuscitation strategies that both used and did not use pulmonary catheters to guide fluid removal and found mixed results.[27–29] In a systematic review and meta-analysis of these trails, a conservative/deresuscitative fluid strategy did not demonstrate a mortality benefit.[30] However, a conservative/deresuscitative fluid strategy was associated with increased ventilator-free days and a shorter ICU length of stay. The combined treatment effect of a conservative deresuscitation on these outcomes was heavily influenced by the inclusion of FACTT trial, which accounted for approximately 50% of the included participants. Other small proof-of-concept RCTs comparing the use of albumin and furosemide versus to placebo or furosemide only suggest that the use of albumin and furosemide may also increase ventilator-free days.[31,32]

The defining trial that tested the effect of conservative fluid strategy in ARDS was the 2006 ARDS Network Fluid and Catheters Treatment Trial.[33] FACTT enrolled 1000 participants with ARDS over 40 hours after admission to the ICU and excluded patients with ongoing shock. The trial randomized participants to a conservative versus liberal fluid strategy that used a strict protocol of active diuresis, fluid bolus, vasopressor, and/or inotrope based on varying ranges of central venous pressure (CVP) and pulmonary artery occlusion pressures (PAOP). Diuresis was held for 12 hours when patients demonstrated evidence of shock and received vasopressors and/or fluid bolus. At 7 days, the trial produced a large difference in the cumulative fluid balance between the conservative and liberal deresuscitation groups (-136 ± 491 mL vs 6992 ± 502 mL; $P<.001$). The daily cumulative fluid balance in the liberal group was similar with prior contemporary ARDS trials (4 L and 6 L by day 4 in ARMA and ALVEOLI, respectively) and consistent with usual care at the time. There was no difference in the primary outcome of 60-day mortality in these groups (25% in conservative strategy vs 28% in liberal strategy, $P=.30$).The conservative strategy group, however, had significantly more ventilator-free days (14.6 ± 0.5 vs 12.1 ± 0.5, $P<.001$) and ICU-free days compared with the liberal strategy group. Despite the aggressive conservative/deresuscitation strategy, which targeted CVP less than 4 mm Hg and a PAOP less than 8 mm Hg, there was no increase in organ failure between the conservative and liberal arms of the study. Moreover, there were no significant differences in the percentage of patients receiving renal replacement therapy (10% in conservative vs 14% in liberal, $P=.06$) or the average number of days of renal support. These findings suggest that active deresuscitation may mitigate the lung injury associated with excess intravenous fluids without compromising organ perfusion.

In the FACTT protocol, deresuscitation was held when enrolled patients developed shock for any reason. When the results were further analyzed to compare the impact of conservative and liberal fluid strategies in baseline shock versus nonshock patients, 60-day hospital mortality was lower in the conservative arm than liberal arm in nonshock patients (19% vs 24%), but higher in the conservative arm than liberal arm in shock patients (39% vs 37%). However, a test for interaction of baseline shock and the treatment effect of fluid therapy was not significant for these outcomes.

Since this landmark study, fluid management in ARDS has undergone a clear paradigm shift from liberal to conservative/deresuscitative strategy among clinicians managing critically ill patients with ARDS. However, many concerns about the use of a conservative/deresuscitative strategy remain. It is important to note that this paradigm shift has occurred largely because of this single trial. Although FACTT suggests a conservative strategy may liberate patients from the ventilator earlier without evidence of harm, the clinical implications of conservative/deresuscitative strategy for ARDS patients with shock are not known. In addition, the secondary outcome findings of FACTT have not been prospectively validated in an RCT that evaluates a conservative/resuscitation strategy with ventilator-free days as the primary outcome. Subsequent prospective trials have failed to show mortality benefit of conservative/deresuscitative strategy, although most of these trials are limited by their small sample size.[27-29] Importantly, and perhaps because of the lack of a strong evidence base, most of the guidelines for ARDS management (ATS/ESICM/SCCM) do not recommend specific fluid management strategies, and the British Thoracic Society (BTS) and Japanese Society of Respiratory Care Medicine and the Japanese Society of Intensive Care Medicine (JSRCM/JSICM) make weak recommendations for conservative fluid management.[34-36] The discordance in these guidelines underscores the need for further investigation, including the necessity of identifying subpopulations of ARDS patients with differing responses to fluid administration.

Heterogeneity of Treatment Effect and Acute Respiratory Distress Syndrome Phenotypes

One of the largest challenges facing ARDS research, as well as many other topics in critical care, is the complex heterogeneity of the diseases of interest. Even a rigorously conducted RCT can produce outcomes that do not accurately answer more nuanced clinical questions because of the heterogeneity of participant enrollment. It is crucial to understand that the primary outcome of any study is an average effect estimate across the enrolled study population. Beneficial or harmful effects to specific subgroups from the intervention may be masked within the same RCT.[37] Identification of patient phenotypes may improve understanding of disease syndromes and enable the development of a precision-based approach to clinical trial design. The heterogenous mixture of patients that comprises ARDS may be grouped in many ways. Examples of ARDS phenotypes include severity of hypoxia, precipitating risk factors (eg, sepsis, trauma, pancreatitis, or transfusion), direct versus indirect lung injury, timing of onset (less than or more than 48 hours from admission), radiographic appearance, genotypes, biomarkers, and hyperinflammatory versus non- or hypoinflammatory.[38] Identifying such phenotypes and assessing the treatment effects in specific phenotypes have the potential to lead to meaningful and clinically applicable results. This is evidenced by the Prone Positing in Severe Acute Respiratory Distress Syndrome (PROSEVA) trial, where the investigators demonstrated that prone positioning reduced mortality in severely hypoxic patients with Pao_2/Fio_2 ratio less than 150 mm Hg.[39]

Latent class analysis is a form of mixture modeling that uses available data to identify unmeasured or latent subgroups in a heterogeneous population.[40] LCA attempts to identify the optimal number of subgroups that best fit a population. Two distinct phenotypes of ARDS have been identified using the latent class analysis, which are hypoinflammatory and hyperinflammatory.[41–45] The hypoinflammatory and hyperin-flammatory phenotypes were derived in a secondary analysis from 2 large ARDS RCTs (ARMA and ALVEOLI) and demonstrated different treatment effects in mortality, ventilator-free days, and organ failure-free days when exposed to different ventilation strategies.[41] Famous and colleagues used FACTT and LCA to assess the mortality outcomes of a conservative versus liberal fluid strategy among the subphenotypes.[42] Their revised secondary analysis of the FACTT cohort found that the hyperinflammatory group had higher 60- and 90-day mortality and fewer ventilator-free days when compared with the hypoinflammatory group. There was no significant difference in 60-day mortality rates between conservative and liberal fluid strategies in each group. Their data show that most ARDS patients are classified as the hypoinflammatory sub-phenotype (73%) compared with the hyperinflammatory subphenotype (23%); howev-er, their 30+ factor model that includes novel biomarkers makes clinical identification of these phenotypes currently not feasible. Subsequent work is exploring a more parsimonious 3-variable model consisting of IL-8, bicarbonate and protein C to facil-itate the clinical integration of subphenotype identification.[46] With the predominance of ARDS patients belonging to the hypoinflammatory subphenotype, and until classi-fication becomes clinically feasible, many clinicians will continue to manage ARDS pa-tients with diuresis and try to achieve even or negative fluid balance.

Precision Based Medicine as Future Treatment of Acute Respiratory Distress Syndrome

Clinical trials often require significant investments of time and money to complete. It is important to invest the limited time and resources available in trials that maximize the probability of detecting clinically meaningful treatment effects. One may accomplish this by identifying relevant subphenotypes and then targeting treatment toward specific patient populations most likely to benefit.[47,48] Robust research design in the fields of ge-nomics, proteomics, and metabolomics is dedicated to identifying biomarkers and deriving biological phenotypes.[49,50] Additionally, machine learning has the potential to identify and study the various phenotypes of ARDS through unsupervised learning methods that may uncover associations in data that are not intuitive to researchers.[51] The ongoing evolution of ARDS phenotypes and the utilization of machine learning and adaptive trial platforms hold great promise for the future of enhanced clinical trial design. This in turn will allow for the evaluation of targeted therapies in ARDS and further under-standing of how one should best use intravenous fluids to treat patients with ARDS.

CLINICS CARE POINTS

- Fluid management is an important component in management of critically ill patients; however the optimal fluid management for ARDS remains unknown.
- Although no prospective, RCTs have shown mortality benefit, it is suggested that conservative fluid management improves outcomes related to ICU stay and mechanical ventilation days.
- Further studies addressing differential responses to fluid management in ARDS phenotypes will help guide fluid management for optimal outcomes.

DISCLOSURE

The authors have nothing to disclose.

REFERENCES

1. Eworuke E, Major JM, Gilbert McClain LI. National incidence rates for acute respiratory distress syndrome (ARDS) and ARDS cause-specific factors in the United States (2006-2014). J Crit Care 2018;47:192–7.
2. Matthay MA, Zemans RL, Zimmerman GA, et al. Acute respiratory distress syndrome. Nat Rev Dis Primers 2019;5(1):18.
3. Ashbaugh DG, Bigelow DB, Petty TL, et al. Acute respiratory distress in adults. Lancet 1967;2(7511):319–23.
4. Bernard GR, Artigas A, Brigham KL, et al. The American-European Consensus Conference on ARDS. Definitions, mechanisms, relevant outcomes, and clinical trial coordination. Am J Respir Crit Care Med 1994;149(3 Pt 1):818–24.
5. ARDS Definition Task Force, Ranieri VM, Rubenfeld GD, et al. Acute respiratory distress syndrome: the Berlin definition. JAMA 2012;307(23):2526–33.
6. Villar J, Blanco J, Kacmarek RM. Current incidence and outcome of the acute respiratory distress syndrome. Curr Opin Crit Care 2016;22(1):1–6.
7. Máca J, Jor O, Holub M, et al. Past and present ARDS mortality rates: a systematic review. Respir Care 2017;62(1):113–22.
8. Huppert LA, Matthay MA, Ware LB. Pathogenesis of acute respiratory distress syndrome. Semin Respir Crit Care Med 2019;40(1):31–9.
9. Derwall M, Martin L, Rossaint R. The acute respiratory distress syndrome: pathophysiology, current clinical practice, and emerging therapies. Expert Rev Respir Med 2018;12(12):1021–9.
10. Ware LB, Matthay MA. The acute respiratory distress syndrome. N Engl J Med 2000;342(18):1334–49.
11. Frank JA, Wray CM, McAuley DF, et al. Alveolar macrophages contribute to alveolar barrier dysfunction in ventilator-induced lung injury. Am J Physiol Lung Cell Mol Physiol 2006;291(6):L1191–8.
12. Martin C, Papazian L, Payan MJ, et al. Pulmonary fibrosis correlates with outcome in adult respiratory distress syndrome. A study in mechanically ventilated patients. Chest 1995;107(1):196–200.
13. Hyers TM. ARDS: the therapeutic dilemma. Chest 1990;97(5):1025.
14. Schuller D, Mitchell JP, Calandrino FS, et al. Fluid balance during pulmonary edema. Is fluid gain a marker or a cause of poor outcome? Chest 1991;100(4):1068–75.
15. Hudson LD. Fluid management strategy in acute lung injury. Am Rev Respir Dis 1992;145(5):988–9 [published correction appears in Am Rev Respir Dis 1992 Aug;146(2):540] [published correction appears in Am Rev Respir Dis 1992 Sep;146(3):808].
16. Schuster DP. The case for and against fluid restriction and occlusion pressure reduction in adult respiratory distress syndrome. New Horiz 1993;1(4):478–88.
17. Simmons RS, Berdine GG, Seidenfeld JJ, et al. Fluid balance and the adult respiratory distress syndrome. Am Rev Respir Dis 1987;135(4):924–9.
18. Acute Respiratory Distress Syndrome Network, Brower RG, Matthay MA, et al. Ventilation with lower tidal volumes as compared with traditional tidal volumes for acute lung injury and the acute respiratory distress syndrome. N Engl J Med 2000;342(18):1301–8.
19. Brower RG, Lanken PN, MacIntyre N, et al. Higher versus lower positive end-expiratory pressures in patients with the acute respiratory distress syndrome. N Engl J Med 2004;351(4):327–36.

20. Humphrey H, Hall J, Sznajder I, et al. Improved survival in ARDS patients associated with a reduction in pulmonary capillary wedge pressure. Chest 1990;97(5): 1176–80.
21. Mitchell JP, Schuller D, Calandrino FS, et al. Improved outcome based on fluid management in critically ill patients requiring pulmonary artery catheterization. Am Rev Respir Dis 1992;145(5):990–8.
22. Chang DW, Huynh R, Sandoval E, et al. Volume of fluids administered during resuscitation for severe sepsis and septic shock and the development of the acute respiratory distress syndrome. J Crit Care 2014;29(6):1011–5.
23. Licker M, de Perrot M, Spiliopoulos A, et al. Risk factors for acute lung injury after thoracic surgery for lung cancer. Anesth Analg 2003;97(6):1558–65.
24. Jia X, Malhotra A, Saeed M, et al. Risk factors for ARDS in patients receiving mechanical ventilation for > 48 h. Chest 2008;133(4):853–61.
25. Ahmed AH, Litell JM, Malinchoc M, et al. The role of potentially preventable hospital exposures in the development of acute respiratory distress syndrome: a population-based study. Crit Care Med 2014;42(1):31–9.
26. Self WH, Semler MW, Bellomo R, et al. Liberal versus restrictive intravenous fluid therapy for early septic shock: rationale for a randomized trial. Ann Emerg Med 2018;72(4):457–66.
27. Hu W, Lin CW, Liu BW, et al. Extravascular lung water and pulmonary arterial wedge pressure for fluid management in patients with acute respiratory distress syndrome. Multidiscip Respir Med 2014;9(1):3.
28. Wang L, Long X, Lv M. Effect of different liquid management strategies on the prognosis of acute respiratory distress syndrome. J Dalian Med Univ 2014;36: 140–3.
29. Zhang Z, Ni H, Qian Z. Effectiveness of treatment based on PiCCO parameters in critically ill patients with septic shock and/or acute respiratory distress syndrome: a randomized controlled trial. Intensive Care Med 2015;41(3):444–51.
30. Silversides JA, Major E, Ferguson AJ, et al. Conservative fluid management or deresuscitation for patients with sepsis or acute respiratory distress syndrome following the resuscitation phase of critical illness: a systematic review and meta-analysis. Intensive Care Med 2017;43(2):155–70.
31. Martin GS, Mangialardi RJ, Wheeler AP, et al. Albumin and furosemide therapy in hypoproteinemic patients with acute lung injury. Crit Care Med 2002;30(10): 2175–82.
32. Martin GS, Moss M, Wheeler AP, et al. A randomized, controlled trial of furosemide with or without albumin in hypoproteinemic patients with acute lung injury. Crit Care Med 2005;33(8):1681–7.
33. National Heart, Lung, and Blood Institute Acute Respiratory Distress Syndrome (ARDS) Clinical Trials Network, Wiedemann HP, Wheeler AP, et al. Comparison of two fluid-management strategies in acute lung injury. N Engl J Med 2006; 354(24):2564–75.
34. Schmidt GA, Girard TD, Kress JP, et al. Official executive summary of an American Thoracic Society/American College of Chest Physicians clinical practice guideline: liberation from mechanical ventilation in critically ill adults. Am J Respir Crit Care Med 2017;195(1):115–9.
35. Griffiths MJD, McAuley DF, Perkins GD, et al. Guidelines on the management of acute respiratory distress syndrome. BMJ Open Respir Res 2019;6(1):e000420.
36. Hashimoto S, Sanui M, Egi M, et al. The clinical practice guideline for the management of ARDS in Japan. J Intensive Care 2017;5:50.

37. Iwashyna TJ, Burke JF, Sussman JB, et al. Implications of heterogeneity of treatment effect for reporting and analysis of randomized trials in critical care. Am J Respir Crit Care Med 2015;192(9):1045–51.
38. Reilly JP, Calfee CS, Christie JD. Acute respiratory distress syndrome phenotypes. Semin Respir Crit Care Med 2019;40(1):19–30.
39. Guérin C, Reignier J, Richard JC, et al. Prone positioning in severe acute respiratory distress syndrome. N Engl J Med 2013;368(23):2159–68.
40. Kongsted A, Nielsen AM. Latent class analysis in health research. J Physiother 2017;63(1):55–8.
41. Calfee CS, Delucchi K, Parsons PE, et al. Subphenotypes in acute respiratory distress syndrome: latent class analysis of data from two randomised controlled trials. Lancet Respir Med 2014;2(8):611–20.
42. Famous KR, Delucchi K, Ware LB, et al. Acute respiratory distress syndrome subphenotypes respond differently to randomized fluid management strategy. Am J Respir Crit Care Med 2017;195(3):331–8 [published correction appears in Am J Respir Crit Care Med. 2018 Dec 15;198(12):1590] [published correction appears in Am J Respir Crit Care Med. 2019 Sep 1;200(5):649].
43. Bos LD, Schouten LR, van Vught LA, et al. Identification and validation of distinct biological phenotypes in patients with acute respiratory distress syndrome by cluster analysis. Thorax 2017;72(10):876–83.
44. Sinha P, Delucchi KL, Thompson BT, et al. Latent class analysis of ARDS subphenotypes: a secondary analysis of the statins for acutely injured lungs from sepsis (SAILS) study. Intensive Care Med 2018;44(11):1859–69.
45. Calfee CS, Delucchi KL, Sinha P, et al. Acute respiratory distress syndrome subphenotypes and differential response to simvastatin: secondary analysis of a randomised controlled trial. Lancet Respir Med 2018;6(9):691–8.
46. Sinha P, Delucchi KL, McAuley DF, et al. Development and validation of parsimonious algorithms to classify acute respiratory distress syndrome phenotypes: a secondary analysis of randomised controlled trials. Lancet Respir Med 2020; 8(3):247–57.
47. Matthay MA, McAuley DF, Ware LB. Clinical trials in acute respiratory distress syndrome: challenges and opportunities. Lancet Respir Med 2017;5(6):524–34.
48. Marshall JC. Why have clinical trials in sepsis failed? Trends Mol Med 2014;20(4): 195–203.
49. Ahmed MU, Saaem I, Wu PC, et al. Personalized diagnostics and biosensors: a review of the biology and technology needed for personalized medicine. Crit Rev Biotechnol 2014;34(2):180–96.
50. Hendrickson CM, Matthay MA. Endothelial biomarkers in human sepsis: pathogenesis and prognosis for ARDS. Pulm Circ 2018;8(2). 2045894018769876.
51. Sinha P, Churpek MM, Calfee CS. Machine learning classifier models can identify acute respiratory distress syndrome phenotypes using readily available clinical data. Am J Respir Crit Care Med 2020;202(7):996–1004.

Pharmacologic Treatments for Acute Respiratory Distress Syndrome

Nida Qadir, MD*, Steven Y. Chang, MD, PhD

KEYWORDS

- ARDS • Neuromuscular blockade • Corticosteroids • Pulmonary vasodilators

KEY POINTS

- The management of acute respiratory distress syndrome is primarily supportive.
- No pharmacologic intervention has yet demonstrated a clear mortality benefit in acute respiratory distress syndrome.
- Improvement in surrogate end points does not necessarily translate into improved survival.
- There is a growing body of evidence suggesting that corticosteroids may improve outcomes in certain subgroups of patients with acute respiratory distress syndrome.
- Further research is needed to assess the impact of investigational therapies such as vitamin C, mesenchymal stromal cells, and granulocyte–macrophage colony stimulating factor.

INTRODUCTION

Over 50 years have passed since the acute respiratory distress syndrome (ARDS) was first described.[1] Despite the passage of more than one-half of a century, almost all of ARDS care continues to be supportive in nature, and mortality remains high at 34% to 45%.[2] As our understanding of ARDS pathophysiology has improved, a number of pharmacologic interventions have been tested, including those targeting ventilator-associated lung injury (VALI), dead space ventilation, inflammation, alveolar epithelial and capillary endothelial injury, and dysfunctional fluid clearance. Although no medications have yet demonstrated a clear mortality benefit in ARDS, a number of therapies are currently being evaluated in clinical trials (**Table 1**). In this article, we review selected pharmacologic treatments for ARDS.

David Geffen School of Medicine at UCLA, 10833 Le Conte Avenue, Room 43-229 CHS, Los Angeles, CA 90095, USA
* Corresponding author.
E-mail address: nqadir@mednet.ucla.edu

Crit Care Clin 37 (2021) 877–893
https://doi.org/10.1016/j.ccc.2021.05.009
0749-0704/21/© 2021 Elsevier Inc. All rights reserved.
criticalcare.theclinics.com

COMMONLY USED THERAPIES

Widely available therapies, and those studied in large clinical trials, include neuromuscular blockade, corticosteroids, and inhaled pulmonary vasodilators. These therapies are frequently used in the clinical setting, despite a lack of strong evidence favoring their use in ARDS. We examine each here, in the context of underlying pathophysiology.

Neuromuscular Blockade

Much of ARDS care is supportive in nature, with lung protective mechanical ventilation as its mainstay. VALI is a well-known occurrence, and approaches to mechanical ventilation are aimed at minimizing it and avoiding its complications. The use of neuromuscular blockade is rationalized as a measure that may decrease the occurrence of VALI, which can be caused by both overdistension (volutrauma, and to a lesser extent, barotrauma) and repeated opening and closing of underrecruited alveoli (atelectrauma). Patients with heterogenous consolidation (**Fig. 1**), often seen in ARDS, are at particularly high risk for both.

The impact of large tidal volumes on lung injury and the protective effect of positive end-expiratory pressure (PEEP) are well-illustrated in a murine model. Dreyfuss and colleagues[3] examined the effects of 5 different ventilator strategies in rats: low pressure–low tidal volume, high pressure–high tidal volume, high pressure–high volume with PEEP, high pressure–low volume (achieved by banding the chest wall), and low pressure–high volume. The rats ventilated with high volumes all had evidence of pulmonary edema.

However, edema was markedly decreased by PEEP. The low-volume groups had an essentially normal lung structure, including the high pressure–low volume group. Intuitively, one would predict that high airway pressures would play a significant role in VALI, but these findings demonstrated that it is actually the transalveolar gradient (intra-alveolar minus pleural pressure) that plays a more substantial role. Additionally, the protective effect of PEEP seen in this model may have been mediated by a decrease in atelectrauma.

Dysfunctional surfactant and gravitational forces resulting in the nonuniform distribution of edema can result in a difficult to recruit lung, regional overdistension, and thus atelectrauma. The application of PEEP can help to mitigate this factor by stenting

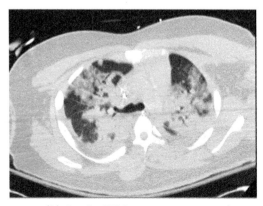

Fig. 1. Heterogenous consolidation in ARDS seen on a computed tomography scan.

open alveoli and preventing the shear forces associated with repeated alveolar opening and collapse.[3]

Large changes in volume can also lead to a disruption of the alveolar epithelial and capillary endothelial interface, with the resultant release of inflammatory mediators, worsening pulmonary edema, further compromise in gas exchange, and, in turn, a perpetual loop of worsening lung injury.[4] Although lung protective ventilator strategies involve low tidal volume ventilation and application of relatively high levels of PEEP,[5,6] current sedation strategies emphasizing daily awakenings and/or light sedation,[7] leading to a fair amount of patient–ventilator interaction. Patients with a high metabolic demand and respiratory drive often attempt to generate higher tidal volumes, which may result in ventilator asynchronies, such as double triggering and even active exhalation, leading to the collapse of alveoli. Repeated collapse and hyperinflation can then in turn lead to worsening lung injury. As such, it may follow that, if a patient is breathing completely passively on the ventilator, there may be a decrease in VALI and an increased potential for healing. Neuromuscular blockade has been used for decades with this rationale in mind.

Although a number of neuromuscular blocking agents have been used for the management of ARDS, the use of older nondepolarizing neuromuscular blocking agents (pancuronium, vecuronium, or atracurium), especially in conjunction with systemic corticosteroids, in critically ill, mechanically ventilated patients has become increasingly limited owing to concerns for critical illness weakness.[8] Hepatic or renal failure, common in these patients, seems to increase the likelihood of persistent weakness substantially. Cisatracurium is a newer nondepolarizing agent that is metabolized via Hoffman degradation to metabolites without neuromuscular blocking activity. It is also associated with a decrease in both pulmonary and systemic inflammatory cytokines,[9] which may be a result not only of minimizing VALI, but also a direct effect of the cisatracurium itself.[10] It is not associated with intensive care unit (ICU)-acquired weakness[11] and, in comparison with vecuronium, cisatracurium is associated with fewer ICU and ventilator days,[12] suggesting that it may be a preferable neuromuscular blocking agent for patients with ARDS.

The usefulness of cisatracurium for the management of ARDS has been assessed in multiple clinical trials (**Table 2**). In the ACURASYS trial, Papazian and colleagues[13] randomized 340 patients with moderate-to-severe ARDS (P/F $\leq$ 150) to either cisatracurium, or placebo (with deep sedation) for 48 hours in a blinded fashion. Although the crude 90-day mortality was not different, after adjustment for baseline oxygenation, Simplified Acute Physiology Score II, and plateau pressure, mortality did seem to be decrease with a hazard ratio of 0.68 (95% confidence interval, 0.48–0.98; $P = .04$). Additionally, there was an increase in the number of ventilator free days both at 28 and 90 days.[13] This trial was criticized because it was underpowered, a mortality benefit was only seen after statistical adjustment, and the control arm consisted of deep sedation to maintain blinding (in contrast with modern practices of daily awakenings or light sedation). Additionally, the assessment of critical care weakness, although performed, was inadequate, and thus remained mostly unresolved. Despite these issues, a prospective, multicenter epidemiologic study showed that 22% of all patients with ARDS and 38% of patients with severe ARDS received neuromuscular blockade.[2] Additionally, a survey of academic intensivists showed that 97% of respondents used paralytics in managing patients with ARDS, and that 40% of intensivists use neuromuscular blockade in more than one-half of their patients.[14] In light of the limitations of ACURASYS, the usefulness of cisatracurium for the management of ARDS was recently reexamined in the Reevaluation of Systemic Early Neuromuscular Blockade (ROSE), a multicenter, randomized, controlled trial comparing early

Table 1
Pharmacologic therapies in ARDS

Therapy	Mechanism of Action	Findings to Date
Neuromuscular blockade[11,13]	Possible ↓ VALI occurrence via ↓ patient-ventilator interaction	No impact on mortality in moderate-to-severe ARDS No impact on incidence of ICU-acquired weakness (specifically with short-term use of cisatracurium)
Corticosteroids[19–26]	↓ Synthesis of proinflammatory mediators	Possible ↓ mortality in early ARDS (<14 d since onset) Possible ↑ mortality in late ARDS (>14 d since onset) ↑ Ventilator-free days
Inhaled pulmonary vasodilators[44–54]	↓ Ventilation–perfusion mismatch	↑ Oxygenation (short term) No known impact on mortality Possible ↑ risk of renal failure (iNO)
Vitamin C[55–61]	↓ Expression of proinflammatory mediators ↓ Microvascular thrombosis Enhancement of epithelial barrier function	Possible ↓ mortality, ICU and hospital days in patients with ARDS + sepsis (exploratory finding)
Beta-agonists[63–67]	↑ Alveolar fluid clearance ↓ Lung vascular permeability	↑ Mortality and ICU days Clinical trial assessing role of inhaled beta agonists for prevention of acute respiratory failure ongoing (NCT04193878)
Statins[68–73]	↓ Synthesis of proinflammatory mediators	No impact on mortality or ventilator-free days Possible benefit in hyperinflammatory subphenotype (exploratory finding)
Mesenchymal Stromal Cells[74–77]	Enhanced epithelial/endothelial repair Improved phagocytosis ↑ Alveolar fluid clearance	Safety established in phase I and IIA studies Multiple clinical trials ongoing (NCT02444455, NCT03608592, NCT03042143, NCT04367077)
GM-CSF[24,78–80]	↓ Oxidative epithelial cell injury Enhanced phagocyte function	Possible ↓ hypoxia and severity of illness (exploratory finding) Clinical trial of inhaled GM-CSF ongoing (NCT02595060)
		(continued on next page)

Table 1
(continued)

Therapy	Mechanism of Action	Findings to Date
Surfactant[87,88]	Replacement of deficient or dysfunctional endogenous surfactant ↓ Alveolar surface tension ↓ Hydrostatic force driving pulmonary edema	No impact on mortality No impact on oxygenation
Interferon β-1a[89]	Prevention of vascular leakage Inhibition of leukocyte recruitment	No impact on mortality No impact on ventilator-free days

neuromuscular blockade to light sedation in ARDS in 1006 patients. One of the biggest differences between the 2 trials were the control arms—a strategy of daily awakenings or light sedation—is known to result in improved outcomes when compared with deep sedation.[7,15] In the ROSE trial, no difference was seen between the 2 groups in hospital mortality, ventilator-free days, ICU-free days, or hospital-free days. The cisatracurium group was less mobile while in the hospital and did have more adverse

Table 2
Comparison of findings from 2 landmark studies on the use of cisatracurium in ARDS

ACURASYS[13]	ROSE[11]	Importance
Multicenter, randomized trial of 340 patients	Multicenter, randomized trial of 1006 patients	ACURASYS was underpowered to detect a mortality difference without statistical adjustment
Double-blind—control group required deep sedation	Unblinded—control group sedation strategy was either to target RASS of –1 to 0, or to perform daily awakenings	Daily awakenings and light sedation have been shown to improve outcomes compared with deep sedation, so there is concern that the control arm in ACURASYS fared more poorly than they would have with modern sedation strategies
Patients enrolled with P/F of <150 on a PEEP of ≥5 cm H_2O	Patients enrolled with P/F of <150 on a PEEP of ≥8 cm H_2O	ROSE may have initially enrolled a more hypoxic cohort
Enrollment allowed up to 48 h after meeting criteria. Median time to enrollment was 16 hours [interquartile range, 6–29 hours]	Enrollment allowed up to 48 h after meeting criteria. Median time to enrollment was 8 hours [interquartile range, 4–16 hours]	ROSE may have enrolled patients who may not have survived to be enrolled in ACURASYS
Ventilatory strategy was low-tidal volume coupled with a conventional PEEP table	Ventilatory strategy was low tidal volume coupled with a moderately high PEEP table	Unclear

cardiovascular events. Importantly, the ROSE trial, in more robust fashion than in ACURASYS, also confirmed that cisatracurium was not associated with ICU-acquired weakness. Although longer term outcomes require further research, the use of neuromuscular blockade was not associated with differences in survival, disability, cognitive function or psychiatric symptoms in the ROSE study. Despite the results of these trials, neuromuscular blockade may have therapeutic value in carefully selected patients with severe ARDS, substantial ventilator asynchrony, and refractory hypoxemia, especially with a Pao_2/Fio_2 of less than 100 mm Hg. However, its routine use cannot be recommended.

Corticosteroids

The pathologic features of ARDS include a marked acute inflammatory response precipitated by alveolar epithelial and capillary endothelial injury.[16] Processes that trigger ARDS, such as sepsis and pancreatitis, are frequently inflammatory themselves, as is VALI, often a consequence of supportive care for ARDS with mechanical ventilation.

Corticosteroids are anti-inflammatory and immunosuppressive. They act by binding to cell-surface receptors, and then translocate to the cell nucleus, where they inhibit the synthesis of proinflammatory mediators, such as cytokines, chemokines, inflammatory enzymes, receptors, and proteins.[17] Corticosteroids are widely administered to patients with ARDS, both for the management of ARDS or for concurrent conditions such as septic shock or pneumonia. In a large US cohort, 44% of patients with moderate-to-severe ARDS received corticosteroids.[18] However, the benefit of steroids in ARDS remains unclear, despite a number of studies assessing their use in ARDS and ARDS-related conditions (**Table 3**).

There has been substantial heterogeneity in steroid dosing, timing, and duration in clinical trials studying steroids in ARDS, and results have been mixed. In 1 trial comparing the early administration of very high-dose methylprednisolone (120 mg/kg over 24 hours in divided doses) with placebo in 99 patients with ARDS, no

Table 3		
Evidence base for the use of corticosteroids in ARDS and ARDS-related conditions		
Patient Population	**Findings to Date**	
ARDS (all causes)[19–26]	Possible ↓ mortality in early ARDS (<14 d since onset) Possible ↑ mortality in late ARDS (>14 d since onset) ↑ Ventilator-free days	
Community-acquired pneumonia[27–33]	↓ Treatment failure ↓ Hospital length of stay ↓ Risk of ARDS	
Influenza[34]	Possible ↑ mortality Possible ↑ hospital-acquired infection Delayed viral clearance	
Middle Eastern respiratory syndrome[36]	No impact on mortality Delayed viral clearance	
Severe acute respiratory syndrome[35]	Unclear impact on mortality Delayed viral clearance	
COVID-19[37–40]	↓ Mortality ↑ Ventilator-free days	

difference was found in the 45-day mortality rate, or in the reversal of ARDS.[19] However, a small subsequent placebo-controlled trial in 24 patients assessing a prolonged course of lower dose methylprednisolone (2 mg/kg/d with tapering over a maximum of 32 days) in unresolving ARDS ($\geq$7 days of mechanical ventilation) reported that steroids were associated with improvements in both physiologic parameters and mortality (ICU and hospital), although there was substantial cross-over in this trial.[20] Similar findings were reported in a larger multicenter, randomized, placebo-controlled trial using even more modest doses of methylprednisolone (1 mg/kg/d with taper, for $\leq$28 days) for early ARDS (within 72 hours of onset), which demonstrated decreased duration of mechanical ventilatory support, ICU length of stay, and mortality (20.6% vs 42.9%; $P = .03$) in patients receiving steroids.[21] Unfortunately, these mortality benefits were not replicated in the Late Steroids Rescue Study (LaSRS) performed by the ARDS Clinical Trials Network.[22] Despite an increase in the number of ventilator-free days and shock-free days in patients with ARDS for more than7 days, the overall mortality rate was not decreased, and there was a concerning increase in 60- and 180-day mortality rates in the subset of patients given steroids more than 2 weeks after onset of ARDS. Some meta-analyses have suggested that steroids may reduce mortality and increase ventilator-free days in ARDS, particularly in patients treated within 14 days of onset,[23-25] indicating that the role of steroids should be further evaluated in early ARDS. Very recently, an unblinded, randomized, controlled trial of 277 patients comparing a 10-day regimen of dexamethasone with placebo in early ARDS (within 30 hours of meeting the Berlin Criteria) was conducted, demonstrating a significant decrease in the primary end point of ventilator-free days at 28 days (12.3 $\pm$ 9.9 vs 7.5 $\pm$ 9.0 days; $P<.0001$), and a secondary end point of all-cause mortality at 60 days (21% vs 36%; $P<.0047$).[26] However, some criticisms of this trial included slow enrollment occurring over 5 years, an inability to complete the planned enrollment, and the exclusion of a large number of patients.

Consistent with the hypothesis that steroids may be beneficial in lung injury, the role of steroids has also been tested in community-acquired pneumonia. Multiple clinical trials have found that steroids improve outcomes in severe community-acquired pneumonia,[27-29] primarily with regard to the resolution of pneumonia, including two multicenter, randomized, double-blind, placebo-controlled trials. The first trial included 304 patients with community-acquired pneumonia and found that dexamethasone decreased the hospital length of stay by 1 day compared with placebo.[30] A subsequent trial of 120 patients with community-acquired pneumonia and high inflammatory response (C-reactive protein of >150 mg/L at admission), found that the use of methylprednisolone decreased treatment failure.[31] These findings have been redemonstrated in recent meta-analyses.[32,33] Similarly, the use of corticosteroids in viral pneumonias has also been evaluated, but with mixed results. Although prior studies evaluating the use of steroids in viral pneumonias have been associated with delayed viral clearance and possible harm,[34-36] there has been marked heterogeneity in these trials. A retrospective review of 774 patients with COVID-19, 90% of whom were receiving oxygen by simple nasal cannula, found that corticosteroid therapy was associated with harm, particularly in those who received high-dose steroids (>200 mg of hydrocortisone or the equivalent) and who received them in the first 3 days of hospitalization.[37] Other clinical trials, however, have found that corticosteroids improved outcomes in patients with COVID-19 with acute hypoxemic respiratory failure.[38-40] The RECOVERY group randomized 2104 patients with COVID-19 to dexamethasone (6 mg/d for $\leq$10 days), and 4321 to usual care. They showed that the use of dexamethasone in these patients resulted in a lower 28-day mortality in those requiring invasive mechanical ventilation (29% vs 41%), as well as in patients receiving supplemental oxygen without invasive mechanical ventilation (23% vs 26%).[40] Patients with COVID-19 ARDS were the focus of the multicenter CoDEX trial, which randomized 299 patients with moderate-to-severe ARDS to high-dose dexamethasone (20 mg/d for 5 days, followed by 10 mg/d for 5 days) or usual care. Patients receiving dexamethasone had more ventilator-free days (6.6 vs 4.0; $P = .04$), although the 28-day mortality was not significantly different (56% vs 62%; $P = .83$).[38] Potential reasons for differences between RECOVERY, CoDEX, and other studies are very possibly related to dosage of steroids, the timing of the administration (early administration may decrease the ability to impair clearance of virus), and severity of illness (increased benefit in those requiring more ventilatory support).[41] A reevaluation of the use of steroids in other viral pneumonias may be warranted, with careful attention to trial design (dose, timing, and severity of illness); this would likely impact the body of evidence for steroids in ARDS.

Inhaled Pulmonary Vasodilators

Vasculopathy in ARDS can contribute to worsening ventilation–perfusion matching and increased dead space ventilation. On a microvascular level, both thromboembolic and endothelial cell injury can result in a decrease in pulmonary blood flow, and hypoxic vasoconstriction also occurs.[42] Together, these phenomena lead to a ventilatory–perfusion mismatch and increased dead space ventilation. An increased dead space fraction is associated with higher mortality in patients with ARDS.[43] Inhaled pulmonary vasodilators such as nitric oxide and prostacyclins are sometimes used as therapeutic agents in ARDS with the goal of improving oxygenation and decreasing dead space.

Inhaled nitric oxide (iNO) diffuses through the alveoli into pulmonary vascular smooth muscle cells where it causes smooth muscle relaxation via an increase in cyclic GMP.[44] Vasodilation results in improved perfusion to ventilated areas of lung, and thus better ventilation–perfusion matching. In a well-designed, multicenter, randomized, blinded, placebo-controlled study of iNO (5 ppm) in 385 patients with ARDS (P/F $\leq$ 250), oxygenation did indeed improve significantly with the use of iNO compared with placebo. Despite this finding, iNO had no impact on either the primary end point of days alive and off assisted ventilation, or the secondary end point of mortality.[45] A subsequent meta-analysis of iNO treatment for ARDS has similarly demonstrated that iNO is associated with improvements in oxygenation, but no significant change in mortality, duration of mechanical ventilation, or ICU length of stay. Improvements in oxygenation also tend to be small and transient, and iNO is associated with an increased incidence of renal failure.[46]

Prostacyclins act on G-protein–coupled receptors in the pulmonary vasculature to increase cyclic adenosine monophosphate, and ultimately vascular smooth muscle relaxation.[47] Like iNO, inhaled prostacyclins have also been shown to improve oxygenation. However, no trials have yet demonstrated an effect on mortality in ARDS.[48–51]

Despite the paucity of evidence supporting their use, inhaled pulmonary vasodilators are used in a small but significant number of patients with ARDS. Their use was reported in 13% of patients with severe ARDS in a large global cohort.[2] Although they may improve right heart function, decrease ventilation–perfusion mismatch, and improve oxygenation,[52–54] pulmonary vasodilators have yet to demonstrate any impact on mortality or other patient-centered outcomes, so their routine use in ARDS cannot be recommended. However, they may be of some usefulness in patients with concurrent right ventricular failure, as a temporizing measure for patients requiring transportation, or as a short-term rescue therapy for patients with refractory hypoxia before the initiation of extracorporeal support. Their utility in other situations requires further research.

Investigational Therapies: Vitamin C

In animal models of sepsis and lung injury, vitamin C has been shown to act on a number of physiologic derangements present in ARDS, including attenuating inflammation, improving epithelial–endothelial function, speeding resolution of pulmonary edema fluid, and decreasing coagulopathy.[55–58] Intravenous vitamin C has also been evaluated in clinical trials of the critically ill. Administration of high-dose vitamin C at 66 mg/kg/h in burn patients has been found to decrease the need for intravenous fluid resuscitation, and potentially decrease respiratory dysfunction.[59] In critically ill patients with sepsis, a phase I study of vitamin C versus placebo demonstrated that high-dose infused vitamin C was safe, and potentially beneficial as reflected in an improved modified Sequential Organ Failure Assessment (mSOFA) scores, a decrease in inflammatory, and a nonstatistically significant decrease in ICU length of stay.[60] Because of these preliminary findings, a multicenter, randomized, double-blind, placebo-controlled trial of 167 patients was conducted to examine the effects of high-dose intravenous vitamin C (50 mg/kg every 6 hours for 96 hours) on the primary outcome measures of mSOFA score and plasma markers of inflammation and vascular injury in patients with ARDS and sepsis. Although the mSOFA scores, biomarkers of inflammation, and vascular injury were not significantly decreased, the secondary outcomes of 28-day mortality, ICU-free days, and hospital-free days did favor the use of vitamin C (**Table 4**).[61] One criticism of the trial was that the mSOFA scores of patients who died or were discharged before the conclusion of the 96-hour study period were excluded from the analysis. In a post hoc analysis incorporating maximum mSOFA scores (20) for patients who were deceased, and minimum scores (0) for those who were discharged alive, a statistically significant improvement of mSOFA score at 96 hours was seen in patients receiving vitamin C.[62] These findings are exploratory and require confirmation in larger randomized controlled trials.

Beta-Agonists

The end result of inflammation, alveolar epithelial–capillary endothelial dysfunction, and dysfunctional fluid clearance is flooding of the alveolar spaces with fluid and pulmonary edema formation. Beta-agonists stimulate alveolar fluid clearance and have been explored as therapeutic agents for ARDS. Their mechanism of action may occur through vectorial transport of sodium from the alveolar space via apical amiloride-sensitive Na channels on alveolar type II cells, and then egress via basolateral Na,

Table 4 Key end points in CITRUS-ALI trial[61]		
Variable	Vitamin C	Placebo
Change in mSOFA at 96 h, mean[a]	3	3.5
All-cause mortality to day 28, %[b]	29.8%	46.3%
Ventilator-free days to day 28, median[b]	13.1	10.6
ICU-free days to day 28, median[b]	10.7	7.7
Hospital-free days to day 28, median[b]	22.6	15.5

[a] Primary end point.
[b] Secondary end point.

K-ATPase pumps.[63] Additionally, beta-agonists may decrease lung vascular permeability.[64]

Despite their theoretic advantages, in a multicenter, randomized controlled trial comparing aerosolized albuterol with placebo in 282 patients with ARDS,[65] patients receiving albuterol had significantly more ICU days but no significant difference in mortality or days of mechanical ventilation. A subsequent randomized controlled trial of 236 patients assessing the effects of intravenous salbutamol on patients with ARDS found that treatment was poorly tolerated and was associated with increased mortality (34% vs 23%; relative risk, 1.47; 95% confidence interval, 1.03–2.08).[66] Routine treatment of established ARDS with beta-agonists should thus be avoided, as it may be associated with harm. However, the combination of beta-agonists with corticosteroids, may have a role in preventing the progression of at-risk patients to ARDS.[67] In a pilot study, 61 patients at risk of developing ARDS based on the presence of at least 1 risk factor and a Lung Injury Prevention Score of 4 or higher were randomized to either placebo or inhaled budesonide and formoterol. Those randomized to the intervention demonstrated improved oxygenation based on the S/F ratio. Additional trials are ongoing, including the Arrest RESpiraTory Failure from PNEUMONIA (ARREST) trial, which examines whether inhaled beta-agonists and corticosteroids can prevent acute respiratory failure in patients with hypoxemia and pneumonia (NCT04193878).

Statins

By inhibiting the conversion of 3-hydroxy-3-methylglutaryl-coenzyme A to L-mevalonate, statins not only inhibit cholesterol synthesis in the liver, but also the production of multiple downstream signaling molecules, which may be the etiology of their anti-inflammatory effects.[68] Statins decrease inflammation and lung injury in murine and human models,[69,70] suggesting a possible role for their use in ARDS. However, both rosuvastatin and simvastatin have been evaluated in multicenter, double-blinded, randomized controlled trials, and neither drug has been shown to decrease mortality or days of mechanical ventilation.[71,72] A secondary analysis of the simvastatin study did, however, reveal a differential response to statins in patients with hypoinflammatory and hyperinflammatory subphenotypes, suggesting its possible value for subsets of patients with a hyperinflammatory ARDS phenotype.[73] Prospective confirmation of these findings is needed in a randomized controlled trial.

Mesenchymal Stromal Cells

Preclinical studies suggest that human mesenchymal stromal cells (MSCs) may have the ability to attenuate inflammation, enhance resolution of lung injury, and facilitate bacterial clearance, and thus hold promise for the treatment of ARDS. MSCs have been found to improve mortality in murine lung injury models, and in ex vivo human lungs.[74] On the basis of these findings, preliminary trials assessing the use of MSCs in patients with moderate-to-severe ARDS have been performed, which have demonstrated that that MSCs are safe and well-tolerated.[74–76] Additionally, an initial report of results from the MUST-ARDS trial, which assessed the use of bone marrow–derived MSCs in patients with moderate to severe ARDS in 30 patients, suggested that the use of MSCs may be associated with decreased mortality, as well as increased ventilator-free days and ICU-free days. However, the primary end point of this study was safety; it was not powered to assess these secondary end points. Although this initial report is promising, further research is needed to determine the efficacy of MSCs, and multiple clinical trials are ongoing (NCT02444455, NCT03608592, NCT03042143, NCT04367077).[77]

Granulocyte–Macrophage Colony Stimulating Factor

Granulocyte–macrophage colony stimulating factor (GM-CSF) plays important roles in surfactant clearance, pulmonary innate immunity, and the growth and survival of alveolar epithelial cells. In animal models, it has been found to prevent hyperoxia-induced lung injury, possibly by limiting epithelial cell injury.[78] Higher concentrations of GM-CSF in the bronchoalveolar lavage fluid from patients with ARDS may also be associated with increased survival.[79] Its use as a therapeutic remains unclear at this time. In a randomized, double-blind, placebo-controlled trial of intravenous GM-CSF in 130 patients with ARDS, there were trends toward lower mortality rates and increased organ failure-free days, but these differences did not achieve statistical significance.[80] A small study of inhalational GM-CSF suggested that its use may improve oxygenation and severity of illness[81]; these findings are being further assessed in a multicenter trial (NCT02595060).

Challenges and Future Directions

The potential reasons why no single pharmacologic treatment has definitively been found to be beneficial in ARDS are manifold. The pathogenesis of ARDS is complex, and involves multiple mechanisms of injury, possibly rendering interventions targeted to single mediators ineffective. There is also substantial heterogeneity in this syndrome—a multitude of etiologies exist, as does a wide spectrum of severity. Variability exists even in the management of ARDS,[18] creating challenges in the evaluation of any single therapy.

In light of these issues, there has been growing interest in the personalization of care in ARDS. A number of strategies have been used to derive homogenous subgroups in ARDS, including categorization based on physiology, etiology, biomarkers, or gene expression.[82] Identifying distinct subsets may increase the likelihood of either response or adverse outcome associated with specific interventions, and as such provide an opportunity for improving patient selection for clinical trials on therapeutics for ARDS.[83,84] As an example, subphenotypes of ARDS with variable levels of inflammation have been identified by using latent class analysis to examine clinical and biological data.[85] These subphenotypes have exhibited divergent clinical outcomes and differential response to specific supportive and pharmacologic therapies.[73,86] Although targeting ARDS therapies to subphenotypes holds promise, another challenge lies in the capability of rapidly identifying such subphenotypes at the bedside. Methods for doing so must first be developed before personalized approaches can be assessed in a meaningful manner.

Additionally, the COVID-19 pandemic has spawned numerous clinical trials, including those involving steroids and immunomodulatory therapies such as IL-1 inhibitors, anti–IL-6 receptor monoclonal antibodies, and interferons. To date, aside from dexamethasone, no agent has yet demonstrated a clear benefit in COVID-19-related ARDS. However, many trials are still ongoing and their impact on ARDS care remains to be seen.

SUMMARY

No pharmacologic interventions have yet demonstrated a clear mortality benefit in ARDS, although some have been associated with improvement in surrogate end points. There is a growing body of evidence suggesting that corticosteroids may be beneficial. Additionally, a number of investigational therapies such as vitamin C, mesenchymal stem cells, and GM-CSF may be promising, but further research is needed.

CLINICS CARE POINTS

- The cornerstone of care for ARDS remains lung protective ventilation, because no definitive pharmacologic therapies have yet been found.
- Currently, the most promising pharmacologic therapy for ARDS is corticosteroid. Timing of administration, however, matters because the benefit has only been seen when initiated in early ARDS. There is no benefit to starting systemic steroid therapy at 7 or more days after the onset of ARDS.
- Although there is no impact on survival, neuromuscular blockade can be of usefulness in carefully selected patients with moderate to severe ARDS.
- We cannot recommend any other pharmacologic interventions at this time given the lack of evidence, although investigations are ongoing for high-dose vitamin C, MSCs, and other potential therapies.

DISCLOSURE

N. Qadir reports no significant conflicts of interest; S.Y. Chang was an advisor for a COVID trial to PureTech Pharmaceuticals in 2020; and was a speaker for La Jolla Pharmaceuticals in 2018.

REFERENCES

1. Ashbaugh DG, Bigelow DB, Petty TL, et al. Acute respiratory distress in adults. Lancet 1967;2:319–23.
2. Bellani G, Laffey JG, Pham T, et al. Epidemiology, patterns of care, and mortality for patients with acute respiratory distress syndrome in intensive care units in 50 countries. J Am Med Assoc 2016;315:788–800.
3. Dreyfuss D, Soler P, Basset G, et al. High inflation pressure pulmonary edema. Respective effects of high airway pressure, high tidal volume, and positive end-expiratory pressure. Am Rev Respir Dis 1988;137:1159–64.
4. Matthay MA, Ware LB, Zimmerman GA. The acute respiratory distress syndrome. J Clin Invest 2012;122:2731–40.
5. Acute Respiratory Distress Syndrome N, Brower RG, Matthay MA, et al. Ventilation with lower tidal volumes as compared with traditional tidal volumes for acute lung injury and the acute respiratory distress syndrome. N Engl J Med 2000;342:1301–8.
6. Meade MO, Cook DJ, Guyatt GH, et al. Ventilation strategy using low tidal volumes, recruitment maneuvers, and high positive end-expiratory pressure for acute lung injury and acute respiratory distress syndrome: a randomized controlled trial. J Am Med Assoc 2008;299:637–45.
7. Kress JP, Pohlman AS, O'Connor MF, et al. Daily interruption of sedative infusions in critically ill patients undergoing mechanical ventilation. N Engl J Med 2000;342:1471–7.
8. Hansen-Flaschen J, Cowen J, Raps EC. Neuromuscular blockade in the intensive care unit. More than we bargained for. Am Rev Respir Dis 1993;147:234–6.
9. Forel JM, Roch A, Marin V, et al. Neuromuscular blocking agents decrease inflammatory response in patients presenting with acute respiratory distress syndrome. Crit Care Med 2006;34:2749–57.
10. Fanelli V, Morita Y, Cappello P, et al. Neuromuscular blocking agent cisatracurium attenuates lung injury by inhibition of nicotinic acetylcholine receptor-alpha1. Anesthesiology 2016;124:132–40.

11. National Heart L, Blood Institute PCTN, Moss M, et al. Early neuromuscular blockade in the acute respiratory distress syndrome. N Engl J Med 2019;380: 1997–2008.
12. Sottile PD, Kiser TH, Burnham EL, et al. An observational study of the efficacy of cisatracurium compared with vecuronium in patients with or at risk for acute respiratory distress syndrome. Am J Respir Crit Care Med 2018;197:897–904.
13. Papazian L, Forel JM, Gacouin A, et al. Neuromuscular blockers in early acute respiratory distress syndrome. N Engl J Med 2010;363:1107–16.
14. Dodia NN, Richert ME, Deitchman AR, et al. A survey of academic intensivists' Use of neuromuscular blockade in subjects with ARDS. Respir Care 2020;65: 362–8.
15. Girard TD, Kress JP, Fuchs BD, et al. Efficacy and safety of a paired sedation and ventilator weaning protocol for mechanically ventilated patients in intensive care (Awakening and Breathing Controlled trial): a randomised controlled trial. Lancet 2008;371:126–34.
16. Ware LB, Matthay MA. The acute respiratory distress syndrome. N Engl J Med 2000;342:1334–49.
17. Barnes PJ. How corticosteroids control inflammation: quintiles prize lecture 2005. Br J Pharmacol 2006;148:245–54.
18. Qadir N, Bartz RR, Cooter ML, et al. Variation in Early Management Practices in Moderate-to-Severe Acute Respiratory Distress Syndrome in the United States. Chest 2021. https://doi.org/10.1016/j.chest.2021.05.047.
19. Bernard GR, Luce JM, Sprung CL, et al. High-dose corticosteroids in patients with the adult respiratory distress syndrome. N Engl J Med 1987;317:1565–70.
20. Meduri GU, Headley AS, Golden E, et al. Effect of prolonged methylprednisolone therapy in unresolving acute respiratory distress syndrome: a randomized controlled trial. J Am Med Assoc 1998;280:159–65.
21. Meduri GU, Golden E, Freire AX, et al. Methylprednisolone infusion in early severe ARDS: results of a randomized controlled trial. Chest 2007;131:954–63.
22. Steinberg KP, Hudson LD, Goodman RB, et al. Efficacy and safety of corticosteroids for persistent acute respiratory distress syndrome. N Engl J Med 2006;354: 1671–84.
23. Peter JV, John P, Graham PL, et al. Corticosteroids in the prevention and treatment of acute respiratory distress syndrome (ARDS) in adults: meta-analysis. BMJ 2008;336:1006–9.
24. Lewis SR, Pritchard MW, Thomas CM, et al. Pharmacological agents for adults with acute respiratory distress syndrome. Cochrane Database Syst Rev 2019;7: Cd004477.
25. Meduri GU, Bridges L, Shih MC, et al. Prolonged glucocorticoid treatment is associated with improved ARDS outcomes: analysis of individual patients' data from four randomized trials and trial-level meta-analysis of the updated literature. Intensive Care Med 2016;42:829–40.
26. Villar J, Ferrando C, Martinez D, et al. Dexamethasone treatment for the acute respiratory distress syndrome: a multicentre, randomised controlled trial. Lancet Respir Med 2020.
27. Confalonieri M, Urbino R, Potena A, et al. Hydrocortisone infusion for severe community- acquired pneumonia: a preliminary randomized study. Am J Respir Crit Care Med 2005;171:242–8.
28. Fernandez-Serrano S, Dorca J, Garcia-Vidal C, et al. Effect of corticosteroids on the clinical course of community-acquired pneumonia: a randomized controlled trial. Crit Care 2011;15:R96.

29. Mikami K, Suzuki M, Kitagawa H, et al. Efficacy of corticosteroids in the treatment of community-acquired pneumonia requiring hospitalization. Lung 2007;185: 249–55.

30. Meijvis SC, Hardeman H, Remmelts HH, et al. Dexamethasone and length of hospital stay in patients with community-acquired pneumonia: a randomised, double-blind, placebo-controlled trial. Lancet 2011;377:2023–30.

31. Torres A, Sibila O, Ferrer M, et al. Effect of corticosteroids on treatment failure among hospitalized patients with severe community-acquired pneumonia and high inflammatory response: a randomized clinical trial. J Am Med Assoc 2015; 313:677–86.

32. Siemieniuk RA, Meade MO, Alonso-Coello P, et al. Corticosteroid therapy for patients hospitalized with community-acquired pneumonia: a systematic review and meta-analysis. Ann Intern Med 2015;163:519–28.

33. Wan YD, Sun TW, Liu ZQ, et al. Efficacy and safety of corticosteroids for community-acquired pneumonia: a systematic review and meta-analysis. Chest 2016;149:209–19.

34. Lansbury LE, Rodrigo C, Leonardi-Bee J, et al. Corticosteroids as adjunctive therapy in the treatment of influenza: an updated Cochrane systematic review and meta- analysis. Crit Care Med 2020;48:e98–106.

35. Lee N, Allen Chan KC, Hui DS, et al. Effects of early corticosteroid treatment on plasma SARS- associated Coronavirus RNA concentrations in adult patients. J Clin Virol 2004;31:304–9.

36. Arabi YM, Mandourah Y, Al-Hameed F, et al. Corticosteroid therapy for critically ill patients with Middle East respiratory syndrome. Am J Respir Crit Care Med 2018; 197:757–67.

37. Liu J, Zhang S, Dong X, et al. Corticosteroid treatment in severe COVID-19 patients with acute respiratory distress syndrome. J Clin Invest 2020;130:6417–28.

38. Tomazini BM, Maia IS, Cavalcanti AB, et al. Effect of dexamethasone on days alive and ventilator-free in patients with moderate or severe acute respiratory distress syndrome and COVID- 19: the CoDEX randomized clinical trial. J Am Med Assoc 2020;324:1307–16.

39. Sterne JAC, Murthy S, Diaz JV, et al. Association between administration of systemic corticosteroids and mortality among critically ill patients with COVID-19: a meta-analysis. J Am Med Assoc 2020;324:1330–41.

40. Horby P, Lim WS, Emberson JR, et al. Dexamethasone in hospitalized patients with Covid-19 - preliminary report. N Engl J Med 2020.

41. Matthay MA, Wick KD. Corticosteroids, COVID-19 pneumonia, and acute respiratory distress syndrome. J Clin Invest 2020;130:6218–21.

42. Tomashefski JF Jr, Davies P, Boggis C, et al. The pulmonary vascular lesions of the adult respiratory distress syndrome. Am J Pathol 1983;112:112–26.

43. Nuckton TJ, Alonso JA, Kallet RH, et al. Pulmonary dead-space fraction as a risk factor for death in the acute respiratory distress syndrome. N Engl J Med 2002; 346:1281–6.

44. Yu B, Ichinose F, Bloch DB, et al. Inhaled nitric oxide. Br J Pharmacol 2019;176: 246–55.

45. Taylor RW, Zimmerman JL, Dellinger RP, et al. Low-dose inhaled nitric oxide in patients with acute lung injury: a randomized controlled trial. J Am Med Assoc 2004; 291:1603–9.

46. Gebistorf F, Karam O, Wetterslev J, et al. Inhaled nitric oxide for acute respiratory distress syndrome (ARDS) in children and adults. Cochrane Database Syst Rev 2016;CD002787.

47. Del Pozo R, Hernandez Gonzalez I, Escribano-Subias P. The prostacyclin pathway in pulmonary arterial hypertension: a clinical review. Expert Rev Respir Med 2017;11:491–503.

48. Afshari A, Bastholm Bille A, Allingstrup M. Aerosolized prostacyclins for acute respiratory distress syndrome (ARDS). Cochrane Database Syst Rev 2017;7: CD007733.

49. Dahlem P, van Aalderen WM, de Neef M, et al. Randomized controlled trial of aerosolized prostacyclin therapy in children with acute lung injury. Crit Care Med 2004;32:1055–60.

50. Walmrath D, Schneider T, Schermuly R, et al. Direct comparison of inhaled nitric oxide and aerosolized prostacyclin in acute respiratory distress syndrome. Am J Respir Crit Care Med 1996;153:991–6.

51. Fuller BM, Mohr NM, Skrupky L, et al. The use of inhaled prostaglandins in patients with ARDS: a systematic review and meta-analysis. Chest 2015;147: 1510–22.

52. Hill NS, Preston IR, Roberts KE. Inhaled therapies for pulmonary hypertension. Respir Care 2015;60:794–802, discussion -5.

53. Siobal M. Aerosolized prostacyclins. Respir Care 2004;49:640–52.

54. Hsu CW, Lee DL, Lin SL, et al. The initial response to inhaled nitric oxide treatment for intensive care unit patients with acute respiratory distress syndrome. Respiration 2008;75:288–95.

55. Mohammed BM, Fisher BJ, Kraskauskas D, et al. Vitamin C: a novel regulator of neutrophil extracellular trap formation. Nutrients 2013;5:3131–51.

56. Fisher BJ, Seropian IM, Kraskauskas D, et al. Ascorbic acid attenuates lipopolysaccharide-induced acute lung injury. Crit Care Med 2011;39:1454–60.

57. Fisher BJ, Kraskauskas D, Martin EJ, et al. Attenuation of sepsis-induced organ injury in mice by vitamin C. JPEN J Parenter Enteral Nutr 2014;38:825–39.

58. Fisher BJ, Kraskauskas D, Martin EJ, et al. Mechanisms of attenuation of abdominal sepsis induced acute lung injury by ascorbic acid. Am J Physiol Lung Cell Mol Physiol 2012;303:L20–32.

59. Tanaka H, Matsuda T, Miyagantani Y, et al. Reduction of resuscitation fluid volumes in severely burned patients using ascorbic acid administration: a randomized, prospective study. Arch Surg 2000;135:326–31.

60. Fowler AA 3rd, Syed AA, Knowlson S, et al. Phase I safety trial of intravenous ascorbic acid in patients with severe sepsis. J Transl Med 2014;12:32.

61. Fowler AA 3rd, Truwit JD, Hite RD, et al. Effect of vitamin C infusion on organ failure and biomarkers of inflammation and vascular injury in patients with sepsis and severe acute respiratory failure: the CITRIS-ALI randomized clinical trial. J Am Med Assoc 2019;322:1261–70.

62. Fowler AA 3rd, Fisher BJ, Kashiouris MG. Vitamin C for sepsis and acute respiratory failure- reply. J Am Med Assoc 2020;323:792–3.

63. Groshaus HE, Manocha S, Walley KR, et al. Mechanisms of beta-receptor stimulation- induced improvement of acute lung injury and pulmonary edema. Crit Care 2004;8:234–42.

64. Basran GS, Hardy JG, Woo SP, et al. Beta-2-adrenoceptor agonists as inhibitors of lung vascular permeability to radiolabelled transferrin in the adult respiratory distress syndrome in man. Eur J Nucl Med 1986;12:381–4.

65. Matthay MA, Brower RG, Carson S, et al. Randomized, placebo-controlled clinical trial of an aerosolized β_2-agonist for treatment of acute lung injury. Am J Respir Crit Care Med 2011;184:561–8.

66. Gao Smith F, Perkins GD, Gates S, et al. Effect of intravenous β-2 agonist treatment on clinical outcomes in acute respiratory distress syndrome (Balti-2): a multicentre, randomised controlled trial. Lancet 2012;379:229–35.

67. Festic E, Carr GE, Cartin-Ceba R, et al. Randomized clinical trial of a combination of an inhaled corticosteroid and beta agonist in patients at risk of developing the acute respiratory distress syndrome. Crit Care Med 2017;45:798–805.

68. Oesterle A, Laufs U, Liao JK. Pleiotropic effects of statins on the cardiovascular system. Circ Res 2017;120:229–43.

69. Jacobson JR, Barnard JW, Grigoryev DN, et al. Simvastatin attenuates vascular leak and inflammation in murine inflammatory lung injury. Am J Physiol Lung Cell Mol Physiol 2005;288:L1026–32.

70. Shyamsundar M, McKeown ST, O'Kane CM, et al. Simvastatin decreases lipopolysaccharide- induced pulmonary inflammation in healthy volunteers. Am J Respir Crit Care Med 2009;179:1107–14.

71. Truwit JD, Bernard GR, Steingrub J, et al. Rosuvastatin for sepsis-associated acute respiratory distress syndrome. N Engl J Med 2014;370:2191–200.

72. McAuley DF, Laffey JG, O'Kane CM, et al. Simvastatin in the acute respiratory distress syndrome. N Engl J Med 2014;371:1695–703.

73. Calfee CS, Delucchi KL, Sinha P, et al. Acute respiratory distress syndrome subphenotypes and differential response to simvastatin: secondary analysis of a randomised controlled trial. Lancet Respir Med 2018;6:691–8.

74. Matthay MA. Therapeutic potential of mesenchymal stromal cells for acute respiratory distress syndrome. Ann Am Thorac Soc 2015;12(Suppl 1):S54–7.

75. Wilson JG, Liu KD, Zhuo H, et al. Mesenchymal stem (stromal) cells for treatment of ARDS: a phase 1 clinical trial. Lancet Respir Med 2015;3:24–32.

76. Yip HK, Fang WF, Li YC, et al. Human umbilical cord-derived mesenchymal stem cells for acute respiratory distress syndrome. Crit Care Med 2020;48:e391–9.

77. Jacono F, Bannard-Smith J, Brealey D, et al. Primary analysis of a phase 1/2 study to assess MultiStem® cell therapy, a regenerative advanced therapy medicinal product (ATMP), in acute respiratory distress syndrome (MUST-ARDS). Am J Respir Crit Care Med 2020;201:A7353.

78. Paine R 3rd, Wilcoxen SE, Morris SB, et al. Transgenic overexpression of granulocyte macrophage-colony stimulating factor in the lung prevents hyperoxic lung injury. Am J Pathol 2003;163:2397–406.

79. Matute-Bello G, Liles WC, Radella F 2nd, et al. Modulation of neutrophil apoptosis by granulocyte colony-stimulating factor and granulocyte/macrophage colony-stimulating factor during the course of acute respiratory distress syndrome. Crit Care Med 2000;28:1–7.

80. Paine R 3rd, Standiford TJ, Dechert RE, et al. A randomized trial of recombinant human granulocyte-macrophage colony stimulating factor for patients with acute lung injury. Crit Care Med 2012;40:90–7.

81. Herold S, Hoegner K, Vadasz I, et al. Inhaled granulocyte/macrophage colony-stimulating factor as treatment of pneumonia-associated acute respiratory distress syndrome. Am J Respir Crit Care Med 2014;189:609–11.

82. Sinha P, Calfee CS. Phenotypes in acute respiratory distress syndrome: moving towards precision medicine. Curr Opin Crit Care 2019;25:12–20.

83. Matthay MA, Arabi YM, Siegel ER, et al. Phenotypes and personalized medicine in the acute respiratory distress syndrome. Intensive Care Med 2020;46:2136–52.

84. Ware LB, Matthay MA, Mebazaa A. Designing an ARDS trial for 2020 and beyond: focus on enrichment strategies. Intensive Care Med 2020;46:2153–6.

85. Sinha P, Churpek MM, Calfee CS. Machine learning classifier models can identify acute respiratory distress syndrome phenotypes using readily available clinical data. Am J Respir Crit Care Med 2020;202:996–1004.

86. Famous KR, Delucchi K, Ware LB, et al. Acute respiratory distress syndrome sub-phenotypes respond differently to randomized fluid management strategy. Am J Respir Crit Care Med 2017;195:331–8.

87. Spragg RG, Taut FJ, Lewis JF, et al. Recombinant surfactant protein C-based sur-factant for patients with severe direct lung injury. Am J Respir Crit Care Med 2011;183:1055–61.

88. Willson DF, Truwit JD, Conaway MR, et al. The adult calfactant in acute respiratory distress syndrome trial. Chest 2015;148:356–64.

89. Ranieri VM, Pettila V, Karvonen MK, et al. Effect of intravenous interferon beta-1a on death and days free from mechanical ventilation among patients with moder-ate to severe acute respiratory distress syndrome: a randomized clinical trial. J Am Med Assoc 2020.

Long-Term Outcomes in Acute Respiratory Distress Syndrome

Epidemiology, Mechanisms, and Patient Evaluation

Jessica A. Palakshappa, MD, MS, Jennifer T.W. Krall, MD,
Lanazha T. Belfield, PhD, D. Clark Files, MD*

KEYWORDS

- Acute lung injury • Physical function • COVID-19 • Cognitive function
- Mental health • Post–intensive care syndrome • Skeletal muscle

KEY POINTS

- Many ARDS survivors experience long-term impairments including limitations in physical and cognitive function, mental health symptoms, and decreased quality of life.
- Premorbid functional status and comorbidities are important contributors to post-ARDS long-term outcomes.
- Given the abrupt rise in ARDS incidence with the COVID-19 pandemic, the prevalence of long-term impairments following ARDS is expected to increase.

INTRODUCTION

Acute respiratory distress syndrome (ARDS) is a clinical syndrome of inflammatory lung injury characterized by the acute onset of hypoxemia, noncardiogenic pulmonary edema, and the need for mechanical ventilation. Since its first description by Ashbaugh and colleagues[1] in 1967, our understanding of its epidemiology, pathogenesis, and long-term impact has grown.[2] Estimates from the early 2000s suggest that ARDS affects more than 190,000 people in the United States each year and results in an estimated 74,500 deaths and 3.6 million hospital days.[3] Over the past 50 years, care has improved for patients with ARDS; for example, randomized trials have provided evidence-based strategies for optimizing mechanical ventilation and fluid therapy.[4,5] There are now a growing number of patients surviving to hospital discharge and

Section of Pulmonary, Critical Care, Allergy and Critical Care, Wake Forest University School of Medicine, 2 Watlington Hall, 1 Medical Center Boulevard, Winston-Salem, NC 27157, USA
* Corresponding author.
E-mail address: Clark.Files@wakehealth.edu

Crit Care Clin 37 (2021) 895–911
https://doi.org/10.1016/j.ccc.2021.05.010
0749-0704/21/© 2021 Elsevier Inc. All rights reserved.

criticalcare.theclinics.com

beyond, an estimated 100,000 patients each year, a number that is expected to rapidly expand during the coronavirus disease 2019 (COVID-19) pandemic.[6,7]

The advent of low tidal volume ventilation at the turn of the century heralded a new era in the management of ARDS.[6] Multiple studies since that time have shown improved mortality and hospital-based outcomes, owing to low tidal volume ventilation and other advances in care.[8–12] Modern management of ARDS may have also led to reduced long-term pulmonary complications, because more recent studies have failed to see the frequency of long-term pulmonary complications reported in the 1980s.[6,13,14] These reductions in short-term mortality and longstanding pulmonary morbidity in survivors opened the door to a focus on other nonpulmonary complications that patients and their families experience as they recover from the acute illness.[6,15] Peer-reviewed publications describing long-term outcomes of ARDS and critical illness have grown substantially from 3 in the 1970s to more than 300 since 2000.[16] Professional and scientific societies, including the American Thoracic Society, Society of Critical Care Medicine, and funding agencies including the National Institutes of Health, have recommended prioritizing research on outcomes of survivors of critical illness, including survivors of ARDS after hospital discharge.[16–20]

Recently, the rapidly emerging COVID-19 pandemic has created a massive surge of ARDS cases in the United States and worldwide. Of those patients hospitalized with COVID-19, approximately one-third develop ARDS.[21] It is unclear what the rates of ARDS will be in 2020 to 2021 worldwide, but it is highly likely that the incidence will be significantly higher than in prior years. Most of the attention during the first 10 months of the pandemic has been focused on the acute management of COVID-19 ARDS and preventing early mortality, of which 60-day mortality estimates for patients with COVID-19 requiring intensive care unit (ICU) care are up to 60%.[22] However, the long-term impairments in survivors of COVID-19 ARDS are likely to contribute to this ongoing major health crisis for years to come, even as the incidence of COVID-19 ARDS declines (**Fig. 1**).

In this review, we discuss the persistent impairments many ARDS survivors face following resolution of their critical illness, including decreased physical and cognitive function, mental health symptoms, and reduced quality of life. Given the high prevalence of these impairments following ARDS, we also discuss the clinical evaluation of the patient post-ARDS, with consideration of the ongoing and evolving knowledge of COVID-19 ARDS.

Impairments in Physical Function Following Acute Respiratory Distress Syndrome

Physical function is defined as the ability to perform basic and instrumental activities of daily living.[23] Physical function is an integrated output from a coordinated response of multiple organ systems. In the ARDS survivor, injury to the pulmonary, neuromuscular, and cardiac systems should be considered as critical organ systems that may influence physical function.

Pulmonary

Patients with ARDS experience severe problems with gas exchange, causing profound hypoxia and necessitating mechanical ventilation. Lung injury resolution is a complex and coordinated response that begins from the onset of injury and has been extensively reviewed by others.[2] When successful, lung injury recovery results in liberation from mechanical ventilation. However, residual pulmonary injuries such as fibrosis and pulmonary diffusion impairments may be present following hospital discharge and may influence a patient's long-term physical function. Through the mid-1990s, research in long-term outcomes following ARDS focused primarily on

Projected Changes in ARDS Landscape Over Time

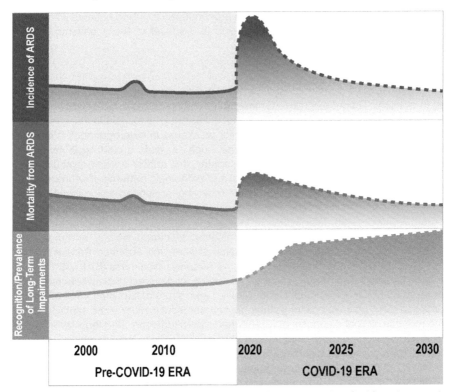

Fig. 1. In the pre-COVID-19 era, declining ARDS mortality was associated with an increase in recognition and prevalence of long-term impairments. In the post-COVID-19 era, there is an anticipated increase in long-term impairments following ARDS even as COVID-19 cases decline.

pulmonary recovery.[13,24,25] In most survivors of ARDS, pulmonary function returns to normal within 6 to 12 months despite severe initial lung injury.[26] Residual pulmonary function impairments are often asymptomatic and include mild restriction or obstruction or mild reduction in diffusing capacity.[14,27,28]

Radiographic evidence of ARDS often persists beyond symptomatic and pulmonary function recovery. In 1999, Desai and colleagues[29] described the acute- and late-phase computed tomographic (CT) scan patterns following ARDS. Ground glass opacification and consolidation are reported in the early phase, whereas a reticular pattern is more common in the late phase and associated with the duration of mechanical ventilation.[29] The Toronto ARDS Outcomes Study Group reported CT imaging findings 5 years after severe ARDS between 1998 and 2001.[30] Pulmonary CT imaging abnormalities were found in most patients (75% of 24 patients) but were generally minor and in the nondependent lung regions. In this study, no correlation was found between radiographic findings and symptoms, pulmonary function tests, or health-related quality of life measures, suggesting that the long-term impairments patients face following ARDS are complicated and are likely not secondary to structural lung disease in most patients.

The long-term pulmonary manifestations of COVID-19 ARDS will be realized as more COVID-19 ARDS survivors are studied in follow-up. Emerging data indicate that many patients experience persistent respiratory complaints.[31] Efforts are under-way worldwide to enroll COVID-19 survivors in long-term follow-up. One such study in the United States, called BLUE CORAL, is prospectively enrolling patients with severe COVID-19 and includes long-term follow-up in a subset of these patients (https://petalnet.org/studies/public/bluecoral).

Neuromuscular

The skeletal muscle system, a major target in ARDS, has often been overlooked as an organ of injury. The loss of muscle mass and function during critical illness has long been recognized since the time of Osler, but it was not until the 1990s that case series emerged reporting profound neuromuscular weakness in heterogeneous cohorts of critically ill patients.[32–38] A variety of terms, such as acute quadriplegic myopathy, thick filament myopathy, critical illness myopathy, and critical illness polyneuropathy, were used to describe the varied electrical and pathologic patterns of neuromuscular injury seen in these patients, often after receiving prolonged mechanical ventila-tion.[39–42] In 2003, a landmark observational study carefully quantified injury to the neuromuscular system in a cohort of critically ill patients on mechanical ventilation for more than 7 days, using a clinical examination, electrophysiology, and muscle bi-opsies.[43] This work coined the term "Intensive Care Unit Acquired Paresis," which later became known as "Intensive Care Unit Acquired Weakness (ICUAW)."[44] In the 25% of patients in this cohort who met the criteria for severe muscle weakness, char-acterized by Medical Research Council (MRC) sum score of less than 48 of 60, all pa-tients had electrophysiologic or pathologic neuromuscular injury. Importantly, patients who met this clinical diagnosis of ICUAW had increased short- and long-term mortal-ity, a finding confirmed in subsequent studies.[45–47] Those who remained severely weak following hospital discharge had an increased risk of death in follow-up, high-lighting ICUAW as a risk factor for subsequent mortality.

The mechanisms driving muscle wasting in ARDS are complex and incompletely understood. However, patients with ARDS universally experience muscle wasting (loss of muscle mass and function) of the limb and respiratory muscles to variable degrees. Electromyography and nerve conduction studies may reveal predominantly neuropathic (critical illness polyneuropathy), myopathic (critical illness myopathy), or mixed (critical illness neuromyopathy) patterns of injury in severe cases.[44] Even in patients who do not exhibit electrophysiological abnormalities, muscle atrophy (loss of muscle mass) is a ubiquitous feature of ARDS, driven by inflammation and disuse.[45,48] Histologically, muscles of patients with ARDS may variably show type 2 myofiber atrophy, myosin loss, or immune cell infiltrates.[48,49] Preclinical and hu-man studies of ARDS-related muscle wasting support the concept that muscles have an imbalance in skeletal muscle homeostasis favoring increased protein degra-dation and decreased protein synthesis.[45,48] Major pathways mediating protein degradation include the ubiquitin proteasome, calpain, and lysosomal pathways.[50] Increasing attention has also been turned to the influence of systemic and muscle metabolism in mediating muscle function in critical illness.[51–53] The area of muscle metabolism may have important implications for nutrient delivery during ARDS and how nutrition may influence skeletal muscle function in the acute and longer-term follow-up.[54–56]

Some ICU exposures may influence the development of ICUAW in ARDS, some of which may be modifiable. Early studies of tight glycemic control in the early 2000s found a reduced incidence of neuromuscular weakness with tight glycemic con-trol.[57–59] The subsequent NICE-SUGAR trial tempered enthusiasm for this approach when a signal for increased mortality emerged.[60] However, glycemic control remains a potentially modifiable risk factor for the development of ICU-acquired weakness in the generally critically ill population, although further study here is needed. The use of corticosteroids and neuromuscular blocking agents has also been variably associated with the development of ICUAW, although confounding by indication for these exposures may limit interpretation in observational cohorts.[61] Importantly, the ROSE randomized controlled trial of cisatracurium versus placebo in early ARDS found no increase in ICUAW incidence through day 28 (47% cisatracurium group vs 39% in placebo group), although missing data for this secondary outcome was common.[62]

Skeletal muscle wasting that occurs during ARDS is likely a major driver of reduced physical function in ARDS survivors observed during long-term follow-up. Certain risk factors and ICU exposures have been variably implicated in the development of muscle weakness in long-term follow-up. In cohorts of patients with acute respiratory failure requiring mechanical ventilation, increased age, severity of illness, comorbid illness, and ICU length of stay have been associated with long-term physical function impairment.[26,63–65] One study suggests that compliance with low tidal volume ventilation reduces long-term mortality, even when adjusting for hospital mortality.[12] Similarly, in a randomized trial of an ICU and hospital-based physical therapy intervention in patients with severe acute respiratory failure, patients randomized to the intervention arm had improved physical function in long-term follow-up, despite no measured benefit at hospital discharge.[66] Collectively these data suggest that ICU exposures during hospitalization with ARDS may influence long-term outcomes such as mortality and physical function.

One interesting observation is that ARDS survivors follow different physical function recovery trajectories. Risk factors such as age, male sex, longer lengths of stay, and hearing or vision loss are more likely to remain functionally impaired.[63,64,67] The mechanisms underlying failed versus successful recovery are incompletely understood, although some clues are emerging. Muscle biopsies from humans with long-term weakness following critical illness show a transcriptomic signature consistent with failed muscle regeneration.[68] Patients with sustained muscle atrophy have decreased muscle stem (satellite) cell content.[69] Future work is needed to better understand potential mechanisms underlying the muscle recovery of ARDS survivors, and this mechanistic work and trajectory analyses will contribute to tailored approaches to study specific ARDS long-term endotypes.

Last, it is important to recognize that not all deficits identified following a critical illness are due to the critical illness itself.[70] Longitudinal cohorts that measured physical function and deficit accumulation before and following critical illness have demonstrated this finding.[71,72] These studies found that many deficits were accumulating before the incident illness. Indeed, these pre–critical illness functional deficits influence mortality and long-term functional impairment.[71,73,74] Failure to recognize pre–critical illness physical function in ARDS survivors results in misattribution and could lead to frustration on the part of both clinicians and patients.

Cardiovascular

Although less well described than pulmonary and muscle injury during ARDS, cardiac injury does occur in a subset of patients and may contribute to long-term morbidity and mortality. Troponin elevation can be found in up to 90% of patients hospitalized with ARDS or sepsis and appears to be correlated with the severity of illness.[75,76] Elevated cardiac biomarkers during critical illness have been associated with long-term mortality.[77] Some patients with ARDS develop echocardiographic evidence of cardiac injury (septic or stress cardiomyopathy), during the critical illness, which may be driven by adverse cardiopulmonary interactions or systemic inflammation.[5,78] Cardiovascular events such as myocardial infarction or stroke are twice as likely in sepsis survivors compared with age-matched controls.[79] Significant interest exists in the relationship of COVID-19 with cardiac complications including acute myocardial injury and myocarditis, arrhythmias, and acute coronary syndrome.[80] Recent data suggest that the angiotensin-converting enzyme 2 receptor, which severe acute respiratory syndrome coronavirus 2 uses for cellular entry, is expressed in the heart.[81] Accumulating data suggest that cardiovascular injury during ARDS likely contributes to reduced functional outcomes in ARDS survivors, although more research is needed in this area.

Cognitive Impairment, Mental Health Symptoms, and Quality of Life Following Acute Respiratory Distress Syndrome

The long-term impact of ARDS extends beyond impairments in physical functioning; observational studies have consistently shown that there are long-term neuropsychiatric impairments in many patients following resolution of the acute lung injury. Long-term cognitive impairment, new or worsening mental health symptoms, and reduced quality of life have all been reported.

Cognitive

Cognitive impairment following ARDS is common, profound, and often persistent. This impairment affects ARDS survivors of all ages. In observational cohort studies of ARDS survivors, the prevalence of cognitive impairment varies based on the subpopulation studied, timing of assessment, and cognitive assessment tool used. In a prospective study by Hopkins and colleagues[82] (n = 106; 62 followed for 1 year), 78% of patients were cognitively impaired on a neuropsychological battery at 1-year follow-up. In a subsequent study (n = 120), participants underwent comprehensive neuropsychological testing at hospital discharge, 1 year, and 2 years. Most participants in this cohort (78%) were impaired at hospital discharge, 46% at 1 year, and 47% at 2 years.[83] In National Heart Lung and Blood Institute ARDSnet studies, longitudinal outcome data also support the conclusion that cognitive impairment following ARDS is common and persistent. In long-term outcome assessments following the Early versus Delayed ENteral feeding (EDEN) trial, 25% of patients were cognitively impaired on the Mini-Mental State Examination Telephone version at 6 months and 21% at 12 months.[56] Following the Statins for Acutely Injured Lungs in Sepsis (SAILS) study, cognitive impairment was present in 37% of ARDS survivors at 6 months and 29% at 12 months.[84] In a large multicenter prospective cohort study of a diverse population of patients in general medical and surgical ICUs, many of whom were intubated and likely had ARDS, one-quarter of patients had cognitive impairment 12 months after critical illness to the degree seen in patients with mild Alzheimer disease and one-third had impairment to the degree seen in patients with moderate traumatic brain injury.[85] In this cohort, impairments were found in a broad range of domains, more than just memory, including executive functioning. Although we do not yet know the prevalence of cognitive impairment following COVID-19 ARDS, early research suggests that neurologic features are often present during acute COVID-19 infection.[85–87] Also, the population at highest risk for severe COVID-19 infection overlaps significantly with those at risk for cognitive decline (advanced age, obesity, diabetes), and we can expect that there may be an increase in long-term cognitive impairment reported following severe COVID-19 in the coming years.[88–90]

Although post-ICU cognitive impairment is commonly reported in ARDS, one challenge in determining the contributory impact of ARDS on cognitive function, particularly in older adults, is that premorbid cognition is generally unknown in observational cohort studies. The development and the duration of delirium are strong predictors of post-ARDS cognitive decline.[85,91,92] Pre-existing cognitive impairment or dementia is a risk factor for the development of delirium in the ICU as well as cognitive decline after critical illness.[85,93] Delirium and cognitive impairment are clearly intertwined; patients who develop delirium during an ARDS hospitalization are a high-risk group for post-ICU cognitive impairment and merit screening postdischarge.[94]

There are multiple pathways by which critical illness may lead to new or worsening cognitive impairment. Hypoxemia is common in patients with ARDS, and the hippocampus is susceptible to hypoxic insults.[95] Neuroimaging studies of ARDS survivors demonstrate accelerated cerebral and hippocampal atrophy.[96] Autopsy studies of patients with ARDS whose critical illness was complicated by delirium have also shown hippocampal hypoxic-ischemic lesions.[97] Damage to the endothelial glycocalyx has been linked with long-term cognitive impairment in a preclinical model and humans with sepsis.[98] Although hippocampal ischemic injury may be an important contributory cause of cognitive impairment, animal studies suggest that cytokine-mediated injury from mechanical ventilation may also play a central role. In a porcine model of ARDS, cytokine-mediated brain damage from lung injury was found to be the major pathophysiological contributor to hippocampal damage, rather than hypoxemia.[99] This finding was supported by a pig model of mechanical ventilation-induced ARDS that found cognitive impairment was greater in the lung injury group (with evidence of more inflammation) compared with the hypoxia-only group.[100] Mechanical ventilation has also been shown to trigger hippocampal apoptosis in mechanically ventilated mice.[101]

Damage to the blood-brain barrier and amyloid-β clearance have also been proposed as potential mechanisms for the cognitive impairment seen following ARDS. Similarities between the pathophysiology of Alzheimer's disease (primarily accumulation of amyloid-β) and the acute sequelae of high-tidal volume mechanical ventilation in mice suggest that there may be a mechanistic link between delirium, Alzheimer's disease, and the underlying cognitive damage reported following ARDS.[102,103] Chronic accumulation of amyloid-β contributes to baseline blood-brain barrier weakening, which, in turn, may result in an increased susceptibility to hippocampal exposure to cytokines and cytokine-mediated damage in patients with underlying cognitive impairment and Alzheimer's disease. Finally, emerging data suggest that bacterial translocation to the brain in sepsis may contribute to delirium and cognitive impairment.[104] Although the causal mechanisms are likely complex, it is clear that there is a link between the lung and brain injury seen in ARDS.

Mental health

Mental health symptoms have been described in a significant proportion of ARDS survivors. Among 629 patients enrolled in 3 ARDSnet trials with at least one psychiatric measure, two-thirds had substantial symptoms in one or more domain during 1-year follow-up.[105] At 6 months, prevalence of substantial symptoms of depression, anxiety, and posttraumatic stress disorder (PTSD) was 36%, 42%, and 24%, respectively. Most survivors (63%) with any psychiatric morbidity had substantial symptoms in 2 or more domains suggesting that co-occurrence of mental health symptoms is common. In this study, severity of illness, mechanical ventilation duration, and ICU length of stay were not associated with worse psychiatric symptoms; younger age, female sex, baseline unemployment, alcohol misuse, and greater in-ICU opioid use were associated with post-ICU psychiatric symptoms. In a systematic review by Davydow and colleagues,[106] the median point prevalence of depression, PTSD, and nonspecific anxiety were similar at 28%, 28%, and 24%, respectively. In a longitudinal cohort of ARDS survivors with 5 year follow-up, 71 of 186 (38%) had a prolonged course (defined as continuous or recurring symptoms) of anxiety; 39 (32%) and 43 (23%) had a prolonged course of depression and PTSD, respectively.[105] Pre-ARDS mental health disorders were strongly and consistently associated with prolonged psychiatric morbidity after ARDS in this cohort as well suggesting that prior psychiatric history is an important risk factor for post-ARDS mental health symptoms.

Quality of life

ARDS survivors have been shown to have reduced post-hospitalization quality of life compared with the US general population.[83,107,108] Although this finding has been consistent, baseline quality of life before the acute illness was not known in these cohort studies. In a prospective, population-based study, decreased quality of life and functional status postdischarge were largely explained by reduced baseline quality of life and functional status before critical illness.[109] In qualitative work with ARDS survivors and their families, ARDS has been described as a life-altering event often resulting in pervasive, persistent disability. It is clear that the recovery process following ARDS is complex and may not be fully captured by general health-related quality of life measures. For example, in this study, patients frequently described delusional traumatic ICU memories that disrupted their families and, at times, led to life-changing repercussions.[110] Predominant memories were related to physical restraints, endotracheal tube suctioning, tracheostomies, and an inability to communicate.

ARDS influences long-term health domains beyond physical and mental health for both patients and families. A multicenter study in the United States found that nearly half of previously employed ARDS survivors were jobless at 12 months following their illness.[111] Those who return to work often experience job loss, occupation change, or worse employment status.[112] Noted barriers to returning to work include persistent fatigue and weakness, poor functional status, work-related stress, and the need for job retraining. Studies have uncovered significant financial burdens on ARDS survivors. One study of survivors found that average costs per patient from years 3 through 5 ranged from $5000 to $6000, close to costs incurred by patients with chronic disease.[113] Cumulative costs were associated with increased coexisting illness at ICU admission. In another cohort of acute respiratory failure survivors, a significant proportion of patients and their family members reported financial stress after discharge; when present, financial stress was associated with symptoms of anxiety and depression and decreased global mental health.[113] In another study following ARDS survivors participating in ARDS Network studies, 40% of patients reported at least one postdischarge hospitalization, with median estimated hospital costs of nearly $19,000.[114]

More than 50% of patients who receive prolonged mechanical ventilation are dependent on caregiver assistance at 1 year follow-up.[115] In a study looking at 1-year outcomes of the caregivers of critically ill patients, caregivers are at higher risk for clinical depression and poorer psychological well-being.[116] In qualitative work with ARDS survivors and their caregivers, the caregivers have endorsed distress by patients' fluctuation in cognition and mental status.[110] The caregivers also describe a lack of support after hospital discharge and significant strain both emotionally and financially with often a new caregiving role. Emerging data suggest that ARDS has a substantial impact on the long-term outcomes of both patients and their families.

One overarching problem with the long-term outcomes field has been a lack of standardization of the assessment tools across different research studies. There has been an attempt to standardize the tools that clinical researchers use to measure long-term outcomes, to bring uniformity to this issue.[117] Investigators designing studies should use these core outcome measures, which can also be found on https://www.improvelto.com/coms/

Clinical Evaluation of the Patient Post–Acute Respiratory Distress Syndrome

Detailed and comprehensive prospective observational studies have greatly impacted critical care and established the basic epidemiology and many of the risk factors for persistent impairments following ARDS.[118] Through the work of a 3-round modified Delphi process, a core set of outcomes now exists for clinical research of acute respiratory failure,[117] which will allow even greater comparison across cohort studies and the incorporation of these important outcomes in ICU and post-ICU clinical trials. Although there is growing consensus around the recommended evaluation of long-term outcomes following ARDS in clinical research, much less is known about the optimal evaluation of patients post-ARDS as part of routine clinical care.

To increase the awareness of long-term consequences of critical illness, the term "post-intensive care syndrome" (PICS) has been used to refer to the physical, cognitive, and/or mental health complications following an ICU stay.[20] The Society of Critical Care Medicine (SCCM) recently published recommendations related to screening tools and timing of assessments to identify long-term impairments after critical illness consistent with PICS that would apply to survivors of ARDS.[94] The recommendations by the SCCM include screening high-risk individuals early and serially for long-term impairments in cognition, mental health, and physical function using a standardized set of tools—the Montreal Cognitive Assessment (MoCA or MoCA-BLIND),[119] the Hospital Anxiety and Depression Scale (HADS),[120] and the 6-minute walk test and/or the EuroQol-5D-5L.[121] The initial assessment is recommended to occur within 2 to 4 weeks of hospital discharge and again with important life or health changes. Although the impact of screening ARDS survivors with these particular tools on longer-term outcomes (such as subsequent morality or improvements in persistent impairments) has not been studied, we agree that these tools serve as a good place to start in the post-ICU evaluation of ARDS survivors. For those patients with subjective complaints of muscle weakness, a global assessment of muscle strength using the MRC scale or handheld dynamometers can also be useful, particularly if following patients longitudinally. Although not included in the SCCM recommendation, the short physical performance battery (SPPB), a tool extensively validated in the geriatric population and with increased use in the post-ICU population, may be a useful adjuvant. The SPPB evaluates lower extremity strength, balance, and gait speed and can be completed in 5 minutes.[122] The SPPB may compliment the 6-minute walk test and provide insight into balance and lower extremity strength, which are key for maintaining functional independence.

Although most patients will have improvement in physical function in the weeks and months following hospital discharge, there will be some who report a persistent impairment in exercise tolerance.[65] In those patients, pulmonary function testing, chest imaging with CT, and echocardiography might be helpful to assess for post-ARDS pulmonary and cardiac injury. Patients who complain of impaired exercise tolerance without a clear cause from this initial evaluation may benefit from a cardiopulmonary exercise test. Finally, physical and mental health impairments have been found to be closely associated with each other in ARDS survivors, and an evaluation of persistent limitations in physical function should also include an assessment of mental health symptoms.[123]

One important point to emphasize in the clinical evaluation of patients with ARDS is the need for standardized assessments, for both cognitive and physical function. In qualitative work, performance-based cognitive tests of memory and attention were not associated with cognitive impairments reported by patients with acute respiratory failure.[124] Patients did not report experiencing cognitive impairment when interviewed but did have memory impairment when compared with population norms, suggesting that patients may not be aware of their deficits, particularly in the domains of memory and executive function. Assessment of physical function through standardized tests such as the SPPB or 6-minute walk distance may assist in guiding a tailored approach to assess deficits in balance, strength, or endurance. Repeat functional testing over time can be useful to gauge recovery or lack thereof over time.

There has been a growing attention to the assessment of long-term outcomes following COVID-19 in patients both with and without ARDS. An International Task Force sponsored by the American Thoracic Society and the European Respiratory Society has suggested that obtaining pulmonary function testing and chest CT scans as well as a transthoracic echo may be useful in the evaluation of patients with post-COVID ARDS and should be obtained for those with persistent symptoms, but there is no evidence at present to support widespread screening with these tests in all patients recovering from COVID-19 or even COVID-19 ARDS.[125] In a more recent publication, the International Task Force recommends rehabilitation for those with persistent limitations and suggests pulmonary rehabilitation as a useful framework.[126] Based on what is known regarding long-term outcomes following ARDS, they also recommend a formal assessment of physical and emotional functioning at 6 to 8 weeks to identify unmet rehabilitation needs.[126] We anticipate that our understanding of the clinical evaluation of patients with ARDS will deepen as we learn from patients recovering from COVID-19 in the coming months.

SUMMARY

Long-term impairments in physical function, cognitive function, mental health, and other domains are common after ARDS. In the pre-COVID-19 era, long-term outcomes from ARDS became apparent as mortality from ARDS decreased. In the post-COVID-19 era, long-term outcomes will become a significant problem owing to the massive increase in ARDS associated with the pandemic. This lasting effect of the COVID-19 pandemic will persist long after the acute illness diminishes. Providers should be prepared to care for the myriad of problems that are of significant importance to patients and families experiencing ARDS.

CLINICS CARE POINTS

- In most patients with ARDS, lung function improves after discharge and returns to normal; deficits in physical and cognitive function are more common.
- Impairments in many organ systems can be seen post-ARDS, and mental health symptoms may present as functional limitations.
- Evaluation of ARDS survivors in the outpatient setting should include standardized assessments, be comprehensive, and include an evaluation of pre-ARDS function when possible.
- Communication between ICU and outpatient providers will be critical to supporting patients and their families as they transition from the ICU back into their communities.

ACKNOWLEDGMENTS

The authors would like to thank Anna Cranford for editorial work and Alice Sanders for graphic design.

DISCLOSURE

Dr J.A. Palakshappa receives support from the Department of Internal Medicine Learning Health System Scholarship and the Center for Healthcare Innovation at Wake Forest School of Medicine. Dr J.T.W. Krall receives support from T32 HL076132-15. Ms L.T. Belfield has no disclosures to report. Dr D.C. Files receives career development support from K08GM123322 related to this work and other funding from the NIH outside the scope of this work. He has worked as a consultant for Cytovale and Medpace, which are outside the scope of this work.

REFERENCES

1. Ashbaugh DG, Bigelow DB, Petty TL, et al. Acute respiratory distress in adults. Lancet 1967;2:319–23.
2. Matthay MA, Ware LB, Zimmerman GA. The acute respiratory distress syndrome. J Clin Invest 2012;122:2731–40.
3. Rubenfeld GD, Caldwell E, Peabody E, et al. Incidence and outcomes of acute lung injury. N Engl J Med 2005;353:1685–93.
4. Brower RG, Matthay MA, Morris A, et al. Ventilation with lower tidal volumes as compared with traditional tidal volumes for acute lung injury and the acute respiratory distress syndrome. N Engl J Med 2000;342:1301–8.
5. Wiedemann HP, Wheeler AP, Bernard GR, et al. Comparison of two fluid-management strategies in acute lung injury. N Engl J Med 2006;354:2564–75.
6. Bernard G. Acute lung failure — our evolving understanding of ARDS. N Engl J Med 2017;377:507–9.
7. del Rio C, Collins LF, Malani P. Long-term health consequences of COVID-19. J Am Med Assoc 2020;324:1723–4.
8. Jardin F, Fellahi JL, Beauchet A, et al. Improved prognosis of acute respiratory distress syndrome 15 years on. Intensive Care Med 1999;25:936–41.
9. Stapleton RD, Wang BM, Hudson LD, et al. Causes and timing of death in patients with ARDS. Chest 2005;128:525–32.
10. Kallet RH, Jasmer RM, Pittet JF, et al. Clinical implementation of the ARDS network protocol is associated with reduced hospital mortality compared with historical controls. Crit Care Med 2005;33:925–9.
11. Chiumello D, Coppola S, Froio S, et al. What's next after ARDS: long-term outcomes. Respir Care 2016;61:689–99.
12. Needham DM, Colantuoni E, Mendez-Tellez PA, et al. Lung protective mechanical ventilation and two year survival in patients with acute lung injury: prospective cohort study. Bmj 2012;344:e2124.
13. Yahav J, Lieberman P, Molho M. Pulmonary function following the adult respiratory distress syndrome. Chest 1978;74:247–50.
14. Ghio AJ, Elliott CG, Crapo RO, et al. Impairment after adult respiratory distress syndrome. An evaluation based on American Thoracic Society recommendations. Am Rev Respir Dis 1989;139:1158–62.
15. Iwashyna TJ. Survivorship will be the defining challenge of critical care in the 21st century. Ann Intern Med 2010;153:204–5.

16. Turnbull AE, Rabiee A, Davis WE, et al. Outcome measurement in ICU survivor-ship research from 1970 to 2013: a scoping review of 425 publications. Crit Care Med 2016;44:1267–77.

17. Angus DC, Carlet J. Surviving intensive care: a report from the 2002 Brussels Roundtable. Intensive Care Med 2003;29:368–77.

18. Angus DC, Mira JP, Vincent JL. Improving clinical trials in the critically ill. Crit Care Med 2010;38:527–32.

19. Spragg RG, Bernard GR, Checkley W, et al. Beyond mortality: future clinical research in acute lung injury. Am J Respir Crit Care Med 2010;181:1121–7.

20. Needham DM, Davidson J, Cohen H, et al. Improving long-term outcomes after discharge from intensive care unit: report from a stakeholders' conference. Crit Care Med 2012;40:502–9.

21. Tzotzos SJ, Fischer B, Fischer H, et al. Incidence of ARDS and outcomes in hospitalized patients with COVID-19: a global literature survey. Crit Care 2020; 24:516.

22. Sixty-day outcomes among patients hospitalized with COVID-19. Ann Intern Med 2021;174:576–8.

23. Garber CE, Greaney ML, Riebe D, et al. Physical and mental health-related correlates of physical function in community dwelling older adults: a cross sectional study. BMC Geriatr 2010;10:6.

24. Matthay MA, Zemans RL, Zimmerman GA, et al. Acute respiratory distress syndrome. Nat Rev Dis Primers 2019;5:18.

25. Klein JJ, van Haeringen JR, Sluiter HJ, et al. Pulmonary function after recovery from the adult respiratory distress syndrome. Chest 1976;69:350–5.

26. Herridge MS, Cheung AM, Tansey CM, et al. One-year outcomes in survivors of the acute respiratory distress syndrome. N Engl J Med 2003;348:683–93.

27. Elliott CG, Rasmusson BY, Crapo RO, et al. Prediction of pulmonary function abnormalities after adult respiratory distress syndrome (ARDS). Am Rev Respir Dis 1987;135:634–8.

28. McHugh LG, Milberg JA, Whitcomb ME, et al. Recovery of function in survivors of the acute respiratory distress syndrome. Am J Respir Crit Care Med 1994; 150:90–4.

29. Desai SR, Wells AU, Rubens MB, et al. Acute respiratory distress syndrome: CT abnormalities at long-term follow-up. Radiology 1999;210:29–35.

30. Wilcox ME, Patsios D, Murphy G, et al. Radiologic outcomes at 5 years after severe ARDS. Chest 2013;143:920–6.

31. Fraser E. Long term respiratory complications of covid-19. BMJ 2020;370: m3001.

32. Leijten FS, De Weerd AW, Poortvliet DC, et al. Critical illness polyneuropathy in multiple organ dysfunction syndrome and weaning from the ventilator. Intensive Care Med 1996;22:856–61.

33. Berek K, Margreiter J, Willeit J, et al. Polyneuropathies in critically ill patients: a prospective evaluation. Intensive Care Med 1996;22:849–55.

34. Witt NJ, Zochodne DW, Bolton CF, et al. Peripheral nerve function in sepsis and multiple organ failure. Chest 1991;99:176–84.

35. Coakley JH, Nagendran K, Honavar M, et al. Preliminary observations on the neuromuscular abnormalities in patients with organ failure and sepsis. Intensive Care Med 1993;19:323–8.

36. Hund E. Myopathy in critically ill patients. Crit Care Med 1999;27:2544–7.

37. Gutmann L, Blumenthal D, Gutmann L, et al. Acute type II myofiber atrophy in critical illness. Neurology 1996;46:819–21.

38. The Principles and practice of medicine designed for the use of practitioners and students of medicine. J Am Med Assoc 1936;106:566.
39. Hirano M, Ott BR, Raps EC, et al. Acute quadriplegic myopathy: a complication of treatment with steroids, nondepolarizing blocking agents, or both. Neurology 1992;42:2082–7.
40. Bolton CF. Neuromuscular manifestations of critical illness. Muscle Nerve 2005; 32:140–63.
41. Lacomis D, Zochodne DW, Bird SJ. Critical illness myopathy. Muscle Nerve 2000;23:1785–8.
42. Latronico N, Bolton CF. Critical illness polyneuropathy and myopathy: a major cause of muscle weakness and paralysis. Lancet Neurol 2011;10:931–41.
43. De Jonghe B, Sharshar T, Lefaucheur JP, et al. Paresis acquired in the intensive care unit: a prospective multicenter study. J Am Med Assoc 2002;288:2859–67.
44. Stevens RD, Marshall SA, Cornblath DR, et al. A framework for diagnosing and classifying intensive care unit-acquired weakness. Crit Care Med 2009;37: S299–308.
45. Files DC, D'Alessio FR, Johnston LF, et al. A critical role for muscle ring finger-1 in acute lung injury-associated skeletal muscle wasting. Am J Respir Crit Care Med 2012;185:825–34.
46. Ali NA, O'Brien JM Jr, Hoffmann SP, et al. Acquired weakness, handgrip strength, and mortality in critically ill patients. Am J Respir Crit Care Med 2008;178:261–8.
47. Hermans G, Van Mechelen H, Clerckx B, et al. Acute outcomes and 1-year mortality of intensive care unit-acquired weakness. A cohort study and propensity-matched analysis. Am J Respir Crit Care Med 2014;190:410–20.
48. Puthucheary ZA, Rawal J, McPhail M, et al. Acute skeletal muscle wasting in critical illness. J Am Med Assoc 2013;310:1591–600.
49. Levine S, Nguyen T, Taylor N, et al. Rapid disuse atrophy of diaphragm fibers in mechanically ventilated humans. N Engl J Med 2008;358:1327–35.
50. Vainshtein A, Sandri M. Signaling pathways that control muscle mass. Int J Mol Sci 2020;21.
51. Gibbs K, Chuang Key CC, Belfied L, et al. Aging influences the metabolic and inflammatory phenotype in an experimental mouse model of acute lung injury. J Gerontol A Biol Sci Med Sci 2020;76(5):770–7.
52. Supinski GS, Schroder EA, Callahan LA. Mitochondria and critical illness. Chest 2020;157:310–22.
53. Puthucheary ZA, Astin R, McPhail MJW, et al. Metabolic phenotype of skeletal muscle in early critical illness. Thorax 2018;73:926–35.
54. Derde S, Vanhorebeek I, Güiza F, et al. Early parenteral nutrition evokes a phenotype of autophagy deficiency in liver and skeletal muscle of critically ill rabbits. Endocrinology 2012;153:2267–76.
55. Casaer MP, Langouche L, Coudyzer W, et al. Impact of early parenteral nutrition on muscle and adipose tissue compartments during critical illness. Crit Care Med 2013;41:2298–309.
56. Needham DM, Dinglas VD, Bienvenu OJ, et al. One year outcomes in patients with acute lung injury randomised to initial trophic or full enteral feeding: prospective follow-up of EDEN randomised trial. Bmj 2013;346:f1532.
57. Van den Berghe G, Wilmer A, Hermans G, et al. Intensive insulin therapy in the medical ICU. N Engl J Med 2006;354:449–61.

58. Hermans G, Schrooten M, Van Damme P, et al. Benefits of intensive insulin therapy on neuromuscular complications in routine daily critical care practice: a retrospective study. Crit Care 2009;13:R5.

59. Van den Berghe G, Wouters P, Weekers F, et al. Intensive insulin therapy in critically ill patients. N Engl J Med 2001;345:1359–67.

60. Intensive versus conventional glucose control in critically ill patients. N Engl J Med 2009;360:1283–97.

61. Jolley SE, Bunnell AE, Hough CL. ICU-acquired weakness. Chest 2016;150: 1129–40.

62. Early neuromuscular blockade in the acute respiratory distress syndrome. N Engl J Med 2019;380:1997–2008.

63. Herridge MS, Chu LM, Matte A, et al. The RECOVER program: disability risk groups and 1-year outcome after 7 or more days of mechanical ventilation. Am J Respir Crit Care Med 2016;194:831–44.

64. Gandotra S, Lovato J, Case D, et al. Physical function Trajectories in survivors of acute respiratory failure. Ann Am Thorac Soc 2019;16:471–7.

65. Fan E, Dowdy DW, Colantuoni E, et al. Physical complications in acute lung injury survivors: a two-year longitudinal prospective study. Crit Care Med 2014;42:849–59.

66. Morris PE, Berry MJ, Files DC, et al. Standardized rehabilitation and hospital length of stay among patients with acute respiratory failure: a randomized clinical trial. J Am Med Assoc 2016;315:2694–702.

67. Ferrante LE, Pisani MA, Murphy TE, et al. Factors associated with functional recovery among older intensive care unit survivors. Am J Respir Crit Care Med 2016;194:299–307.

68. Walsh CJ, Batt J, Herridge MS, et al. Transcriptomic analysis reveals abnormal muscle repair and remodeling in survivors of critical illness with sustained weakness. Scientific Rep 2016;6:29334.

69. Dos Santos C, Hussain SN, Mathur S, et al. Mechanisms of chronic muscle wasting and dysfunction after an intensive care unit stay. A pilot study. Am J Respir Crit Care Med 2016;194:821–30.

70. Iwashyna TJ, Prescott HC. When is critical illness not like an asteroid strike? Am J Respir Crit Care Med 2013;188:525–7.

71. Ferrante LE, Pisani MA, Murphy TE, et al. Functional trajectories among older persons before and after critical illness. JAMA Intern Med 2015;175:523–9.

72. Iwashyna TJ, Netzer G, Langa KM, et al. Spurious inferences about long-term outcomes: the case of severe sepsis and geriatric conditions. Am J Respir Crit Care Med 2012;185:835–41.

73. Iwashyna TJ. Trajectories of recovery and dysfunction after acute illness, with implications for clinical trial design. Am J Respir Crit Care Med 2012;186:302–4.

74. Dinglas VD, Aronson Friedman L, Colantuoni E, et al. Muscle weakness and 5-year survival in acute respiratory distress syndrome survivors. Crit Care Med 2017;45:446–53.

75. Frencken JF, Donker DW, Spitoni C, et al. Myocardial injury in patients with sepsis and its association with long-term outcome. Circ Cardiovasc Qual Outcomes 2018;11:e004040.

76. Metkus TS, Guallar E, Sokoll L, et al. Prevalence and prognostic association of circulating troponin in the acute respiratory distress syndrome. Crit Care Med 2017;45:1709–17.

77. Gayat E, Cariou A, Deye N, et al. Determinants of long-term outcome in ICU survivors: results from the FROG-ICU study. Crit Care 2018;22:8.

78. Beesley SJ, Weber G, Sarge T, et al. Septic cardiomyopathy. Crit Care Med 2018;46:625–34.

79. Yende S, Linde-Zwirble W, Mayr F, et al. Risk of cardiovascular events in survivors of severe sepsis. Am J Respir Crit Care Med 2014;189:1065–74.

80. Krittanawong C, Kumar A, Hahn J, et al. Cardiovascular risk and complications associated with COVID-19. Am J Cardiovasc Dis 2020;10:479–89.

81. Chen L, Li X, Chen M, et al. The ACE2 expression in human heart indicates new potential mechanism of heart injury among patients infected with SARS-CoV-2. Cardiovasc Res 2020;116:1097–100.

82. Hopkins RO, Weaver LK, Pope D, et al. Neuropsychological sequelae and impaired health status in survivors of severe acute respiratory distress syndrome. Am J Respir Crit Care Med 1999;160:50–6.

83. Hopkins RO, Weaver LK, Collingridge D, et al. Two-year cognitive, emotional, and quality-of-life outcomes in acute respiratory distress syndrome. Am J Respir Crit Care Med 2005;171:340–7.

84. Needham DM, Colantuoni E, Dinglas VD, et al. Rosuvastatin versus placebo for delirium in intensive care and subsequent cognitive impairment in patients with sepsis-associated acute respiratory distress syndrome: an ancillary study to a randomised controlled trial. Lancet Respir Med 2016;4:203–12.

85. Pandharipande PP, Girard TD, Jackson JC, et al. Long-term cognitive impairment after critical illness. N Engl J Med 2013;369:1306–16.

86. Mao L, Jin H, Wang M, et al. Neurologic manifestations of hospitalized patients with Coronavirus disease 2019 in Wuhan, China. JAMA Neurol 2020;77:683–90.

87. Helms J, Kremer S, Merdji H, et al. Neurologic features in severe SARS-CoV-2 infection. N Engl J Med 2020;382:2268–70.

88. Baumgart M, Snyder HM, Carrillo MC, et al. Summary of the evidence on modifiable risk factors for cognitive decline and dementia: a population-based perspective. Alzheimers Dement 2015;11:718–26.

89. Cummings MJ, Baldwin MR, Abrams D, et al. Epidemiology, clinical course, and outcomes of critically ill adults with COVID-19 in New York City: a prospective cohort study. Lancet 2020;395:1763–70.

90. Baker HA, Safavynia SA, Evered LA. The 'third wave': impending cognitive and functional decline in COVID-19 survivors. Br J Anaesth 2021;126(1):44–7.

91. Girard TD, Thompson JL, Pandharipande PP, et al. Clinical phenotypes of delirium during critical illness and severity of subsequent long-term cognitive impairment: a prospective cohort study. Lancet Respir Med 2018;6:213–22.

92. Wilcox ME, Brummel NE, Archer K, et al. Cognitive dysfunction in ICU patients: risk factors, predictors, and rehabilitation interventions. Crit Care Med 2013;41:S81–98.

93. Pisani MA, Murphy TE, Van Ness PH, et al. Characteristics associated with delirium in older patients in a medical intensive care unit. Arch Intern Med 2007;167:1629–34.

94. Mikkelsen ME, Still M, Anderson BJ, et al. Society of critical care medicine's international consensus conference on prediction and identification of long-term impairments after critical illness. Crit Care Med 2020;48:1670–9.

95. Kandikattu HK, Deep SN, Razack S, et al. Hypoxia induced cognitive impairment modulating activity of Cyperus rotundus. Physiol Behav 2017;175:56–65.

96. Hopkins RO, Gale SD, Weaver LK. Brain atrophy and cognitive impairment in survivors of acute respiratory distress syndrome. Brain Inj 2006;20:263–71.

97. Janz DR, Abel TW, Jackson JC, et al. Brain autopsy findings in intensive care unit patients previously suffering from delirium: a pilot study. J Crit Care 2010; 25:538.e7-e12.

98. Singer BH. The vasculature in sepsis: delivering poison or remedy to the brain? The J Clin Invest 2019;129:1527-9.

99. Fries M, Bickenbach J, Henzler D, et al. S-100 protein and neurohistopathologic changes in a porcine model of acute lung injury. Anesthesiology 2005;102: 761-7.

100. Bickenbach J, Biener I, Czaplik M, et al. Neurological outcome after experimental lung injury. Respir Physiolo Neurobiol 2011;179:174-80.

101. González-López A, López-Alonso I, Aguirre A, et al. Mechanical ventilation triggers hippocampal apoptosis by vagal and dopaminergic pathways. Am J Respir Crit Care Med 2013;188:693-702.

102. Lahiri S, Regis GC, Koronyo Y, et al. Acute neuropathological consequences of short-term mechanical ventilation in wild-type and Alzheimer's disease mice. Crit Care 2019;23:63.

103. Sasannejad C, Ely EW, Lahiri S. Long-term cognitive impairment after acute respiratory distress syndrome: a review of clinical impact and pathophysiological mechanisms. Crit Care 2019;23:352.

104. Singer BH, Dickson RP, Denstaedt SJ, et al. Bacterial dissemination to the brain in sepsis. Am J Respir Crit Care Med 2018;197:747-56.

105. Bienvenu OJ, Friedman LA, Colantuoni E, et al. Psychiatric symptoms after acute respiratory distress syndrome: a 5-year longitudinal study. Intensive Care Med 2018;44:38-47.

106. Davydow DS, Desai SV, Needham DM, et al. Psychiatric morbidity in survivors of the acute respiratory distress syndrome: a systematic review. Psychosom Med 2008;70:512-9.

107. Schelling G, Stoll C, Vogelmeier C, et al. Pulmonary function and health-related quality of life in a sample of long-term survivors of the acute respiratory distress syndrome. Intensive Care Med 2000;26:1304-11.

108. Weinert CR, Gross CR, Kangas JR, et al. Health-related quality of life after acute lung injury. Am J Respir Crit Care Med 1997;156:1120-8.

109. Biehl M, Kashyap R, Ahmed AH, et al. Six-month quality-of-life and functional status of acute respiratory distress syndrome survivors compared to patients at risk: a population-based study. Crit Care 2015;19:356.

110. Cox CE, Docherty SL, Brandon DH, et al. Surviving critical illness: acute respiratory distress syndrome as experienced by patients and their caregivers. Crit Care Med 2009;37:2702-8.

111. Kamdar BB, Huang M, Dinglas VD, et al. Joblessness and lost earnings after acute respiratory distress syndrome in a 1-year national multicenter study. Am J Respir Crit Care Med 2017;196:1012-20.

112. Kamdar BB, Sepulveda KA, Chong A, et al. Return to work and lost earnings after acute respiratory distress syndrome: a 5-year prospective, longitudinal study of long-term survivors. Thorax 2018;73:125-33.

113. Khandelwal N, Hough CL, Downey L, et al. Prevalence, risk factors, and outcomes of financial stress in survivors of critical illness. Crit Care Med 2018;46: e530-9.

114. Ruhl AP, Huang M, Colantuoni E, et al. Healthcare utilization and costs in ARDS survivors: a 1-year longitudinal national US multicenter study. Intensive Care Med 2017;43:980-91.

115. Chelluri L, Im KA, Belle SH, et al. Long-term mortality and quality of life after prolonged mechanical ventilation. Crit Care Med 2004;32:61–9.
116. Cameron JI, Chu LM, Matte A, et al. One-year outcomes in caregivers of critically ill patients. N Engl J Med 2016;374:1831–41.
117. Needham DM, Sepulveda KA, Dinglas VD, et al. Core outcome measures for clinical research in acute respiratory failure survivors. An international modified Delphi consensus study. Am J Respir Crit Care Med 2017;196:1122–30.
118. Azoulay E, Vincent JL, Angus DC, et al. Recovery after critical illness: putting the puzzle together-a consensus of 29. Crit Care 2017;21:296.
119. Nasreddine ZS, Phillips NA, Bédirian V, et al. The Montreal Cognitive Assessment, MoCA: a brief screening tool for mild cognitive impairment. J Am Geriatr Soc 2005;53:695–9.
120. Zigmond AS, Snaith RP. The hospital anxiety and depression scale. Acta Psychiatr Scand 1983;67:361–70.
121. EuroQol–a new facility for the measurement of health-related quality of life. Health Policy 1990;16:199–208.
122. Bakhru RN, Davidson JF, Bookstaver RE, et al. Physical function impairment in survivors of critical illness in an ICU Recovery Clinic. J Crit Care 2018;45:163–9.
123. Brown SM, Wilson EL, Presson AP, et al. Understanding patient outcomes after acute respiratory distress syndrome: identifying subtypes of physical, cognitive and mental health outcomes. Thorax 2017;72:1094–103.
124. Nelliot A, Dinglas VD, O'Toole J, et al. Acute respiratory failure survivors' physical, cognitive, and mental health outcomes: quantitative measures versus semistructured interviews. Ann Am Thorac Soc 2019;16:731–7.
125. Bai C, Chotirmall SH, Rello J, et al. Updated guidance on the management of COVID-19: from an American Thoracic society/European respiratory society coordinated International Task Force (29 july 2020). Eur Respir Rev 2020;29(157).
126. Spruit MA, Holland AE, Singh SJ, et al. COVID-19: Interim Guidance on Rehabilitation in the Hospital and Post-Hospital Phase from a European Respiratory Society and American Thoracic Society-coordinated International Task Force. Eur Respir J 2020;56(6).

UNITED STATES POSTAL SERVICE ® Statement of Ownership, Management, and Circulation (All Periodicals Publications Except Requester Publications)

1. Publication Title	2. Publication Number	3. Filing Date
CRITICAL CARE CLINICS	000 – 708	9/18/2021

4. Issue Frequency	5. Number of Issues Published Annually	6. Annual Subscription Price
JAN, APR, JUL, OCT	4	$258.00

7. Complete Mailing Address of Known Office of Publication (Not printer) (Street, city, county, state, and ZIP+4®)

ELSEVIER INC.
230 Park Avenue, Suite 800
New York, NY 10169

Contact Person
Malathi Samayan

Telephone (Include area code)
91-44-4299-4507

8. Complete Mailing Address of Headquarters or General Business Office of Publisher (Not printer)

ELSEVIER INC.
230 Park Avenue, Suite 800
New York, NY 10169

9. Full Names and Complete Mailing Addresses of Publisher, Editor, and Managing Editor (Do not leave blank)

Publisher (Name and complete mailing address)

DOLORES MELONI, ELSEVIER INC.
1600 JOHN F KENNEDY BLVD. SUITE 1800
PHILADELPHIA, PA 19103-2899

Editor (Name and complete mailing address)

JOANNA COLLETT, ELSEVIER INC.
1600 JOHN F KENNEDY BLVD. SUITE 1800
PHILADELPHIA, PA 19103-2899

Managing Editor (Name and complete mailing address)

PATRICK MANLEY, ELSEVIER INC.
1600 JOHN F KENNEDY BLVD. SUITE 1800
PHILADELPHIA, PA 19103-2899

10. Owner (Do not leave blank. If the publication is owned by a corporation, give the name and address of the corporation immediately followed by the names and addresses of all stockholders owning or holding 1 percent or more of the total amount of stock. If not owned by a corporation, give the names and addresses of the individual owners. If owned by a partnership or other unincorporated firm, give its name and address as well as those of each individual owner. If the publication is published by a nonprofit organization, give its name and address.)

Full Name	Complete Mailing Address
WHOLLY OWNED SUBSIDIARY OF REED/ELSEVIER, US HOLDINGS	1600 JOHN F KENNEDY BLVD. SUITE 1800 PHILADELPHIA, PA 19103-2899

11. Known Bondholders, Mortgagees, and Other Security Holders Owning or Holding 1 Percent or More of Total Amount of Bonds, Mortgages, or Other Securities. If none, check box ☐ None

Full Name	Complete Mailing Address
N/A	

12. Tax Status (For completion by nonprofit organizations authorized to mail at nonprofit rates) (Check one)
The purpose, function, and nonprofit status of this organization and the exempt status for federal income tax purposes:
☒ Has Not Changed During Preceding 12 Months
☐ Has Changed During Preceding 12 Months (Publisher must submit explanation of change with this statement)

PS Form 3526, July 2014 (Page 1 of 4 (see instructions page 4)) PSN 7530-01-000-9931 PRIVACY NOTICE: See our privacy policy on www.usps.com.

13. Publication Title	14. Issue Date for Circulation Data Below
CRITICAL CARE CLINICS	JULY 2021

15. Extent and Nature of Circulation			Average No. Copies Each Issue During Preceding 12 Months	No. Copies of Single Issue Published Nearest to Filing Date
a. Total Number of Copies (Net press run)			286	262
b. Paid Circulation (By Mail and Outside the Mail)	(1)	Mailed Outside-County Paid Subscriptions Stated on PS Form 3541 (Include paid distribution above nominal rate, advertiser's proof copies, and exchange copies)	171	162
	(2)	Mailed In-County Paid Subscriptions Stated on PS Form 3541 (Include paid distribution above nominal rate, advertiser's proof copies, and exchange copies)	0	0
	(3)	Paid Distribution Outside the Mails Including Sales Through Dealers and Carriers, Street Vendors, Counter Sales, and Other Paid Distribution Outside USPS®	69	63
	(4)	Paid Distribution by Other Classes of Mail Through the USPS (e.g. First-Class Mail®)	0	0
c. Total Paid Distribution (Sum of 15b (1), (2), (3), and (4))		▶	240	225
d. Free or Nominal Rate Distribution (By Mail and Outside the Mail)	(1)	Free or Nominal Rate Outside-County Copies included on PS Form 3541	30	21
	(2)	Free or Nominal Rate In-County Copies Included on PS Form 3541	0	0
	(3)	Free or Nominal Rate Copies Mailed at Other Classes Through the USPS (e.g. First-Class Mail)	0	0
	(4)	Free or Nominal Rate Distribution Outside the Mail (Carriers or other means)	0	0
e. Total Free or Nominal Rate Distribution (Sum of 15d (1), (2), (3) and (4))		▶	30	21
f. Total Distribution (Sum of 15c and 15e)		▶	270	246
g. Copies not Distributed (See Instructions to Publishers #4 (page #3))		▶	16	16
h. Total (Sum of 15f and g)		▶	286	262
i. Percent Paid (15c divided by 15f times 100)			88.88%	91.46%

* If you are claiming electronic copies, go to line 16 on page 3. If you are not claiming electronic copies, skip to line 17 on page 3.

PS Form 3526, July 2014 (Page 2 of 4)

16. Electronic Copy Circulation		Average No. Copies Each Issue During Preceding 12 Months	No. Copies of Single Issue Published Nearest to Filing Date
a. Paid Electronic Copies	▶		
b. Total Paid Print Copies (Line 15c) + Paid Electronic Copies (Line 16a)	▶		
c. Total Print Distribution (Line 15f) + Paid Electronic Copies (Line 16a)	▶		
d. Percent Paid (Both Print & Electronic Copies) (16b divided by 16c × 100)	▶		

☒ I certify that 50% of all my distributed copies (electronic and print) are paid above a nominal price.

17. Publication of Statement of Ownership

☒ If the publication is a general publication, publication of this statement is required. Will be printed in the OCTOBER 2021 issue of this publication. ☐ Publication not required.

18. Signature and Title of Editor, Publisher, Business Manager, or Owner

Malathi Samayan - Distribution Controller

Malathi Samayan   Date 9/18/2021

I certify that all information furnished on this form is true and complete. I understand that anyone who furnishes false or misleading information on this form or who omits material or information requested on the form may be subject to criminal sanctions (including fines and imprisonment) and/or civil sanctions (including civil penalties).

PS Form 3526, July 2014 (Page 3 of 4) PRIVACY NOTICE: See our privacy policy on www.usps.com

Moving?

Make sure your subscription moves with you!

To notify us of your new address, find your **Clinics Account Number** (located on your mailing label above your name), and contact customer service at:

Email: journalscustomerservice-usa@elsevier.com

800-654-2452 (subscribers in the U.S. & Canada)
314-447-8871 (subscribers outside of the U.S. & Canada)

Fax number: 314-447-8029

Elsevier Health Sciences Division
Subscription Customer Service
3251 Riverport Lane
Maryland Heights, MO 63043

Printed and bound by CPI Group (UK) Ltd, Croydon, CR0 4YY

03/10/2024

01040405-0003